Updates in Management of SARS-CoV-2 Infection

Updates in Management of SARS-CoV-2 Infection

Editor

Robert Flisiak

MDPI • Basel • Beijing • Wuhan • Barcelona • Belgrade • Manchester • Tokyo • Cluj • Tianjin

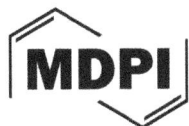

Editor
Robert Flisiak
Medical University of
Bialystok
Bialystok, Poland

Editorial Office
MDPI
St. Alban-Anlage 66
4052 Basel, Switzerland

This is a reprint of articles from the Special Issue published online in the open access journal *Journal of Clinical Medicine* (ISSN 2077-0383) (available at: https://www.mdpi.com/journal/jcm/special_issues/SARS-CoV-2_Infection).

For citation purposes, cite each article independently as indicated on the article page online and as indicated below:

LastName, A.A.; LastName, B.B.; LastName, C.C. Article Title. *Journal Name* **Year**, *Volume Number*, Page Range.

ISBN 978-3-0365-5389-4 (Hbk)
ISBN 978-3-0365-5390-0 (PDF)

© 2022 by the authors. Articles in this book are Open Access and distributed under the Creative Commons Attribution (CC BY) license, which allows users to download, copy and build upon published articles, as long as the author and publisher are properly credited, which ensures maximum dissemination and a wider impact of our publications.

The book as a whole is distributed by MDPI under the terms and conditions of the Creative Commons license CC BY-NC-ND.

Contents

About the Editor ix

Robert Flisiak, Dorota Zarebska-Michaluk, Marta Flisiak-Jackiewicz and Piotr Rzymski
Updates in Management of SARS-CoV-2 Infection
Reprinted from: *J. Clin. Med.* **2022**, *11*, 4472, doi:10.3390/jcm11154472 1

Rodrigo San-Cristobal, Roberto Martín-Hernández, Omar Ramos-Lopez, Diego Martinez-Urbistondo, Víctor Micó, Gonzalo Colmenarejo, Paula Villares Fernandez, Lidia Daimiel and Jose Alfredo Martínez
Longwise Cluster Analysis for the Prediction of COVID-19 Severity within 72 h of Admission: COVID-DATA-SAVE-LIFES Cohort
Reprinted from: *J. Clin. Med.* **2022**, *11*, 3327, doi:10.3390/jcm11123327 5

Stefania Principe, Amelia Grosso, Alida Benfante, Federica Albicini, Salvatore Battaglia, Erica Gini, Marta Amata, Ilaria Piccionello, Angelo Guido Corsico and Nicola Scichilone
Comparison between Suspected and Confirmed COVID-19 Respiratory Patients: What Is beyond the PCR Test
Reprinted from: *J. Clin. Med.* **2022**, *11*, 2993, doi:10.3390/jcm11112993 21

Jarosław Janc, Michał Suchański, Magdalena Mierzchała-Pasierb, Ewa Woźnica-Niesobska, Lidia Łysenko and Patrycja Leśnik
Does the Serum Concentration of Angiotensin II Type 1 Receptor Have an Effect on the Severity of COVID-19? A Prospective Preliminary Observational Study among Healthcare Professionals
Reprinted from: *J. Clin. Med.* **2022**, *11*, 1769, doi:10.3390/jcm11071769 29

Robert Flisiak, Piotr Rzymski, Dorota Zarebska-Michaluk, Magdalena Rogalska, Marta Rorat, Piotr Czupryna, Beata Lorenc, Przemysław Ciechanowski, Dorota Kozielewicz, Anna Piekarska, Maria Pokorska-Śpiewak, Katarzyna Sikorska, Magdalena Tudrujek, Beata Bolewska, Grzegorz Angielski, Justyna Kowalska, Regina Podlasin, Włodzimierz Mazur, Barbara Oczko-Grzesik, Izabela Zaleska, Aleksandra Szymczak, Paulina Frańczak-Chmura, Małgorzata Sobolewska-Pilarczyk, Krzysztof Kłos, Magdalena Figlerowicz, Piotr Leszczyński, Izabela Kucharek and Hubert Grabowski
Demographic and Clinical Overview of Hospitalized COVID-19 Patients during the First 17 Months of the Pandemic in Poland
Reprinted from: *J. Clin. Med.* **2022**, *11*, 117, doi:10.3390/jcm11010117 43

Maria Pokorska-Śpiewak, Ewa Talarek, Anna Mania, Małgorzata Pawłowska, Jolanta Popielska, Konrad Zawadka, Magdalena Figlerowicz, Katarzyna Mazur-Melewska, Kamil Faltin, Przemysław Ciechanowski, Joanna Łasecka-Zadrożna, Józef Rudnicki, Barbara Hasiec, Martyna Stani, Paulina Frańczak-Chmura, Izabela Zaleska, Leszek Szenborn, Kacper Toczyłowski, Artur Sulik, Barbara Szczepańska, Ilona Pałyga-Bysiecka, Izabela Kucharek, Adam Sybilski, Małgorzata Sobolewska-Pilarczyk, Urszula Dryja, Ewa Majda-Stanisławska, Sławomira Niedźwiecka, Ernest Kuchar, Bolesław Kalicki, Anna Gorczyca and Magdalena Marczyńska
Clinical and Epidemiological Characteristics of 1283 Pediatric Patients with Coronavirus Disease 2019 during the First and Second Waves of the Pandemic—Results of the Pediatric Part of a Multicenter Polish Register SARSTer
Reprinted from: *J. Clin. Med.* **2021**, *10*, 5098, doi:10.3390/jcm10215098 55

Frane Paštrovic, Marko Lucijanic, Armin Atic, Josip Stojic, Mislav Barisic Jaman, Ida Tjesic Drinkovic, Marko Zelenika, Marko Milosevic, Barbara Medic, Jelena Loncar, Maja Mijic, Tajana Filipec Kanizaj, Dominik Kralj, Ivan Lerotic, Lucija Virovic Jukic, Neven Ljubicic, Kresimir Luetic, Dora Grgic, Matea Majerovic, Rajko Ostojic, Zeljko Krznaric, Ivica Luksic, Nevenka Piskac Zivkovic, Tatjana Keres, Vlatko Grabovac, Jasminka Persec, Bruno Barsic and Ivica Grgurevic
Prevalence and Prognostic Impact of Deranged Liver Blood Tests in COVID-19: Experience from the Regional COVID-19 Center over the Cohort of 3812 Hospitalized Patients
Reprinted from: *J. Clin. Med.* **2021**, *10*, 4222, doi:10.3390/jcm10184222 . . . . **67**

Omar Ramos-Lopez, Rodrigo San-Cristobal, Diego Martinez-Urbistondo, Víctor Micó, Gonzalo Colmenarejo, Paula Villares-Fernandez, Lidia Daimiel and J. Alfredo Martinez
Proinflammatory and Hepatic Features Related to Morbidity and Fatal Outcomes in COVID-19 Patients
Reprinted from: *J. Clin. Med.* **2021**, *10*, 3112, doi:10.3390/jcm10143112 . . . . **83**

Patrícia Moniz, Sérgio Brito and Pedro Póvoa
SARS-CoV-2 and Cytomegalovirus Co-Infections—A Case Series of Critically Ill Patients
Reprinted from: *J. Clin. Med.* **2021**, *10*, 2792, doi:10.3390/jcm10132792 . . . . **95**

Ysaline Seynaeve, Justine Heylen, Corentin Fontaine, François Maclot, Cécile Meex, Anh Nguyet Diep, Anne-Françoise Donneau, Marie-Pierre Hayette and Julie Descy
Evaluation of Two Rapid Antigenic Tests for the Detection of SARS-CoV-2 in Nasopharyngeal Swabs
Reprinted from: *J. Clin. Med.* **2021**, *10*, 2774, doi:10.3390/jcm10132774 . . . . **101**

Dorota Zarebska-Michaluk, Jerzy Jaroszewicz, Magdalena Rogalska, Beata Lorenc, Marta Rorat, Anna Szymanek-Pasternak, Anna Piekarska, Aleksandra Berkan-Kawińska, Katarzyna Sikorska, Magdalena Tudrujek-Zdunek, Barbara Oczko-Grzesik, Beata Bolewska, Piotr Czupryna, Dorota Kozielewicz, Justyna Kowalska, Regina Podlasin, Krzysztof Kłos, Włodzimierz Mazur, Piotr Leszczyński, Bartosz Szetela, Katarzyna Reczko and Robert Flisiak
Impact of Kidney Failure on the Severity of COVID-19
Reprinted from: *J. Clin. Med.* **2021**, *10*, 2042, doi:10.3390/jcm10092042 . . . . **111**

Álvaro Tamayo-Velasco, Pedro Martínez-Paz, María Jesús Peñarrubia-Ponce, Ignacio de la Fuente, Sonia Pérez-González, Itziar Fernández, Carlos Dueñas, Esther Gómez-Sánchez, Mario Lorenzo-López, Estefanía Gómez-Pesquera, María Heredia-Rodríguez, Irene Carnicero-Frutos, María Fe Muñoz-Moreno, David Bernardo, Francisco Javier Álvarez, Eduardo Tamayo and Hugo Gonzalo-Benito
HGF, IL-1α, and IL-27 Are Robust Biomarkers in Early Severity Stratification of COVID-19 Patients
Reprinted from: *J. Clin. Med.* **2021**, *10*, 2017, doi:10.3390/jcm10092017 . . . . **125**

Robert Flisiak, Jerzy Jaroszewicz, Magdalena Rogalska, Tadeusz Łapiński, Aleksandra Berkan-Kawińska, Beata Bolewska, Magdalena Tudrujek-Zdunek, Dorota Kozielewicz, Marta Rorat, Piotr Leszczyński, Krzysztof Kłos, Justyna Kowalska, Paweł Pabjan, Anna Piekarska, Iwona Mozer-Lisewska, Krzysztof Tomasiewicz, Małgorzata Pawłowska, Krzysztof Simon, Joanna Polanska and Dorota Zarebska-Michaluk
Tocilizumab Improves the Prognosis of COVID-19 in Patients with High IL-6
Reprinted from: *J. Clin. Med.* **2021**, *10*, 1583, doi:10.3390/jcm11154472 . . . . **139**

Alberto Enrico Maraolo, Anna Crispo, Michela Piezzo, Piergiacomo Di Gennaro, Maria Grazia Vitale, Domenico Mallardo, Luigi Ametrano, Egidio Celentano, Arturo Cuomo, Paolo A. Ascierto and Marco Cascella
The Use of Tocilizumab in Patients with COVID-19: A Systematic Review, Meta-Analysis and Trial Sequential Analysis of Randomized Controlled Studies
Reprinted from: *J. Clin. Med.* **2021**, *10*, 4935, doi:10.3390/jcm10214935 . . . . **153**

Paweł Jemioło, Dawid Storman and Patryk Orzechowski
Artificial Intelligence for COVID-19 Detection in Medical Imaging—Diagnostic Measures and Wasting—A Systematic Umbrella Review
Reprinted from: *J. Clin. Med.* **2022**, *11*, 2054, doi:10.3390/jcm11072054 . . . . **171**

About the Editor

Robert Flisiak

Robert Flisiak is head of the Department of Infectious Diseases and Hepatology of the Medical University of Bialystok, Poland, as well as previous Dean (2005–2008) and vice-Rector (2008–2012) at this University. He earned his medical education at the Medical University of Bialystok and completed training there in internal medicine (1988) and infectious diseases (1991). From 1991–1992 he completed research training at Mount Sinai School of Medicine in New York and additional clinical training in London and Salzburg. Professor Robert Flisiak is current President of Polish Association of Epidemiology and Infectious Diseases, President of the Central European Hepatologic Collaboration, President of the Polish Expert Group for HBV and the past President of the Polish Association for the Study of Liver. He is also Editor-in-Chief of *Clinical and Experimental Hepatology*, editor and author of chapters in several handbooks, including the editor of the Polish edition of *Harrison's Infectious Diseases* and a recently published four-volume handbook *Infectious and Parasitic Diseases*. The scientific activity of Prof. Flisiak focuses on infectious diseases and hepatology, and his scientific achievements include 414 publications registered in the Web of Science Core Collection (h-index: 43, 15 000 citations). Prof. Flisiak participated in almost 200 clinical trials as principal investigator, country coordinator or world leading investigator. He was a coordinator of a number of multicenter, investigator-initiated clinical studies focused on Viral Hepatitis and COVID-19.

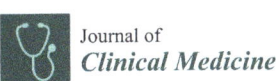

Editorial

Updates in Management of SARS-CoV-2 Infection

Robert Flisiak [1,*], Dorota Zarębska-Michaluk [2], Marta Flisiak-Jackiewicz [3] and Piotr Rzymski [4]

1. Department of Infectious Diseases and Hepatology, Medical University of Białystok, 15-540 Białystok, Poland
2. Department of Infectious Diseases, Jan Kochanowski University, 25-317 Kielce, Poland; dorota1010@tlen.pl
3. Department of Pediatrics, Gastroenterology, Hepatology, Nutrition and Allergology, Medical University of Białystok, 15-247 Białystok, Poland; m_flisiak@op.pl
4. Department of Environmental Medicine, Poznan University of Medical Sciences, 60-806 Poznań, Poland; rzymskipiotr@ump.edu.pl
* Correspondence: robert.flisiak1@gmail.com

1. Introduction

Severe acute respiratory syndrome coronavirus 2 (SARS-CoV-2) has spread worldwide since the beginning of 2020 [1]. Its infections are mostly asymptomatic or mild, but some patients may develop COVID-19 (coronavirus disease 2019) with a severe or critical course leading to pneumonia, acute respiratory distress syndrome, and multi-organ failure. Apart from the virus-related damage to the lungs, pathomechanism of the disease seems to be linked to thromboembolism and inflammation accompanied by overproduction of proinflammatory cytokines [2]. Since developing new therapeutic molecules, dedicated strictly to targeting a particular virus is time-consuming [3], scientists and physicians have started to test and repurpose old medications in clinical practice [4]. Despite the introduction of antiviral drugs and immunomodulators, after two and a half years of pandemics, there is still a lack of optimal therapy. A major issue is also insufficient knowledge on predictors of the severe or deadly course of the disease, which could also help to switch from one therapeutic option to another. Due to many gaps in the management of COVID-19, there is a need for accumulating new data, particularly from real-world experience which could be applicable to practice guidelines. The objective of this Special Issue of the Journal of Clinical Medicine was to provide an update on the management for the diagnostic workup and therapy of SARS-CoV-2 infection. The issue includes fourteen original articles covering problems related to the diagnosis, clinic, and treatment of COVID-19, with an emphasis on predictors of severity of the disease.

2. Clinical Picture

The study based on the SARSTer database analyzed the data of 5199 COVID-19 patients hospitalized in 30 Polish centers in periods of dominance of various SARS-CoV-2 variants [5]. It showed some shifts in SARS-CoV-2 pathogenicity between March 2020 and July 2021 in the Polish cohort of hospitalized patients. A share of patients presenting respiratory, systemic, and gastrointestinal symptoms was higher in the later phase of a pandemic than in the first three months. Interestingly there was no shift in the age of admitted patients and patients who died throughout the studied period. No gender difference in fatality rate was seen, although the age of males who died was significantly lower. It is also plausible that other factors had influenced the shift in disease severity and outcome throughout the considered period as a separate analysis of the SARSTer database has shown the relationship between patients' exposure to increased levels of air pollution and inflammation, need for oxygen therapy, and odds of death due to COVID-19 [6]. Data in the pediatric population from the initial period of the pandemic are presented in the study by Pokorska-Śpiewak et al. [7]. The authors showed that the characteristics of pediatric patients infected with SARS-CoV-2 and the clinical presentation of COVID-19 are age-related. Younger children were more frequently infected by close relatives, and

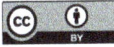

they more often suffered from pneumonia and gastrointestinal symptoms and require hospitalization. The results of these two studies can be considered as a reference for further analyses conducted under the dominance of new SARS-CoV-2 variants [5,7].

Based on data from 455 patients with previously diagnosed kidney failure, Zarębska-Michaluk et al. [8] showed that this population was characterized by significantly older age and a more severe clinical course of COVID-19. The age, baseline SpO2, need for oxygen therapy, neutrophil and platelet count, estimated glomerular filtration rate, C-reactive protein concentration, and some comorbidities were the independent predictors of 28-day mortality in this population. This analysis clearly showed that underlying kidney disease in patients with COVID-19 should be considered one of the leading factors associated with a higher risk of severe clinical presentation and mortality.

Moniz et al. [9] presented a case series of five patients coinfected with cytomegalovirus (CMV) admitted to the intensive care unit due to respiratory failure related to COVID-19. The authors speculate that the reason for the reactivation was the immunosuppression possibly associated with COVID-19. However, they emphasize the importance of multiple confounding factors usually associated with immunosuppression, such as the clinical profile of older patients with multiple comorbidities, the critical illness itself, or immunosuppressive treatments should also be considered.

3. Diagnostics

The article by Seynaeve Y. et al. [10] published in June 2021 documents research on the usefulness of antigen tests in the diagnosis of COVID-19. It was a time of confusion related to the appearance of a large number of such tests, often of poor quality, which undermined the credibility of this diagnostic method. Thanks to such works, only antigen tests with diagnostic effectiveness similar to the RT-PCR technique remained in use, and the speed and convenience caused a real revolution in diagnostic and epidemiological procedures. Of course, the RT-PCR technique remains the standard for the diagnosis, but technical difficulties often require supporting the diagnosis with other methods. The work of Principe et al. [11] proved that the genetic test should be combined with pulmonary CT scans, clinical pictures, and some inflammatory blood tests, to increase the accuracy of the diagnosis of COVID-19.

Since the beginning of the COVID-19 pandemic, medical imaging has been assigned a key role in the diagnosis of the disease. However, a question arose if and to which extent automated tools could be included in clinical diagnosis. Artificial intelligence, has started to play an increasing role in medicine, including COVID-19. Jemioło et al. [12] investigated the methodological quality of the reviews on artificial intelligence techniques to diagnose COVID-19 in medical images. Unfortunately, the authors found that most of the reviews included less than 10% of available studies, which makes it difficult to collect and organize knowledge.

4. Predictors of the Outcome

A significant part of the publications included in the Special Issue were works devoted to the search for predictors of the clinical course of COVID-19. Tamayo-Velasco et al. [13] investigated the role of inflammatory cytokines using the 45-plex Human XL Cytokine Luminex Performance Panel and found that three of them may be predictive. High levels of hepatocyte growth factor and interleukin-1α accompanied with low levels of interleukin-27 at admission can predict clinical outcomes. Of course, the predictive value depends on the availability of the methodology in laboratories. Therefore, in another work, Ramos-Lopez et al. [14] focused on simple indicators of liver and proinflammatory features as determinants of COVID-19 morbidity and fatal outcomes. They found the predictive values of ROC curves for FIB-4, aminotransferases (AST/ALT) ratio, C-reactive protein, Charlson Comorbidity Index, neutrophils, and platelets concerning intensive care and death outcomes. In turn, Pastrovic et al. [15] showed that patients with more severe liver injury more frequently experienced higher rates of intensive care unit admission, mechanical ventilation, and mortality.

Due to the fact that SARS-CoV-2 uses angiotensin-converting enzyme 2 (ACE-2) as a receptor enabling human infection, research has been undertaken on a possible relationship between angiotensin 1 receptor (AT1R) levels in the serum and the course of the disease. However, Janc et al. [16] did not show the effect of AT1R on the severity of symptoms associated with COVID-19 among healthcare professionals and any prognostic significance. On the other hand, San-Cristobal et al. [17], based on the analysis of clinical and biochemical variables obtained in the first 72 h of hospitalization from 1039 COVID-19 patients, specified three clusters with different clinical severity outcomes. These clusters displayed mortality from below 2% (cluster A), through around 15% (B) to as much as 40% (C) in patients with multi-organ lesions and significantly altered inflammatory and immune responses.

5. Treatment

The pathogenesis of COVID-19 includes, in addition to direct viral effect and coagulopathy, an overproduction of proinflammatory cytokines termed a cytokine storm, which is responsible for organ damage and is considered a major reason for death due to COVID-19. Tocilizumab, an antagonist of the interleukine-6 receptor, has emerged as a promising therapeutic choice, especially for the severe form of the disease. A systematic review and meta-analysis by Maraolo et al. [18] confirmed this view, pointing to the need for further studies to consolidate these findings and to identify the populations that benefit most from treatment with tocilizumab. Such a population was indicated in another study published in this Special Issue. Tocilizumab was found to be a therapeutic option to significantly reduce mortality and speed up clinical improvement in patients with a baseline concentration of interleukin-6 over 100 pg/mL, particularly if they need oxygen supplementation due to SpO2 values below 90% [19].

6. Conclusions

This editorial highlights the key findings of the research published in this Special Issue of the Journal of Clinical Medicine. We strongly encourage you to read particular papers for a detailed understanding of the reported results. The articles were published between April 2021 and May 2022; therefore, reading them, you must be aware of how quickly our knowledge of COVID-19 has changed. Nevertheless, most of the information in these publications is still valid and influences the management of patients

Author Contributions: Conceptualization, R.F.; methodology, R.F.; formal analysis, R.F.; writing—original draft preparation, R.F., D.Z.-M., M.F.-J. and P.R.; writing—review and editing, R.F., D.Z.-M., M.F.-J. and P.R.; supervision, R.F.; project administration, R.F. All authors have read and agreed to the published version of the manuscript.

Funding: This research received no external funding.

Conflicts of Interest: The authors declare no conflict of interest.

References

1. Cucinotta, D.; Vanelli, M. WHO Declares COVID-19 a Pandemic. *Acta Biomed.* **2020**, *91*, 157–160. [PubMed]
2. Robba, C.; Battaglini, D.; Pelosi, P.; Rocco, P.R.M. Multiple Organ Dysfunction in SARS-CoV-2: MODS-CoV-2. *Expert Rev. Respir. Med.* **2020**, *14*, 865–868. [CrossRef] [PubMed]
3. Rahmah, L.; Abarikwu, S.O.; Arero, A.G.; Jibril, A.T.; Fal, A.; Flisiak, R.; Makuku, R.; Marquez, L.; Mohamed, K.; Ndow, L.; et al. Oral Antiviral Treatments for COVID-19: Opportunities and Challenges. *Pharmacol. Rep.* **2022**. [CrossRef] [PubMed]
4. Cusinato, J.; Cau, Y.; Calvani, A.M.; Mori, M. Repurposing Drugs for the Management of COVID-19. *Expert Opin. Ther. Pat.* **2021**, *31*, 295–307. [CrossRef] [PubMed]
5. Flisiak, R.; Rzymski, P.; Zarębska-Michaluk, D.; Rogalska, M.; Rorat, M.; Czupryna, P.; Lorenc, B.; Ciechanowski, P.; Kozielewicz, D.; Piekarska, A.; et al. Demographic and Clinical Overview of Hospitalized COVID-19 Patients during the First 17 Months of the Pandemic in Poland. *J. Clin. Med.* **2021**, *11*, 117. [CrossRef] [PubMed]

6. Rzymski, P.; Poniedziałek, B.; Rosińska, J.; Rogalska, M.; Zarębska-Michaluk, D.; Rorat, M.; Moniuszko-Malinowska, A.; Lorenc, B.; Kozielewicz, D.; Piekarska, A.; et al. The Association of Airborne Particulate Matter and Benzo[a]Pyrene with the Clinical Course of COVID-19 in Patients Hospitalized in Poland. *Environ. Pollut.* **2022**, *306*, 119469. [CrossRef] [PubMed]
7. Pokorska-Śpiewak, M.; Talarek, E.; Mania, A.; Pawłowska, M.; Popielska, J.; Zawadka, K.; Figlerowicz, M.; Mazur-Melewska, K.; Faltin, K.; Ciechanowski, P.; et al. Clinical and Epidemiological Characteristics of 1283 Pediatric Patients with Coronavirus Disease 2019 during the First and Second Waves of the Pandemic-Results of the Pediatric Part of a Multicenter Polish Register SARSTer. *J. Clin. Med.* **2021**, *10*, 5098. [CrossRef] [PubMed]
8. Zarębska-Michaluk, D.; Jaroszewicz, J.; Rogalska, M.; Lorenc, B.; Rorat, M.; Szymanek-Pasternak, A.; Piekarska, A.; Berkan-Kawińska, A.; Sikorska, K.; Tudrujek-Zdunek, M.; et al. Impact of Kidney Failure on the Severity of COVID-19. *J. Clin. Med.* **2021**, *10*, 2042. [CrossRef] [PubMed]
9. Moniz, P.; Brito, S.; Póvoa, P. SARS-CoV-2 and Cytomegalovirus Co-Infections-A Case Series of Critically Ill Patients. *J. Clin. Med.* **2021**, *10*, 2792. [CrossRef] [PubMed]
10. Seynaeve, Y.; Heylen, J.; Fontaine, C.; Maclot, F.; Meex, C.; Diep, A.N.; Donneau, A.-F.; Hayette, M.-P.; Descy, J. Evaluation of Two Rapid Antigenic Tests for the Detection of SARS-CoV-2 in Nasopharyngeal Swabs. *J. Clin. Med.* **2021**, *10*, 2774. [CrossRef] [PubMed]
11. Principe, S.; Grosso, A.; Benfante, A.; Albicini, F.; Battaglia, S.; Gini, E.; Amata, M.; Piccionello, I.; Corsico, A.G.; Scichilone, N. Comparison between Suspected and Confirmed COVID-19 Respiratory Patients: What Is beyond the PCR Test. *J. Clin. Med.* **2022**, *11*, 2993. [CrossRef] [PubMed]
12. Jemioło, P.; Storman, D.; Orzechowski, P. Artificial Intelligence for COVID-19 Detection in Medical Imaging-Diagnostic Measures and Wasting-A Systematic Umbrella Review. *J. Clin. Med.* **2022**, *11*, 2054. [CrossRef] [PubMed]
13. Tamayo-Velasco, Á.; Martínez-Paz, P.; Peñarrubia-Ponce, M.J.; de la Fuente, I.; Pérez-González, S.; Fernández, I.; Dueñas, C.; Gómez-Sánchez, E.; Lorenzo-López, M.; Gómez-Pesquera, E.; et al. HGF, IL-1α, and IL-27 Are Robust Biomarkers in Early Severity Stratification of COVID-19 Patients. *J. Clin. Med.* **2021**, *10*, 2017. [CrossRef] [PubMed]
14. Ramos-Lopez, O.; San-Cristobal, R.; Martinez-Urbistondo, D.; Micó, V.; Colmenarejo, G.; Villares-Fernandez, P.; Daimiel, L.; Martinez, J.A. Proinflammatory and Hepatic Features Related to Morbidity and Fatal Outcomes in COVID-19 Patients. *J. Clin. Med.* **2021**, *10*, 3112. [CrossRef] [PubMed]
15. Paštrovic, F.; Lucijanic, M.; Atic, A.; Stojic, J.; Barisic Jaman, M.; Tjesic Drinkovic, I.; Zelenika, M.; Milosevic, M.; Medic, B.; Loncar, J.; et al. Prevalence and Prognostic Impact of Deranged Liver Blood Tests in COVID-19: Experience from the Regional COVID-19 Center over the Cohort of 3812 Hospitalized Patients. *J. Clin. Med.* **2021**, *10*, 4222. [CrossRef] [PubMed]
16. Janc, J.; Suchański, M.; Mierzchała-Pasierb, M.; Woźnica-Niesobska, E.; Łysenko, L.; Leśnik, P. Does the Serum Concentration of Angiotensin II Type 1 Receptor Have an Effect on the Severity of COVID-19? A Prospective Preliminary Observational Study among Healthcare Professionals. *J. Clin. Med.* **2022**, *11*, 1769. [CrossRef] [PubMed]
17. San-Cristobal, R.; Martín-Hernández, R.; Ramos-Lopez, O.; Martinez-Urbistondo, D.; Micó, V.; Colmenarejo, G.; Villares Fernandez, P.; Daimiel, L.; Martínez, J.A. Longwise Cluster Analysis for the Prediction of COVID-19 Severity within 72 h of Admission: COVID-DATA-SAVE-LIFES Cohort. *J. Clin. Med.* **2022**, *11*, 3327. [CrossRef] [PubMed]
18. Maraolo, A.E.; Crispo, A.; Piezzo, M.; Di Gennaro, P.; Vitale, M.G.; Mallardo, D.; Ametrano, L.; Celentano, E.; Cuomo, A.; Ascierto, P.A.; et al. The Use of Tocilizumab in Patients with COVID-19: A Systematic Review, Meta-Analysis and Trial Sequential Analysis of Randomized Controlled Studies. *J. Clin. Med.* **2021**, *10*, 4935. [CrossRef] [PubMed]
19. Flisiak, R.; Jaroszewicz, J.; Rogalska, M.; Łapiński, T.; Berkan-Kawińska, A.; Bolewska, B.; Tudrujek-Zdunek, M.; Kozielewicz, D.; Rorat, M.; Leszczyński, P.; et al. Tocilizumab Improves the Prognosis of COVID-19 in Patients with High IL-6. *J. Clin. Med.* **2021**, *10*, 1583. [CrossRef] [PubMed]

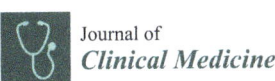

Article

Longwise Cluster Analysis for the Prediction of COVID-19 Severity within 72 h of Admission: COVID-DATA-SAVE-LIFES Cohort

Rodrigo San-Cristobal [1,*,†], Roberto Martín-Hernández [2,†], Omar Ramos-Lopez [3], Diego Martinez-Urbistondo [4], Víctor Micó [1], Gonzalo Colmenarejo [2], Paula Villares Fernandez [4], Lidia Daimiel [5] and Jose Alfredo Martínez [1,6]

1. Precision Nutrition and Cardiometabolic Health Researh Program, Institute on Food and Health Sciences (Institute IMDEA Food), 28049 Madrid, Spain; victor.mico@imdea.org (V.M.); jalfredo.martinez@imdea.org (J.A.M.)
2. Biostatistics & Bioinformatics Unit, Madrid Institute for Advanced Studies (IMDEA) Food, CEI UAM + CSIS, 28049 Madrid, Spain; roberto.martin@imdea.org (R.M.-H.); gonzalo.colmenarejo@imdea.org (G.C.)
3. Medicine and Psychology School, Autonomous University of Baja California, Tijuana 22390, Baja California, Mexico; oscar.omar.ramos.lopez@uabc.edu.mx
4. Internal Medicine Department, Hospital Universitario HM Sanchinarro, 28050 Madrid, Spain; dmurbistondo@gmail.com (D.M.-U.); pvillares@hmhospitales.com (P.V.F.)
5. Nutritional Control of the Epigenome Group, IMDEA Food Institute, CEI UAM + CSIS, 28049 Madrid, Spain; lidia.daimiel@imdea.org
6. CIBERobn Physiopathology of Obesity and Nutrition, Institute of Health Carlos III (ISCIII), 28029 Madrid, Spain
* Correspondence: rodrigo.sancristobal@imdea.org
† These authors contributed equally to this work.

Abstract: The use of routine laboratory biomarkers plays a key role in decision making in the clinical practice of COVID-19, allowing the development of clinical screening tools for personalized treatments. This study performed a short-term longitudinal cluster from patients with COVID-19 based on biochemical measurements for the first 72 h after hospitalization. Clinical and biochemical variables from 1039 confirmed COVID-19 patients framed on the "COVID Data Save Lives" were grouped in 24-h blocks to perform a longitudinal k-means clustering algorithm to the trajectories. The final solution of the three clusters showed a strong association with different clinical severity outcomes (OR for death: Cluster A reference, Cluster B 12.83 CI: 6.11–30.54, and Cluster C 14.29 CI: 6.66–34.43; OR for ventilation: Cluster-B 2.22 CI: 1.64–3.01, and Cluster-C 1.71 CI: 1.08–2.76), improving the AUC of the models in terms of age, sex, oxygen concentration, and the Charlson Comorbidities Index (0.810 vs. 0.871 with $p < 0.001$ and 0.749 vs. 0.807 with $p < 0.001$, respectively). Patient diagnoses and prognoses remarkably diverged between the three clusters obtained, evidencing that data-driven technologies devised for the screening, analysis, prediction, and tracking of patients play a key role in the application of individualized management of the COVID-19 pandemics.

Keywords: COVID-19; Charlson Comorbidities Index; cluster analysis; longitudinal cluster; individualized management

1. Introduction

The Severe Acute Respiratory Syndrome Coronavirus 2 (SARS-CoV-2) appeared around December 2019 in Wuhan (China) and has been spreading all around the globe thenceforth [1,2]. The World Health Organization (WHO) declared the disease (COVID-19) caused by SARS-CoV-2 as a pandemic in March 2020, based on the incidence growths due to the high contagiousness and high levels of lethality presented [3]. The major challenge for clinicians and practitioners has been the wide clinical presentation form of the disease and requiring the decision of intensive care unit (ICU) admission, together with the use of mechanical ventilation. Patients with COVID-19 could present as asymptomatic or with milder symptoms (including fever, sore throat, dry cough, dyspnea, myalgia, headache, or diarrhea) or with more severe symptoms, such as chest pain, hypoxemia, pneumonia, and other complications [4]. Since the appearance of this pandemic, several authors have tried to stratify the patients depending on the symptoms, oxygen saturation, or the chest computed tomography in order to predict the severity of the patients, aiming to facilitate decision making in the clinical practice [5].

COVID-19 infection displays a mean incubation period between 6 and 7 days from the initial infection, followed by a viremic phase from the 8th day to the 10th day. However, the delay between symptom onset and hospitalization could vary from 2.6 to 9.7 days, depending on the country and the age of patients [6]. The delay of detection and hospitalization has a large impact on the concurrent inflammatory stage, and, thus, on the prognosis and the fatality of the disease [7]. These manifestations are accompanied by microvascular damages caused by the cytokine "storm" [8], and often, the pathophysiological COVID-19 condition is also associated with bacterial infections [9] and with body metabolic impairments [10,11], where prescribed anti-inflammatory medications also may play a role [12].

With all of this, the use of routine laboratory biomarkers is the key monitoring tool to predict the prognosis of the disease. There are several studies that have focused their research on a limited number of these markers or have uniquely performed cross-sectional analyses at the baseline and their relationship with the prognosis of these patients [13,14]. Thus, the identification of patients that are more likely to develop severe illness after diagnosis is a critical *checkpoint* in order to decrease mortality rates, as well as to avoid the collapse of medical care within the hospitals [15]. Therefore, taking into account the time evolution of comorbidities and potential organ injuries throughout the course of severe COVID-19 is crucial in the precise clinical management of patients, influencing treatment approaches and recovery rates [16] where inflammation has a very strong role [17], as well as immunity and hematological alterations [18] and liver dysfunctions [19]. All of this emphasizes the need for a clustered clinical management of this disease and one that would lead to achieve more personalized and effective interventions [20].

In this regard, understanding the short-term longitudinal variation and the specific profiles of these biomarkers based on the severity of disease progression would allow the development of stratification tools [21] to characterize distinctive phenotypes concerning patients with COVID-19 that predict their potential prognosis [22]. In this regard, the use of data science methods to identify underlying patterns or profiles present in patients with COVID-19 could shed light on the mechanisms that occur and would allow for the prescription of personalized treatments through the determination of clusters of patients attending objectively measured variables [5]. Based on this background, the present study aimed to explore data from patients admitted to all HM private hospitals in the Madrid region during the first pandemic peak reported in Spain, in order to find clusters of patients based on the biochemical measurements for the first 72 h of attendance and further implication in their prognosis.

2. Materials and Methods

2.1. Patients Database

The data used for the present analysis were framed on the "COVID Data Save Lives" (COVIDDSL) initiative carried out by the *HM Hospitales*. This initiative made freely available an anonymous dataset containing the information from the Electronic Health Record (EHR) system of the HM Hospitales (information available at https://www.hmhospitales.com/coronavirus/covid-data-save-lives/english-version (accessed on 20 July 2020)). The anonymized information contains the records of 2310 patients that were admitted with a diagnosis of COVID-19 between 26 December 2019 and 10 June 2020. Multicenter longitudinal information from this EHR comprise different datasets corresponding to the main clinical characteristics of different domains. Each patient was identified by an anonymized unique admission code. The datasets include information about the COVID-19 treatment process, including complete information on admission and diagnoses, treatments, ICU admissions, diagnostic imaging tests, laboratory results, drug administration, and cause of discharge or death). This study was conducted according to the guidelines of the Declaration of Helsinki and approved by the Ethics Committee of the HM hospitals consortium (CEI HM Hospitales Ref No. 20.05.1627-GHM).

2.2. Data Collection and Definitions

The data sets were preprocessed considering only adult patients with confirmed COVID-19. Both clinical and biochemical variables were selected and grouped in blocks of 24 h to 72 h from the patients' admission to the hospital. In those patients that presented more than one measure per day, the median value was used to avoid the potential effect of extreme values for these variables. Additionally, patients were categorized according to the cause of discharge or admission to the ICU and the administration of mechanical ventilation. Reported death and mechanical ventilation variables were used to test the prognostic value of the current exploratory analysis.

Data included for the exploratory analysis were patient's age, sex, clinical history of previous diseases, vital signs and tests performed throughout the hospitalization, and the medications administered until the discharge. The vital sign variables included for the analysis were oxygen saturation (%), body temperature (°C), heart rate (beats/min), and systolic and diastolic blood pressure (mmHg). The following parameters were selected from the different tests collected: white cell proportions including leukocytes (1000/µL), basophil (%), eosinophils (%), lymphocyte (%), monocyte (%), and neutrophils (%); red cell markers including red cell distribution width (RDW, in %), hemoglobin (g/dL), hematocrit (%), mean corpuscular hemoglobin (pg/cell), mean corpuscular hemoglobin concentration (g/dL), and mean corpuscular volume (fL); platelets and prothrombin markers such as mean platelet volume (%), platelet count (1000/µL), the international normalized ratio (INR), prothrombin activity (%), and prothrombin time (seconds); metabolic markers and electrolytes including glucose (mg/dL), Gamma-glutamil transferase (GGT, in IU/L), aspartate aminotransferase (AST, in IU/L), alanine aminotransferase (ALT, in IU/L), sodium (mmol/L), and potassium (mmol/L); and finally, inflammatory and catabolic markers such as C-Reactive Protein (CRP, in mg/L), D-Dimer (ng/mL), lactate dehydrogenase (IU/L), creatinine (mg/dL), and urea (mg/dL).

Additionally, International Statistical Classification of Disease and Related Health Problems (ICD-10) coding tables with clinical records of diseases and procedures, as well as medications classified by ATC5/ATC7, for each patient and time point were also condensed in categories and activity of medications, respectively. The coded information was used to carried out complementary descriptive analysis. Additionally, clinical variables were encoded following the criteria of the Charlson comorbidity index (CCI) categories [23] to adjust the logistic regression models and measure the effect in the models of concomitant diseases as a potential confounder in the prognosis of these patients.

2.3. Statistical Analysis

Patients with less than 50% of missing values for the selected variables during the first 4 blocks of 24 h were selected to conduct the present analysis. Patients were categorized, by the median number of comorbidities at the baseline (by CCI), patients with 3 or less comorbidities and those with more than 3 comorbidities at the baseline, to carry out the descriptive analysis, including means and standard deviations (SD) for quantitative variables and absolute value with percentages for categorical variables. Student's t tests for continuous variables and chi-squared tests for categorical variables were used to assess differences between patients from both comorbidity groups.

The longitudinal unsupervised clustering was performed by using the *Kml3d* library, which provided a longitudinal implementation of the widely used k-means algorithms [24]. The technique used for this study was an unsupervised non-parametric cluster analysis that classifies the trajectories of the patients by simultaneously providing the 33 routine biochemical parameters from the first 72 h after the admission of the patients. This technique implements a path expectation-maximization algorithm by alternating different initialization methods to obtain the most stable solution for the clusters, and it can feature groups of patients associated with specific disease risks. Clustering approaches are not ultimately predictive, but they are descriptive and contribute to identify patterns concerning hidden structural data, which do not demand a formal hypothesis. Indeed, clustering analysis can feature groups of patients associated with specific disease risks. Clustering permits targeting patients in a cost-effective feasible nature and relevant clinical impact. Cluster analysis has been used to characterize risk factors associated with diseases [25] and may require further regression analysis to predict other related variables [26]. This library was used to specifically cluster patients based on the joint trajectories of the selected clinical and biochemical variables throughout the 24-h time periods during the first 72 h of hospitalization. A range of 2 to 10 clusters was assayed to fit the most adequate solution for the model, based on the lowest Bayesian information criterion (BIC) and the clinical relevance of clustering solutions (measured by the severity of outcomes related to the cluster using logistic regression), resulting in a final best solution of 3 clusters. Principal component analysis was conducted to visualize the categorization of the patients. The relative importance of the variables and the time periods was estimated through variable/time permutation to gain a better understanding of the most important variables and times in the clusters obtained. ANOVA analysis was carried out to compare clinical characteristics among clusters, and a Tukey *post hoc* analysis was applied to compare individual groups.

A multivariable logistic regression model was used afterwards to estimate the gain upon inclusion of the clusters previously obtained as independent variables for the prediction of two outcome variables, namely death and administration of mechanical ventilation during hospitalization. Three different models were developed to evaluate the effect of the inclusion of the cluster assignment, in addition to the main factors that impacted the COVID prognosis. Model 1 used age-independent CCI, sex, and age as predictor variables; model 2 was additionally adjusted by temperature and oxygen saturation at admission; and the final model 3 was additionally adjusted by the cluster assignments. Area under the curve (AUC) from receiver operating characteristic curves (ROC) was estimated to evaluate the predictive value of each model. All the statistical analyses were performed using R statistical software version 4.0.1 (R Project for Statistical Computing) within RStudio statistical software version 1.4 (Rstudio Team. Rstudio: Integrated Development Environment for R. Boston, MA, USA).

3. Results

3.1. Study Sample Description

The cleaned dataset (Table 1) contained 1039 confirmed COVID-19 patients, 60% male and 40% female, with a global age mean of 68.5 years. The mean days of hospitalization were 10.1, with 5.4% of the patients admitted to ICU and 62.6% receiving mechanical ventilation during the hospitalization. The main cause of medical discharge was home referral (78.5% of patients), while the referral to other centers corresponded to 6.2% of the hospitalization, and death represented 11.5% of the patients. The patients presented an average CCI of 3.6 at hospitalization. As expected, when the patients were categorized by CCI with a cut-off of 3 points (Table 1), those above the cutoff were older and evidenced worse health status concerning hospitalization features and higher death, and they suffered more comorbidities including cardiovascular events, liver diseases, diabetes, and cancer; however, a significant association with sex was observed.

Table 1. Baseline and outcome characteristics of COVID-19 patients from DATA SAVE LIVES categorized by the Charlson comorbidity index.

	Overall	≤3 Points	>3 Points	p
n	1039	533	506	
Age	68.5 (15.5)	58.0 (11.9)	79.5 (10.3)	<0.001
Sex (male (%))	626 (60.3)	328 (61.5)	298 (58.9)	0.419
Hospitalization (days)	10.1 (8.6)	8.9 (7.7)	11.3 (9.3)	<0.001
ICU stay (yes (%))	56 (5.4)	29 (5.4)	27 (5.3)	1
Mechanical ventilation (yes (%))	650 (62.6)	295 (55.3)	355 (70.2)	<0.001
Cause of discharge (%)				<0.001
Voluntary discharge	1 (0.1)	0 (0.0)	1 (0.2)	
Home	816 (78.5)	476 (89.3)	340 (67.2)	
Death	120 (11.5)	15 (2.8)	105 (20.8)	
Health center transfer	31 (3.0)	3 (0.6)	28 (5.5)	
Hospital transfer	33 (3.2)	19 (3.6)	14 (2.8)	
Not registered	38 (3.7)	20 (3.8)	18 (3.6)	
CCI	3.58 (2.53)	1.58 (1.11)	5.68 (1.81)	<0.001
Myocardial infarction (yes (%))	79 (7.6)	3 (0.6)	76 (15.0)	<0.001
Congestive heart failure (yes (%))	54 (5.2)	1 (0.2)	53 (10.5)	<0.001
Peripheral vascular disease (yes (%))	32 (3.1)	0 (0.0)	32 (6.3)	<0.001
Cerebrovascular accident (yes (%))	22 (2.1)	1 (0.2)	21 (4.2)	<0.001
Dementia (yes (%))	42 (4.0)	1 (0.2)	41 (8.1)	<0.001
COPD (yes (%))	131 (12.6)	30 (5.6)	101 (20.0)	<0.001
Connective tissue disease (yes (%))	13 (1.3)	4 (0.8)	9 (1.8)	0.226
Peptic ulcer disease (yes (%))	2 (0.2)	0 (0.0)	2 (0.4)	0.456
Liver disease (yes (%))	35 (3.4)	2 (0.4)	33 (6.5)	<0.001
Diabetes mellitus (yes (%))	194 (18.7)	36 (6.8)	158 (31.2)	<0.001
Hemiplegia (yes (%))	2 (0.2)	1 (0.2)	1 (0.2)	1
Moderate to severe CKD (yes (%))	153 (14.7)	4 (0.8)	149 (29.4)	<0.001
Solid tumor (yes (%))	44 (4.2)	1 (0.2)	43 (8.5)	<0.001
Lymphoma (yes (%))	16 (1.5)	0 (0.0)	16 (3.2)	<0.001
Leukemia (yes (%))	8 (0.8)	0 (0.0)	8 (1.6)	0.01
AIDS (yes (%))	2 (0.2)	0 (0.0)	2 (0.4)	0.456

p-value: t-test for continuous variables and chi-square for categorical variables. ICU: intensive care unit; CCI: Charlson comorbidity index; COPD: chronic obstructive pulmonary disease; CKD: chronic kidney disease; AIDS: acquired immune deficiency syndrome.

3.2. Patient Clusterization

The cluster analysis was developed to categorize the sample based on the longitudinal evolution of multiple vital signs and laboratory tests (see Section 2). The best clustering was obtained with three clusters. Supplementary Figure S1b displays a PCA with all these variables, colored by the three clusters obtained. We can see the good separation of the patients achieved by this longitudinal clustering. In addition, in order to interpret the clustering, we estimated the relative importance of the different variables and times by permutation-based feature/time importance analyses. The resulting ranked importance of variables and times are displayed in Supplementary Figure S1c, where it can be seen that monocytes, GGT, neutrophils, prothrombin time, and urea were the most remarkable variable contributors to the clustering, and the first 24 h is the most important time of all.

In addition, in Table 2, we analyzed the association of these clusters with different baseline and outcome variables, in order have an idea of the clinical profiles of the three clusters. In this way, Cluster A encompassed patients with lower hospitalization, ICU stay, and clinical complication rates, displaying a death rate of only 1.6%; Cluster B showed an intermediate prevalence of chronic diseases with a fatality incidence of 14.4%; and Cluster C showed the eldest group of patients, with a mortality rate of 37.4% and a higher clinical morbidity prevalence.

Table 2. Baseline and outcome characteristics of COVID-19 patients from DATA SAVE LIVES categorized by cluster.

	Stratified by Cluster			
	A	B	C	p
n	496	403	147	
Age	66.1 (15.8)	66.1 (13.7)	83.1 (9.9)	<0.001
Sex (male (%))	252 (50.8)	287 (71.2)	92 (62.6)	<0.001
Hospitalization (days)	7.6 (5.6)	13.7 (11.9)	10.1 (7.9)	<0.001
ICU stay (yes (%))	0.10 (1.57)	1.36 (5.08)	0.17 (1.51)	<0.001
Mechanical ventilation (yes (%))	258 (52.0)	287 (71.2)	112 (76.2)	<0.001
Cause of discharge (%)				<0.001
Voluntary discharge	0 (0.0)	1 (0.2)	0 (0.0)	
Home	433 (87.3)	313 (77.7)	75 (51.0)	
Death	8 (1.6)	58 (14.4)	55 (37.4)	
Health center transfer	18 (3.6)	3 (0.7)	10 (6.8)	
Hospital transfer	14 (2.8)	16 (4.0)	3 (2.0)	
Not registered	23 (4.6)	12 (3.0)	4 (2.7)	
CCI	3.2 (2.4)	3.1 (2.2)	6.2 (2.2)	<0.001
Myocardial infarction (yes (%))	40 (8.1)	17 (4.3)	22 (15.1)	<0.001
Congestive heart failure (yes (%))	19 (3.8)	11 (2.8)	24 (16.4)	<0.001
Peripheral vascular disease (yes (%))	18 (3.6)	3 (0.8)	11 (7.5)	<0.001
Cerebrovascular accident (yes (%))	8 (1.6)	5 (1.3)	9 (6.2)	0.001
Dementia (yes (%))	23 (4.6)	8 (2.0)	11 (7.5)	0.01
COPD (yes (%))	67 (13.5)	35 (8.8)	29 (19.9)	0.002
Connective tissue disease (yes (%))	8 (1.6)	1 (0.3)	4 (2.7)	0.041
Peptic ulcer disease (yes (%))	1 (0.2)	0 (0.0)	1 (0.7)	0.271
Liver disease (yes (%))	17 (3.4)	16 (4.0)	2 (1.4)	0.314
Diabetes mellitus (yes (%))	89 (18.0)	59 (14.8)	46 (31.5)	<0.001
Hemiplegia (yes (%))	1 (0.2)	1 (0.3)	0 (0.0)	0.837
Moderate to severe CKD (yes (%))	44 (8.9)	46 (11.6)	63 (43.2)	<0.001
Solid tumor (yes (%))	12 (2.4)	15 (3.8)	17 (11.6)	<0.001
Lymphoma (yes (%))	8 (1.6)	5 (1.3)	3 (2.1)	0.784
Leukemia (yes (%))	4 (0.8)	2 (0.5)	2 (1.4)	0.586
AIDS (yes (%))	0 (0.0)	2 (0.5)	0 (0.0)	0.199

p-value: ANOVA for continuous variables and chi-square for categorical variables. ICU: intensive care unit; CCI: Charlson comorbidity index; COPD: chronic obstructive pulmonary disease; CKD: chronic kidney disease; AIDS: acquired immune deficiency syndrome.

Additionally, clinical variables evolved during the initial 72 h after hospital admission according to different cluster profiles, as can be seen in Figure 1, where the time evolution of these variables is displayed for the three classes, color coded in reference to recommended values (above, within, below). In general, Cluster C presented the most altered medical variables in comparison with the other two clusters, while Cluster B showed a mildly severe inflammatory condition. More specifically, the patients in Cluster B showed the lowest eosinophil levels and the highest levels of GGT, AST, ALT, C-reactive protein, and lactate dehydrogenase during the 72 h compared to the other clusters. Meanwhile, Cluster C presented the lowest lymphocyte levels and prothrombin activity, as well as the most elevated levels for prothrombin time, INR, glucose, D-dimer, creatinine, and urea (Figure 1).

Vital signs (Supplementary Figure S2) indicated that, while Cluster A presented less unhealthy symptoms, Cluster B and C displayed significantly worse clinical outcomes maintained throughout all time points (0–72 h). When white blood cell count was observed (Supplementary Figure S3), Cluster A involved fewer biological abnormalities. Specifically, lower levels of eosinophils were detected in the three clusters at all-time points, while only Cluster B and Cluster C had lymphocyte counts below the laboratory references. Curiously, Cluster A presented high levels of monocyte count. Those cluster differences were present across the 72-h measured course (Figure 1 and Supplementary Figure S3). Red blood cell levels, despite some significant cluster differences, were not different to normalized values (Figure 1 and Supplementary Figure S4).

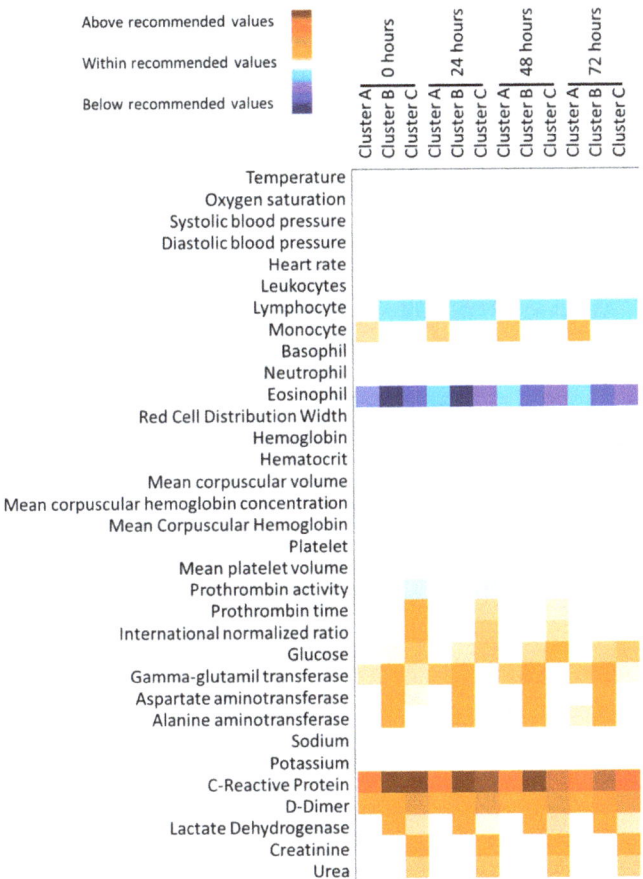

Figure 1. Heatmap plot of adequacy to reference values for clinical variables included in the cluster analysis. White means that the mean value for the cluster was within the recommended values; meanwhile, blue and orange intensity represent the deviation from the recommended values below and above, respectively.

Regarding blotting (prothrombin activity and time besides international normalized ratio) and hepatic related enzymes (ALT, AST, and GGT), Cluster C had altered high levels of those indications, while the other two cluster were closer to reference normality (Figure 1 and Supplementary Figures S5 and S6). Finally, inflammation (C-reactive protein) and thrombosis (D-Dimer) examinations, as well as lactate dehydrogenase, were impaired in all the clusters, with a greater severity in Cluster B and C compared to Cluster A, while renal functionality assessed by creatinine and urea were only altered in Cluster C (Figure 1 and Supplementary Figure S7).

3.3. Logistic Regression Models to Predict Severe Outcomes

Finally, a logistic regression model was fitted to discern the capacity of the modeled clusters to predict the disease fatality (Table 3, Figure 2). The first model, including the age-independent CCI, sex, and age as predictors, showed only age and sex with significant *p*-values and an AUROC of 0801. A second model, which added oxygen saturation and temperature (the former significant but not the latter) to the previous one, had a negligible increase of AUROC to 0.81. However, the inclusion of the cluster variable in the third model (green line in Figure 2) resulted in a large boost of the AUROC, up to 0.87. The third model presented the highest value of AUC, showing the better capacity of death prediction (p-value obtained by parametric bootstrapping for differences between Model 1 vs. Model 3 and Model 2 vs. Model 3, <0.001 and <0.001, respectively).

Table 3. Logistic regression model for the risk of death.

	OR	(95% CI)	p	AUC
Model 1				0.801
Age-independent CCI	1.09	(0.97–1.21)	0.126	
Sex (male)	2.66	(1.69–4.25)	0.000	
Age	1.09	(1.07–1.11)	0.000	
Model 2				0.810
Age-independent CCI	1.10	(0.98–1.23)	0.087	
Oxygen saturation	0.94	(0.9–0.98)	0.007	
Temperature	1.12	(0.82–1.54)	0.469	
Sex (male)	2.55	(1.63–4.09)	0.000	
Age	1.09	(1.07–1.11)	0.000	
Model 3				0.871
Cluster (Cluster B)	12.83	(6.11–30.54)	0.000	
Cluster (Cluster C)	14.29	(6.66–34.43)	0.000	
Age-independent CCI	1.05	(0.93–1.18)	0.431	
Oxygen saturation	0.96	(0.92–1)	0.071	
Temperature	0.81	(0.58–1.13)	0.231	
Sex (male)	2.12	(1.31–3.52)	0.003	
Age	1.08	(1.06–1.11)	0.000	

OR: Odds Ratio; CI: Confidence interval; AUC: area under the curve; CCI: Charlson comorbidity index.

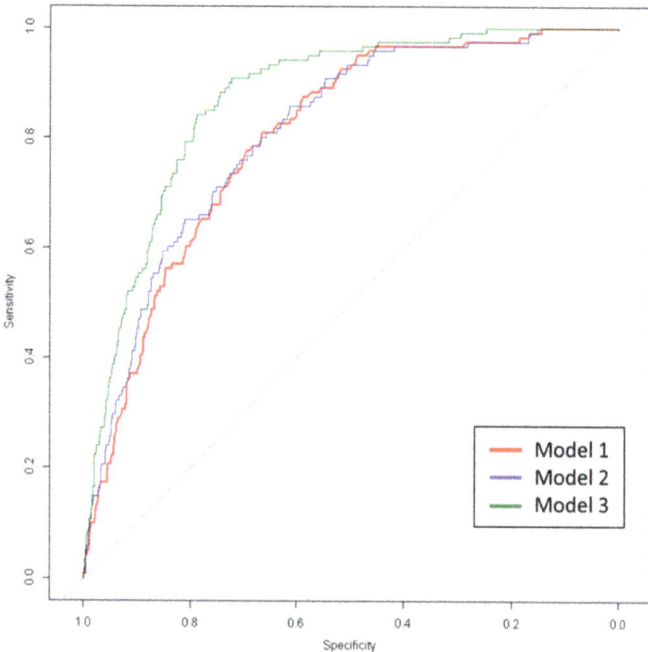

Figure 2. ROC curve of logistic regression for the three models.

A similar analysis was performed to predict the risk of mechanical ventilation using these models (Table 4). The obtained results were similar, with a better predictive capacity in Model 3 compared to the other two models (Figure 3), confirming the utility of patients' clusterization (p-value obtained by parametric bootstrapping for differences between Model 1 vs. Model 3 and Model 2 vs. Model 3 = 0.023 and <0.001, respectively).

Table 4. Logistic regression model for the risk of mechanical ventilation.

	OR (95% CI)		p	AUC
Model 1				0.775
Age-independent CCI	1.18	(1.08–1.29)	0.000	
Sex (male)	1.17	(0.9–1.53)	0.246	
Age	1.02	(1.01–1.03)	0.000	
Model 2				0.749
Age-independent CCI	1.20	(1.1–1.32)	0.000	
Oxygen saturation	1.01	(0.98–1.05)	0.467	
Temperature	1.49	(1.22–1.83)	0.000	
Sex (male)	1.16	(0.88–1.51)	0.291	
Age	1.02	(1.01–1.03)	0.000	
Model 3				0.807
Cluster (Cluster B)	2.22	(1.64–3.01)	0.000	
Cluster (Cluster C)	1.71	(1.08–2.76)	0.024	
Age-independent CCI	1.21	(1.1–1.33)	0.000	
Oxygen saturation	1.02	(0.99–1.06)	0.205	
Temperature	1.28	(1.04–1.59)	0.021	
Sex (male)	1.00	(0.75–1.32)	0.980	
Age	1.02	(1.01–1.03)	0.000	

AUC: area under the curve; CCI: Charlson comorbidity index.

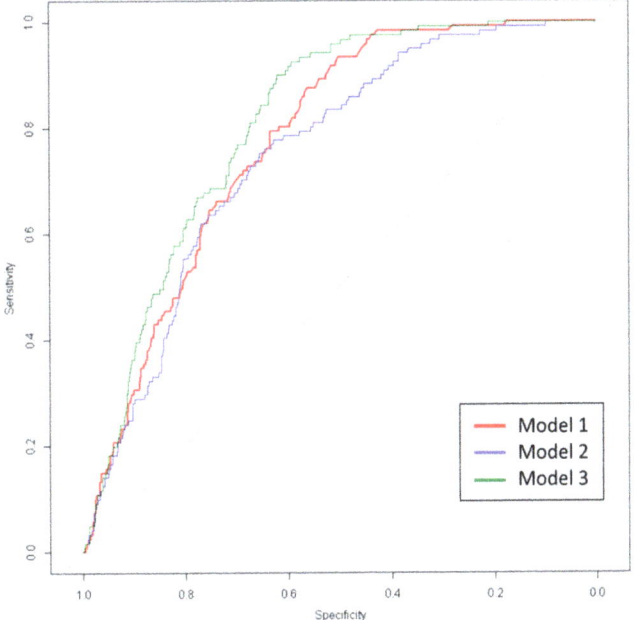

Figure 3. ROC curve of logistic regression for the three models.

4. Discussion

Coronavirus disease has affected all nations and territories, while several investigations are now being conducted to seek personalized clinical prescriptions and provide epidemiological surveillance to control this pandemic [15,27]. Indeed, research concerning the early symptomatic identification and assessing specific traits involving clinical manifestations, medical outcomes, and epidemiological estimates with machine learning models offers huge opportunities for precision medicine despite some limitations and challenges [28]. In this context, the COVID-19 disease presents a unique prospect to understand whether there are distinct phenotypes of COVID-19 outcomes, whose knowledge will provide important benefits not only for the personalized management of infected patients, but also for optimizing health care systems and for devising public health policies [29] by considering phenotypical plus family and clinical history backgrounds, as well as individual lifestyle factors [30].

The implementation of multivariate statistical and bioinformatic instruments to provide valid information for clinical purposes includes hierarchical cluster analysis, principal component analysis, random forest, discriminant analysis, support vector machine algorithms, and neural network-based deep learning methods, with value on disease characterization, diagnosis, and treatment [20]. In this context, a longitudinal cluster analysis was implemented on the "COVID Data Save Lives" (COVIDDSL) dataset to unhidden statistically significant clinical variables and the internal structure, as performed elsewhere with COVID-19 infected patients [31].

In our clinical setting, regarding a group of Spanish public/private hospitals, applying longitudinal cluster analyses enabled three distinctive COVID-19 medical phenotypes to emerge: Cluster A characterized by including patients' mild inflammatory symptoms and low death occurrence (1.6%), Cluster B featuring important immune-inflammatory distress and specific liver dysfunctions with a rate of 14.4% mortality, while Cluster C encompassed specific coagulation disorders and renal alterations, in addition to inflammatory and immunocompetence abnormalities with a fatality prevalence of 37.4% of the patients. Thus, survival times across clusters notably differed in the three groups of patients, which is key for ameliorating disease management and outcomes by considering individualized patient profiling, predictive personalized models, and precision cost-effective risks, alleviating procedures as previously described in the palliative treatment of liver tumors using unsupervised artificial intelligence [32]. Moreover, the age and number of comorbidities, as associated with increased risk of mortality in patients with COVID-19, need to be accounted for [33], as delineated in the three A, B, and C clusters.

In this scenario, analyses concerning longitudinal COVID-19 disease trajectories were able to recognize vulnerable population clusters that would particularly benefit from specific health resources and provide insights for public health targets in order to manage the COVID-19 infectious pandemic. Thus, tuberculosis and HIV/AIDS, hepatitis, cardiomyopathies, and diabetes were consistently associated with an increased risk to be found in a more vulnerable cluster [34]. Furthermore, a comprehensive measurement of dysfunction severity of six organ systems based on the Sequential Organ Failure Assessment (SOFA) score revealed that cardiovascular, central nervous system, coagulation, liver, renal, and respiration pathobiology were able to identify distinct strata of COVID-19 patients, as defined by the baseline post-intubation SOFA. This includes findings suggestive of inflammation as a mechanism involving differential COVID-19 disease severity outcomes, as well as a heterogeneous physiopathological lung illness [29], which is in accordance with some of our findings, given that inflammatory responses, clothing, hepatic/renal alterations, and impaired immunocompetence were markers involved in cluster discrimination

Another study developed with machine learning tools and based on a decision tree model to anticipate COVID-19 outcomes from a list of 132,939 recovered COVID-19 subjects evidenced that mortality prevalence was specifically clustered among males, older cases, and hospital admission history as predictors of case fatality [35]. In addition, a database study encompassing hospitalized COVID-19 patients over 24 and 48 h in the Mount

Sinai Health System predicted intubation, intensive care unit transfer, and mortality and was able to identify important features, such as pulse oximetry with clinical importance in the outcome [36]. Results from the current analyses confirm trends during the 72-h outcomes among the three clusters, with some differential responses concerning PCR, hemoglobin, and coagulation indicators, while the fitted logistic regression model for the risk of mechanical ventilation and death considered both variables independently influenced by cluster allocation.

Another analysis devised to generate an accurate diagnosis model of COVID-19 based on routine tests and clinical symptoms by applying machine learning to COVID-19 data found several associations between clinical variables, such as having idiosyncratic levels of circulating lymphocytes and neutrophils, suggesting that COVID-19 patients could be clustered into several phenotype subtypes based on immune cells, gender, and declared symptoms, which could overcome the influence of a low testing capacity or the concurrent impact of other bacterial or viral infections [37]. Indeed, our cluster model demonstrated discrimination abilities associated with lymphocyte, monocyte, and eosinophil counts among then and during the 72 h after hospitalization.

Noteworthy, anemia and iron deficiency may play a role in the Coronavirus disease, as shown in a systematic review and associated meta-analyses, where hemoglobin levels were lower with older age but higher in subjects with diabetes, hypertension, and overall comorbidities and those admitted to intensive care [38], which is independently categorized by Cluster C in our model

The severe proinflammatory state commonly reported in COVID-19 patients has been associated with the activation of coagulation pathways and thrombosis [39], as well as by a characteristic coagulopathy and procoagulant endothelial phenotype [40]. The current clustered model for COVID-19 patients classified prothrombin activity and time, specifically in Cluster C, and also demonstrated some stratification competences in Dimer-D measurements, but not in increased platelet consumption. Interestingly, thrombocytopenia is relatively uncommon in COVID-19, being estimated that the dysregulated immune system responses as coordinated by inflammatory cytokines, lymphocyte cell death, and endothelial damage are involved [41]. Thus, patients with COVID-19 may suffer coagulation and thrombotic abnormalities, stimulating a hypercoagulable condition and increasing thromboembolic incidence [42].

Associations between blood biomarkers such as the neutrophil-to-lymphocyte ratio with the severity of COVID-19 lesions have been established, as well as with other specific and unspecific proinflammatory markers, such as CRP and other measures commonly analyzed for COVID-19, such as hemoglobin, D-dimers, and eosinophils counts [18], which should orientate the clinician for infected patients' management being eased by the existence of algorithms and cluster categorization. Further statistical analyses indicated that inflammatory CRP and D-dimer levels were increased and can assist as early indicators of severe COVID-19 cerebrovascular problems [27].

In these circumstances, exacerbated innate and adaptive immune responses are crucial in foreseeing the development and progression of NAFLD in COVID-19 patients [19]. A specific implication of severe COVID-19 in NAFLD patients putatively mediated by immunocompetence status is highlighted in the B cluster, where transaminases and liver health markers showed abnormal values and may drive personalized medicine approaches, as prompted by the allocation to a cluster with related measurements uncovering therapeutic targets. In a previous report, patients concerning this COVID-DATA-SAFE-LIFES cohort were categorized following conventional criteria to explain disease severity and deaths, which verified that liver and proinflammatory features are important determinants of COVID-19 morbidity and mortality in order to ameliorate the understanding of morbid manifestations of COVID-19, besides to help the therapy decision-making protocols under a personalized medicine scope [11]. Indeed, the liver health and coagulation axis appears as a relevant surrogate for elucidating some COVID-19 outcomes linked to systemic inflammation [43], as well as thrombotic and fibrinolytic disturbances [44], which were deciphered in the currently emerged three clusters, including some markers of global health such as lactate dehydrogenase or creatinine/urea measurements [45], as particularly discriminated in Cluster C. Interestingly, hemoglobin and prothrombin values evidenced divergent patterns after the following 72-h period, which represent a worth for a cluster monitor. Indeed, our results provide a tool in the early management of COVID-19 patients, in contrast to other related papers in COVID where it has been taken into account with cardiac biomarkers [46] or other more complex techniques, such as imaging-based prognosis or gene/protein expression [47,48].

This research had some limitations and strengths. Thus, as a multipurpose cohort, the aims and hypotheses were assigned after the database was closed, and this was partly overcome by the large number of collected clinical determinations and the relatively high sample size. In addition, the initial uncertainties about the clinical management guidelines and concurrent morbid conditions/medications in COVID-19 patients may have an impact on data interpretation, although we provided information about pharmacological treatments (Supplementary Table S2) and several diseases at admission.

The identification of subgroups of COVID-19 patients through the longwise cluster analysis performed in this study allowed the identification of latent profiles of COVID-19 patients to shed light on the most appropriate treatment focused on objective routine blood markers commonly used in clinical practice, unlike other articles that only study a single marker follow-up [27], cross-sectional analyses [14], composite index [29], or non-objective markers [13]. Moreover, a model using machine learning was able to predict case fatality in the elderly population, with a large history of hospital admission, which increases the rate of COVID-19 death [35]. Novel aspects of this analysis concerned the discrimination of patients by clustering routine determinations and being able to forecast death rates and associated comorbidities in the first 72 h. Previous studies have focused on exploring the value of these bioinformatic tools for coronavirus diagnosis and treatment [20], including image processing [49]. These results have been reinforced in systematic and metanalysis, which described clinical subgroups, while other researchers using result-driven technologies implemented the screening, analyses, and predictors of data tracking to confirm death cases [50]. Furthermore, the longitudinal follow up for 72 h allowed the confirmation of trends and alignments, giving support to the interest of multiple clinical analytical measurements at entrance. Actually, healthcare provision necessitates the backing of innovative skills and strategies, including artificial intelligence (AI), Big Data, and machine learning approaches to combat and project actions against new diseases such as COVID and other complex syndromes. Identifying the pool of cases and predicting where this viral infection and associated comorbidities will move in future interventions require collecting clinical information and bioinformatically analyzing available preceding data [50].

5. Conclusions

Summing up the current cohort, by applying a longwise cluster analysis of the first 72 h enabled to materialize three discriminated COVID-19 clinical clustered phenotypes: Cluster A, featuring patients mainly displaying mild inflammatory abnormalities and a low fatal occurrence below 2%; Cluster B, involving specific immune-inflammatory and explicit liver dysfunctions, with a mortality incidence around 15%; and Cluster C exhibiting hemoglobin, prothrombin, and renal impairments, together with importantly altered inflammatory and immune responses, resulting in about 40% of deaths in this group. Indeed, patient diagnoses and prognoses remarkably diverged in the three clusters, which is relevant for considering predictive patient alignment, tailored precision clinical prescriptions, personalized cost-effective engagements, and alleviating epidemiological measures, as pioneers reported in diverse communicable and non-communicable diseases using artificial intelligence and machine learning instruments. Actually, medical-driven technologies devised for the proper screening, analysis, prediction, and tracking of SARS-

CoV-2 infected patients are partaking significant developments and applications for the precision and individualized management of the COVID-19 pandemics.

Supplementary Materials: The following supporting information can be downloaded at: https://www.mdpi.com/article/10.3390/jcm11123327/s1, Supplementary Table S1: Reference values for clinical variables included in the cluster analysis; Supplementary Table S2: Drug use by cluster and time (drugs with overall frequency n > 100); Supplementary Figure S1: A Principal component plot of the 2 main components from the cluster analysis; Supplementary Figure S2: Vital signs within the first 72 h of patients categorized by cluster; Supplementary Figure S3: White cells proportions within the first 72 h of patients categorized by cluster; Supplementary Figure S4: Red cells markers within the first 72 h of patients categorized by cluster; Supplementary Figure S5: Platelets and prothrombin markers within the first 72 h of patients categorized by cluster; Supplementary Figure S6: Metabolic markers and electrolytes within the first 72 h of patients categorized by cluster; Supplementary Figure S7: Inflammation and catabolic markers within the first 72 h of patients categorized by cluster.

Author Contributions: Conceptualization, R.S.-C., O.R.-L., D.M.-U., L.D. and J.A.M.; methodology, R.S.-C., R.M.-H., G.C. and J.A.M.; investigation, R.S.-C., R.M.-H., O.R.-L., D.M.-U., G.C., V.M., P.V.F., L.D. and J.A.M.; data Curation and formal analysis, R.S.-C., V.M., L.D. and R.M.-H.; writing—original draft preparation, R.S.-C., R.M.-H. and O.R.-L.; writing—review and editing, R.S.-C., R.M.-H., D.M.-U., V.M., G.C., P.V.F., L.D. and J.A.M. All authors have read and agreed to the published version of the manuscript.

Funding: This research was funded by the Community of Madrid and the European Union, through the European Regional Development Fund (ERDF)-REACT-EU resources of the Madrid Operational Program 2014–2020, in the action line of R + D + i projects in response to COVID 19 (REACT EU Program "FACINGLCOVID-CM"). J.A.M. acknowledges financial support from Synergic R&D Projects in New and Emerging Scientific Areas on the Frontier of Science and Interdisciplinary Nature of The Community of Madrid (METAINFLAMATION-Y2020/BIO-6600). The support from CIBERobn is also credited.

Institutional Review Board Statement: The study was conducted in accordance with the Declaration of Helsinki and was approved by the Ethics Committee of the HM hospitals consortium (CEI HM Hospitales Ref No. 20.05.1627-GHM).

Informed Consent Statement: Informed consent was obtained from all subjects involved in the study.

Data Availability Statement: HM Hospitales makes this clinical dataset available to researchers from academic, university and healthcare institutions who request it and whose project is approved. The content is expected to be expanded and updated periodically, and its update will not be completed until this pandemic is terminated. To obtain the data, it will be necessary to send the following request to the email coviddatasavelives@hmhospitales.com or data_science@hmhospitales.com in order to be evaluated by the Data Science Commission and, where appropriate, by the Research Ethics Committee of HM Hospitales or any other accredited research ethics committee.

Acknowledgments: R.S.-C. acknowledges financial support from the Juan de la Cierva Programme Training Grants of the Spanish State Research Agency of the Spanish Ministerio de Ciencia e Innovación y Ministerio de Universidades (FJC2018-038168- I). Authors thank HM hospitals for access to the COVID-DATA-SAFE-LIFES database.

Conflicts of Interest: The authors declare no conflict of interest.

References

1. Zhu, N.; Zhang, D.; Wang, W.; Li, X.; Yang, B.; Song, J.; Zhao, X.; Huang, B.; Shi, W.; Lu, R.; et al. A Novel Coronavirus from Patients with Pneumonia in China, 2019. *N. Engl. J. Med.* **2020**, *382*, 727–733. [CrossRef] [PubMed]
2. Wu, F.; Zhao, S.; Yu, B.; Chen, Y.M.; Wang, W.; Song, Z.G.; Hu, Y.; Tao, Z.W.; Tian, J.H.; Pei, Y.Y.; et al. A new coronavirus associated with human respiratory disease in China. *Nature* **2020**, *579*, 265–269. [CrossRef] [PubMed]
3. Bedford, J.; Enria, D.; Giesecke, J.; Heymann, D.L.; Ihekweazu, C.; Kobinger, G.; Lane, H.C.; Memish, Z.; Oh, M.D.; Sall, A.A.; et al. COVID-19: Towards controlling of a pandemic. *Lancet* **2020**, *395*, 1015–1018. [CrossRef]
4. Menni, C.; Valdes, A.M.; Freidin, M.B.; Sudre, C.H.; Nguyen, L.H.; Drew, D.A.; Ganesh, S.; Varsavsky, T.; Cardoso, M.J.; El-Sayed Moustafa, J.S.; et al. Real-time tracking of self-reported symptoms to predict potential COVID-19. *Nat. Med.* **2020**, *26*, 1037–1040. [CrossRef] [PubMed]

5. Sudre, C.H.; Lee, K.A.; Lochlainn, M.N.; Varsavsky, T.; Murray, B.; Graham, M.S.; Menni, C.; Modat, M.; Bowyer, R.C.E.; Nguyen, L.H.; et al. Symptom clusters in COVID-19: A potential clinical prediction tool from the COVID Symptom Study app. *Sci. Adv.* **2021**, *7*, eabd4177. [CrossRef]
6. Faes, C.; Abrams, S.; Van Beckhoven, D.; Meyfroidt, G.; Vlieghe, E.; Hens, N.; Belgian Collaborative Group on COVID-19 Hospital Surveillance. Time between Symptom Onset, Hospitalisation and Recovery or Death: Statistical Analysis of Belgian COVID-19 Patients. *Int. J. Environ. Res. Public Health* **2020**, *17*, 7560. [CrossRef]
7. Pellis, L.; Scarabel, F.; Stage, H.B.; Overton, C.E.; Chappell, L.H.K.; Fearon, E.; Bennett, E.; Lythgoe, K.A.; House, T.A.; Hall, I.; et al. Challenges in control of COVID-19: Short doubling time and long delay to effect of interventions. *Philos. Trans. R. Soc. Lond. B Biol. Sci.* **2021**, *376*, 20200264. [CrossRef]
8. Martinez-Urbistondo, M.; Mora-Vargas, A.; Exposito-Palomo, E.; Castejon, R.; Citores, M.J.; Rosado, S.; de Mendoza, C.; Banos, I.; Fernandez-Cruz, A.; Daimiel, L.; et al. Inflammatory-Related Clinical and Metabolic Outcomes in COVID-19 Patients. *Mediat. Inflamm.* **2020**, *2020*, 2914275. [CrossRef]
9. Moreno-Torres, V.; de Mendoza, C.; de la Fuente, S.; Sanchez, E.; Martinez-Urbistondo, M.; Herraiz, J.; Gutierrez, A.; Gutierrez, A.; Hernandez, C.; Callejas, A.; et al. Bacterial infections in patients hospitalized with COVID-19. *Intern. Emerg. Med.* **2021**, *17*, 431–438. [CrossRef]
10. Martinez Urbistondo, M.; Mora Vargas, A.; Exposito Palomo, E.; Aparicio de Miguel, M.; Castejon Diaz, R.; Daimiel, L.; Ramos Lopez, O.; San Cristobal, R.; Martinez, J.A.; Vargas Nunez, J.A. Evolution of patients infected with SARS-CoV-2 according to previous metabolic status. *Nutr. Hosp.* **2021**, *38*, 1068–1074. [CrossRef]
11. Ramos-Lopez, O.; San-Cristobal, R.; Martinez-Urbistondo, D.; Mico, V.; Colmenarejo, G.; Villares-Fernandez, P.; Daimiel, L.; Martinez, J.A. Proinflammatory and Hepatic Features Related to Morbidity and Fatal Outcomes in COVID-19 Patients. *J. Clin. Med.* **2021**, *10*, 3112. [CrossRef] [PubMed]
12. Yokota, S.; Miyamae, T.; Kuroiwa, Y.; Nishioka, K. Novel Coronavirus Disease 2019 (COVID-19) and Cytokine Storms for More Effective Treatments from an Inflammatory Pathophysiology. *J. Clin. Med.* **2021**, *10*, 801. [CrossRef] [PubMed]
13. Giacomelli, A.; Pezzati, L.; Conti, F.; Bernacchia, D.; Siano, M.; Oreni, L.; Rusconi, S.; Gervasoni, C.; Ridolfo, A.L.; Rizzardini, G.; et al. Self-reported Olfactory and Taste Disorders in Patients with Severe Acute Respiratory Coronavirus 2 Infection: A Cross-sectional Study. *Clin. Infect. Dis.* **2020**, *71*, 889–890. [CrossRef] [PubMed]
14. Pan, L.; Mu, M.; Yang, P.; Sun, Y.; Wang, R.; Yan, J.; Li, P.; Hu, B.; Wang, J.; Hu, C.; et al. Clinical Characteristics of COVID-19 Patients with Digestive Symptoms in Hubei, China: A Descriptive, Cross-Sectional, Multicenter Study. *Am. J. Gastroenterol.* **2020**, *115*, 766–773. [CrossRef] [PubMed]
15. Moradian, N.; Ochs, H.D.; Sedikies, C.; Hamblin, M.R.; Camargo, C.A., Jr.; Martinez, J.A.; Biamonte, J.D.; Abdollahi, M.; Torres, P.J.; Nieto, J.J.; et al. The urgent need for integrated science to fight COVID-19 pandemic and beyond. *J. Transl. Med.* **2020**, *18*, 205. [CrossRef]
16. Crisci, C.D.; Ardusso, L.R.F.; Mossuz, A.; Muller, L. A Precision Medicine Approach to SARS-CoV-2 Pandemic Management. *Curr. Treat. Options Allergy* **2020**, *7*, 422–440. [CrossRef]
17. Russell, S.M.; Alba-Patino, A.; Baron, E.; Borges, M.; Gonzalez-Freire, M.; de la Rica, R. Biosensors for Managing the COVID-19 Cytokine Storm: Challenges Ahead. *ACS Sens.* **2020**, *5*, 1506–1513. [CrossRef]
18. Man, M.A.; Rajnoveanu, R.M.; Motoc, N.S.; Bondor, C.I.; Chis, A.F.; Lesan, A.; Puiu, R.; Lucaciu, S.R.; Dantes, E.; Gergely-Domokos, B.; et al. Neutrophil-to-lymphocyte ratio, platelets-to-lymphocyte ratio, and eosinophils correlation with high-resolution computer tomography severity score in COVID-19 patients. *PLoS ONE* **2021**, *16*, e0252599. [CrossRef]
19. Lamadrid, P.; Alonso-Pena, M.; San Segundo, D.; Arias-Loste, M.; Crespo, J.; Lopez-Hoyos, M. Innate and Adaptive Immunity Alterations in Metabolic Associated Fatty Liver Disease and Its Implication in COVID-19 Severity. *Front. Immunol.* **2021**, *12*, 651728. [CrossRef]
20. Garip Ustaoglu, S.; Kaygusuz, H.; Bilgin, M.D.; Severcan, F. Novel approaches for COVID-19 diagnosis and treatment: A nonsystematic review. *Turk. J. Biol.* **2021**, *45*, 358–371. [CrossRef]
21. Guan, J.; Wei, X.; Qin, S.; Liu, X.; Jiang, Y.; Chen, Y.; Chen, Y.; Lu, H.; Qian, J.; Wang, Z.; et al. Continuous tracking of COVID-19 patients' immune status. *Int. Immunopharmacol.* **2020**, *89*, 107034. [CrossRef] [PubMed]
22. Falzone, L.; Gattuso, G.; Tsatsakis, A.; Spandidos, D.A.; Libra, M. Current and innovative methods for the diagnosis of COVID19 infection (Review). *Int. J. Mol. Med.* **2021**, *47*, 100. [CrossRef] [PubMed]
23. Charlson, M.E.; Pompei, P.; Ales, K.L.; MacKenzie, C.R. A new method of classifying prognostic comorbidity in longitudinal studies: Development and validation. *J. Chronic. Dis.* **1987**, *40*, 373–383. [CrossRef]
24. Genolini, C.; Pingault, J.B.; Driss, T.; Cote, S.; Tremblay, R.E.; Vitaro, F.; Arnaud, C.; Falissard, B. KmL3D: A non-parametric algorithm for clustering joint trajectories. *Comput. Methods Programs Biomed.* **2013**, *109*, 104–111. [CrossRef]
25. Chatterjee, A.; Gerdes, M.W.; Martinez, S.G. Identification of Risk Factors Associated with Obesity and Overweight-A Machine Learning Overview. *Sensors* **2020**, *20*, 2734. [CrossRef]
26. DeGregory, K.W.; Kuiper, P.; DeSilvio, T.; Pleuss, J.D.; Miller, R.; Roginski, J.W.; Fisher, C.B.; Harness, D.; Viswanath, S.; Heymsfield, S.B.; et al. A review of machine learning in obesity. *Obes. Rev.* **2018**, *19*, 668–685. [CrossRef]
27. Alzoughool, F.; Alanagreh, L.; Abumweis, S.; Atoum, M. Cerebrovascular comorbidity, high blood levels of C-reactive protein and D-dimer are associated with disease outcomes in COVID-19 patients. *Clin. Hemorheol. Microcirc.* **2021**, *77*, 311–322. [CrossRef]

28. Chahar, S.; Roy, P.K. COVID-19: A Comprehensive Review of Learning Models. *Arch. Comput. Methods Eng.* **2021**, *29*, 1915–1940. [CrossRef]
29. Su, C.; Xu, Z.; Hoffman, K.; Goyal, P.; Safford, M.M.; Lee, J.; Alvarez-Mulett, S.; Gomez-Escobar, L.; Price, D.R.; Harrington, J.S.; et al. Identifying organ dysfunction trajectory-based subphenotypes in critically ill patients with COVID-19. *Sci. Rep.* **2021**, *11*, 15872. [CrossRef]
30. Ramos-Lopez, O.; Milton-Laskibar, I.; Martinez, J.A.; Collaborators Rodrigo, S.-C.; Maria, P.P. Precision nutrition based on phenotypical traits and the (epi)genotype: Nutrigenetic and nutrigenomic approaches for obesity care. *Curr. Opin. Clin. Nutr. Metab. Care* **2021**, *24*, 315–325. [CrossRef]
31. Chaudhary, L.; Singh, B. Community detection using unsupervised machine learning techniques on COVID-19 dataset. *Soc. Netw. Anal. Min.* **2021**, *11*, 28. [CrossRef] [PubMed]
32. Goldstein, E.; Yeghiazaryan, K.; Ahmad, A.; Giordano, F.A.; Frohlich, H.; Golubnitschaja, O. Optimal multiparametric set-up modelled for best survival outcomes in palliative treatment of liver malignancies: Unsupervised machine learning and 3 PM recommendations. *EPMA J.* **2020**, *11*, 505–515. [CrossRef] [PubMed]
33. Senia, P.; Vella, F.; Mucci, N.; Dounias, G.; Trovato, A.; Marconi, A.; Ledda, C.; Rapisarda, V.; Vitale, E. Survey on COVID-19-related mortality associated with occupational infection during the first phase of the pandemic: A systematic review. *Exp. Ther. Med.* **2022**, *23*, 10. [CrossRef] [PubMed]
34. Vahabi, N.; Salehi, M.; Duarte, J.D.; Mollalo, A.; Michailidis, G. County-level longitudinal clustering of COVID-19 mortality to incidence ratio in the United States. *Sci. Rep.* **2021**, *11*, 3088. [CrossRef] [PubMed]
35. Migrino, J.R., Jr.; Batangan, A.R.U. Using machine learning to create a decision tree model to predict outcomes of COVID-19 cases in the Philippines. *West. Pac. Surveill. Response J.* **2021**, *12*, 56–64. [CrossRef]
36. Wanyan, T.; Honarvar, H.; Jaladanki, S.K.; Zang, C.; Naik, N.; Somani, S.; De Freitas, J.K.; Paranjpe, I.; Vaid, A.; Zhang, J.; et al. Contrastive learning improves critical event prediction in COVID-19 patients. *Patterns* **2021**, *2*, 100389. [CrossRef]
37. Li, W.T.; Ma, J.; Shende, N.; Castaneda, G.; Chakladar, J.; Tsai, J.C.; Apostol, L.; Honda, C.O.; Xu, J.; Wong, L.M.; et al. Using machine learning of clinical data to diagnose COVID-19: A systematic review and meta-analysis. *BMC Med. Inform. Decis. Mak.* **2020**, *20*, 247. [CrossRef]
38. Taneri, P.E.; Gomez-Ochoa, S.A.; Llanaj, E.; Raguindin, P.F.; Rojas, L.Z.; Roa-Diaz, Z.M.; Salvador, D., Jr.; Groothof, D.; Minder, B.; Kopp-Heim, D.; et al. Anemia and iron metabolism in COVID-19: A systematic review and meta-analysis. *Eur. J. Epidemiol.* **2020**, *35*, 763–773. [CrossRef]
39. Rostami, M.; Mansouritorghabeh, H. D-dimer level in COVID-19 infection: A systematic review. *Expert. Rev. Hematol.* **2020**, *13*, 1265–1275. [CrossRef]
40. Wool, G.D.; Miller, J.L. The Impact of COVID-19 Disease on Platelets and Coagulation. *Pathobiology* **2021**, *88*, 15–27. [CrossRef]
41. Iba, T.; Levy, J.H.; Levi, M.; Thachil, J. Coagulopathy in COVID-19. *J. Thromb. Haemost.* **2020**, *18*, 2103–2109. [CrossRef] [PubMed]
42. Ortega-Paz, L.; Capodanno, D.; Montalescot, G.; Angiolillo, D.J. Coronavirus Disease 2019-Associated Thrombosis and Coagulopathy: Review of the Pathophysiological Characteristics and Implications for Antithrombotic Management. *J. Am. Heart Assoc.* **2021**, *10*, e019650. [CrossRef]
43. Hartl, L.; Jachs, M.; Simbrunner, B.; Bauer, D.J.M.; Semmler, G.; Gompelmann, D.; Szekeres, T.; Quehenberger, P.; Trauner, M.; Mandorfer, M.; et al. Cirrhosis-Associated RAS-Inflammation-Coagulation Axis Anomalies: Parallels to Severe COVID-19. *J. Pers. Med.* **2021**, *11*, 1264. [CrossRef] [PubMed]
44. Hanff, T.C.; Mohareb, A.M.; Giri, J.; Cohen, J.B.; Chirinos, J.A. Thrombosis in COVID-19. *Am. J. Hematol.* **2020**, *95*, 1578–1589. [CrossRef] [PubMed]
45. Mertoglu, C.; Huyut, M.T.; Arslan, Y.; Ceylan, Y.; Coban, T.A. How do routine laboratory tests change in coronavirus disease 2019? *Scand. J. Clin. Lab. Investig.* **2021**, *81*, 24–33. [CrossRef]
46. Oikonomou, E.; Paraskevas, T.; Velissaris, D. Cardiac biomarkers alterations in patients with SARS-CoV-2 infection. *Rom. J. Intern. Med.* **2022**, *60*, 6–13. [CrossRef] [PubMed]
47. Caruso, F.P.; Scala, G.; Cerulo, L.; Ceccarelli, M. A review of COVID-19 biomarkers and drug targets: Resources and tools. *Brief. Bioinform.* **2021**, *22*, 701–713. [CrossRef]
48. Carobene, A.; Milella, F.; Famiglini, L.; Cabitza, F. How is test laboratory data used and characterised by machine learning models? A systematic review of diagnostic and prognostic models developed for COVID-19 patients using only laboratory data. *Clin. Chem. Lab. Med.* **2022**. [CrossRef]
49. Bhargava, A.; Bansal, A.; Goyal, V. Machine learning-based automatic detection of novel coronavirus (COVID-19) disease. *Multimed. Tools Appl.* **2022**, *81*, 13731–13750. [CrossRef]
50. Vaishya, R.; Javaid, M.; Khan, I.H.; Haleem, A. Artificial Intelligence (AI) applications for COVID-19 pandemic. *Diabetes Metab. Syndr.* **2020**, *14*, 337–339. [CrossRef]

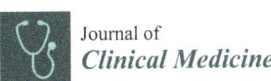

Journal of Clinical Medicine

Article

Comparison between Suspected and Confirmed COVID-19 Respiratory Patients: What Is beyond the PCR Test

Stefania Principe [1,2], Amelia Grosso [3], Alida Benfante [1], Federica Albicini [3], Salvatore Battaglia [1], Erica Gini [3], Marta Amata [1], Ilaria Piccionello [1], Angelo Guido Corsico [3] and Nicola Scichilone [1,*]

1. Department of Pulmonology–Palermo (PA) (Italy), AOUP Policlinico Paolo Giaccone, University of Palermo, 90127 Palermo, Italy; stefania.principe@unipa.it (S.P.); alida.benfante@unipa.it (A.B.); salvatore.battaglia@unipa.it (S.B.); marta.amata@gmail.com (M.A.); ilaria.piccionello@virgilio.it (I.P.)
2. Department of Respiratory Medicine–Amsterdam, Amsterdam UMC, University of Amsterdam, 1105 AZ Amsterdam, The Netherlands
3. Department of Pulmonology, Fondazione IRCCS Policlinico San Matteo, 27100 Pavia, Italy; amelia.grosso@gmail.com (A.G.); federica.albicini@gmail.com (F.A.); erica.gini@gmail.com (E.G.); corsico@unipv.it (A.G.C.)
* Correspondence: nicola.scichilone@unipa.it

Abstract: COVID-19 modified the healthcare system. Nasal-pharyngeal swab (NPS), with real-time reverse transcriptase-polymerase (PCR), is the gold standard for the diagnosis; however, there are difficulties related to the procedure that may postpone it. The study aims to evaluate whether other elements than the PCR-NPS are reliable and confirm the diagnosis of COVID-19. This is a cross-sectional study on data from the Lung Unit of Pavia (confirmed) and at the Emergency Unit of Palermo (suspected). COVID-19 was confirmed by positive NPS, suspected tested negative. We compared clinical, laboratory and radiological variables and performed Logistic regression to estimate which variables increased the risk of COVID-19. The derived ROC-AUCcurve, assessed the accuracy of the model to distinguish between COVID-19 suspected and confirmed. We selected 50 confirmed and 103 suspected cases. High Reactive C-Protein (OR: 1.02; CI95%: 0.11–1.02), suggestive CT-images (OR: 11.43; CI95%: 3.01–43.3), dyspnea (OR: 10.48; CI95%: 2.08–52.7) and respiratory failure (OR: 5.84; CI95%: 1.73–19.75) increased the risk of COVID-19, whereas pleural effusion decreased the risk (OR: 0.15; CI95%: 0.04–0.63). ROC confirmed the discriminative role of these variables between suspected and confirmed COVID-19 (AUC 0.91). Clinical, laboratory and imaging features predict the diagnosis of COVID-19, independently from the NPS result.

Keywords: COVID-19; PCR test; COVID-19 diagnosis

Citation: Principe, S.; Grosso, A.; Benfante, A.; Albicini, F.; Battaglia, S.; Gini, E.; Amata, M.; Piccionello, I.; Corsico, A.G.; Scichilone, N. Comparison between Suspected and Confirmed COVID-19 Respiratory Patients: What Is beyond the PCR Test. *J. Clin. Med.* **2022**, *11*, 2993. https://doi.org/10.3390/jcm11112993

Academic Editor: Robert Flisiak

Received: 30 April 2022
Accepted: 24 May 2022
Published: 25 May 2022

Publisher's Note: MDPI stays neutral with regard to jurisdictional claims in published maps and institutional affiliations.

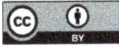

Copyright: © 2022 by the authors. Licensee MDPI, Basel, Switzerland. This article is an open access article distributed under the terms and conditions of the Creative Commons Attribution (CC BY) license (https://creativecommons.org/licenses/by/4.0/).

1. Introduction

In December 2019, a new Coronavirus, named SARS-CoV-2, was isolated in the respiratory tract cells of humans [1]. On 11 March 2020, the WHO declared the first SARS-CoV-2 outbreak in China as an international public health emergency [2], starting the beginning of the COVID-19 pandemic. COVID-19 infection causes mild or moderate symptoms such as cough, fever, asthenia and sometimes headache and gastrointestinal symptoms, such as vomiting and diarrhea [3]. However, a great proportion of individuals also experienced respiratory symptoms such as dyspnea and respiratory failure suggestive of severe pneumonia that led to access to the Intensive Care Unit or death.

The virus has been isolated in biological respiratory fluids, both through oronasal swabs and bronchoalveolar lavage [4]. The analysis of the nasal-pharyngeal swab (NPS), which uses the real-time reverse transcriptase-polymerase chain reaction (RT-PCR), is considered the gold standard for the diagnosis of COVID-19. The sensitivity and specificity of the RT-PCR technique have been discussed in several studies; Dramé et al. [5], showed that the sensitivity of NPS was under 40% and suggested performing NPSs repeatedly over time, in correlation with patients' symptoms and other diagnostic tests to avoid missing diagnosis. Conversely, Xiang et al. considered the SARS-CoV-2 antibody tests IgM and IgG as a better diagnostic investigation than the swab [6]. However, during the pandemic, NPS appeared to be the simplest and fastest technique, despite the limitations that could be linked to non-optimal management of the sample or the difficulties related to the procedure. As a matter of fact, NPS can give false-positive and false-negative results. This could be the consequence of various factors, such as cross-contamination with other viruses, unsuitable laboratories and inexperienced operators, but also the viral load, which depends on the days of illness that have passed [7]. Moreover, a systematic review by Rodriguez et al. pointed out the need to perform repeated tests in subjects with a strong suspicion of infection, considering that 54% of COVID-19 positive patients showed a false negative result on the first test with the RT-PCR method [8].

During the COVID-19 pandemic, Italy was one of the most affected countries and the positivity rate and the management of screening tests were heterogeneous among regions, especially during the first outbreak [9,10]. The management of a suspected patient i.e., those who, in addition to typical symptoms, reported a close contact with a positive COVID-19 patient or who were living or traveled through areas at a greater risk of infection (defined as a "red zone"), represented the area of uncertainty leading to the lack of a unified policy to face the emergency [9]. As an example, patients with respiratory symptoms and features of COVID-19 disease that accessed the hospital were transferred to the so-called "grey areas", in which they received prompt assistance while waiting for the NPS results [11]. This system was established to avoid the spread of COVID-19 in non-COVID-19 units.

Even though the vaccination campaign curbed the spread of SARS-CoV-2 infection, the COVID-19 pandemic steadily continues, and it is arduous to make a prevision about its end. Although the severity of the disease and the number of hospital admissions could potentially be reduced by promoting vaccination strategies, the management of the hospital admissions of COVID-19 patients is still unclear and needs to be further implemented in the long term. An early diagnosis, isolation systems and quarantine of suspected patients are fundamental to controlling the spread of the infection [12]. The introduction in the decision-making of the clinical, radiological and laboratory features to increase the risk of COVID-19 could facilitate the diagnosis and reduce the permanence in the "grey areas". Assuming that the negative result of the RT-PCR NPS cannot completely rule out COVID-19 diagnosis, we aimed to investigate whether clinical, laboratory and imaging characteristics can improve the reliability of the NPS in differentiating suspected from ascertained COVID-19 cases.

2. Materials and Methods

2.1. Study Population

This is a retrospective, cross-sectional, multicenter study. The population was divided in confirmed and suspected COVID-19 cases. In the first group, the disease was confirmed by the positivity of NPS from the upper respiratory tract by RT-PCR. In the second group, patients with clinical, radiological and laboratory features suggestive of SARS-CoV-2 infection and negative NPS were included. Data were collected from March to May 2020. Suspected COVID-19 cases were selected from medical records of the Emergency Care Unit of the University Hospital of Palermo, Italy, whereas confirmed COVID-19 cases were retrieved from medical records of the Lung Unit of the Fondazione IRCCS Policlinico San Matteo, University of Pavia, Italy. The study obtained the approval of the Ethical Board of both institutions.

2.2. Data Collection

Demographic characteristics, respiratory signs and symptoms at admissions, such as fever, dyspnea and cough, clinical laboratory tests with complete blood count and serum biochemical tests (lactic dehydrogenase (LDH), D-dimer and C-reactive protein (CPR)) were extracted from medical electronic records at the time of the admission to the Emergency Care Unit for suspected COVID-19 cases and at the time of the admission to the

Lung Unit for COVID-19-confirmed cases. Chest computed tomographic (CT) scans were carried out for all the patients and were considered suggestive of SARS-CoV-2 infection if they reported the following characteristics: evidence of focal unilateral or diffuse bilateral ground-glass opacities with or without co-existed consolidations [13,14]. Respiratory failure was classified according to blood gas abnormalities [15]. In both units, a PCR-NPS test was performed on all the patients at the moment of the admission. Suspected cases were considered negative for SARS-CoV-2 infection after at least two negative PCR-NPS tests within 48–72 h as well as their consequent admission to a non-COVID Unit.

2.3. Statistical Analysis

Clinical, laboratory and radiological variables were summarized using means and Standard Deviations (SD). Normality was assessed by visual inspection of histograms and q-q plots. Continuous baseline variables judged to follow a non-normal distribution were summarized using medians and interquartile ranges. A comparison of those characteristics was performed using Chi-squared or *t*-test for categorical and continuous variables, respectively. A logistic regression model was performed after the selection of the variables considered statistically different (with a *p*-value <0.05) between the two groups to evaluate which exploratory variables were considered to increase or reduce the risk of SARS-CoV-2 diagnosis. The Wald test was used to assess the accuracy of the logistic regression classification. Afterward, a prediction model was performed and, according to the predicted classification, the confusion matrix of the dataset was generated to calculate the sensitivity and specificity of the overall predictive values. From the results of the prediction model, we constructed a receiver operating characteristic (ROC) curve and calculated the area under the curve (AUC) to assess the overall accuracy. A *p*-value < 0.05 was considered statistically significant. The analysis was performed using R studio version 1.1.463 (R Studio Inc., Boston, MA, USA) and R version 3.5.1 (The R Foundation for Statistical Computing, Vienna, Austria).

3. Results

We included a total of 153 subjects: 50 belonged to the group of confirmed COVID-19 cases and 103 to the suspected COVID-19 cases. A summary of the general characteristics and the comparison between groups is presented in Table 1. Significant differences were found between suspected and confirmed COVID-19 patients in terms of smoking history, physiological parameters and symptoms, such as the presence/absence of fever, dyspnea, respiratory failure, as well as radiological findings (presence/absence of pleural effusion, CT scan suggestive of SARS-CoV-2 infection) and laboratory exams (CPR, Lymphocytes (%), LDH).

A total of four logistic regression models were performed: the first model included all symptoms and physiological features that resulted in significantly different between the two groups (Supplementary Table S1). In this model, the presence of dyspnea (OR 12.59; CI95%: 1.7–93; *p*-value: 0.013) and the evidence of respiratory failure (OR 8.42; CI95%: 1.32–53.62; *p*-value: 0.024) increased the risk of diagnosis of COVID-19. The second model (Supplementary Table S2), which included only radiological findings, showed that the presence of a CT scan indicative of SARS-CoV-2 infection increased the risk of COVID-19 diagnosis (OR 3.73; CI95%: 1.68–8.28; *p*-value: 0.001), while the presence of pleural effusion reduced the risk (OR 0.24; CI95%: 0.09–0.63; *p*-value: 0.002). In the third model (Supplementary Table S3), which collected laboratory findings, we demonstrated that only CPR could be considered as a potential risk factor for COVID-19 diagnosis (OR 1.02; CI95%: 0.11–1.03; *p*-value: <0.001). A fourth logistic regression model was performed bringing the above-mentioned variables together as it is shown in Table 2.

Table 1. General characteristics and comparison of the two study groups. CT: Computed Tomography; CPR: C-Reactive Protein; LDH: lactic dehydrogenase. Comorbidities are defined as any chronic disease or medical condition.

	COVID-19 Confirmed	COVID-19 Suspected	p-Value
N	50	103	
Age (mean (SD))	67.02 (10.98)	66.68 (17.52)	0.900
Sex = M/F n (%)	33/17 (66.0/34.0)	57/46 (55.3/44.7)	0.279
Smoking n (%)			<0.001
Never	18 (47.4)	33 (63.5)	
Former	1 (2.6)	12 (23.1)	
Active	19 (50.0)	7 (13.5)	
Comorbidities = N/Y n (%)	12/38 (24.0/76.0)	18/85 (17.5/82.5)	0.462
Fever = N/Y n (%)	4/46 (8.0/92.0)	70/33 (68.0/32.0)	<0.001
Temperature (°C) (mean (SD))	37.36 (0.82)	36.69 (0.90)	<0.001
Dyspnea = N/Y n (%)	7/43 (14.0/86.0)	41/62 (39.8/60.2)	0.002
Cough = N/Y n (%)	27/23 (54.0/46.0)	69/34 (67.0/33.0)	0.167
CT positive = N/Y n (%)	11/39 (22.0/78.0)	57/46 (55.3/44.7)	<0.001
Pleural effusion = N/Y n (%)	44/6 (88.0/12.0)	61/42 (59.2/40.8)	0.001
D-dimer (ng/mL) (median [IQR])	558.50 [503.50, 1010.25]	1360.00 [770.00, 3285.50]	0.375
Lymphocytes (%) (median [IQR])	10.30 [5.10, 14.20]	13.70 [8.00, 22.55]	0.006
CPR (mg/L) (median [IQR])	136.70 [76.15, 203.10]	21.82 [3.56, 67.16]	<0.001
LDH (mu/mL) (median [IQR])	436.00 [356.50, 523.75]	257.00 [208.25, 373.50]	<0.001
Respiratory Failure = N/Y n (%)	20/30 (40.0/60.0)	70/33 (68.0/32.0)	0.002

Table 2. Logistic regression model. OR: Odd ratio; CI(95%): Confidence interval at 95%. CPR: C-Reactive Protein; CT: Chest-Tomography.

	OR	CI(95%)	p-Value
CPR	1.02	0.11, 1.02	<0.001
CT positive	11.43	3.01, 43.3	<0.001
Pleural effusion	0.15	0.04, 0.63	0.009
Dyspnea	10.48	2.08, 52.7	0.004
Respiratory Failure	5.84	1.73, 19.75	0.002

Those characteristics were able to discriminate between COVID-19-confirmed and COVID-19-suspected cases with a sensitivity of 0.60, specificity of 0.90 and high accuracy, represented with an ROC-AUC curve of 0.91 (Figure 1).

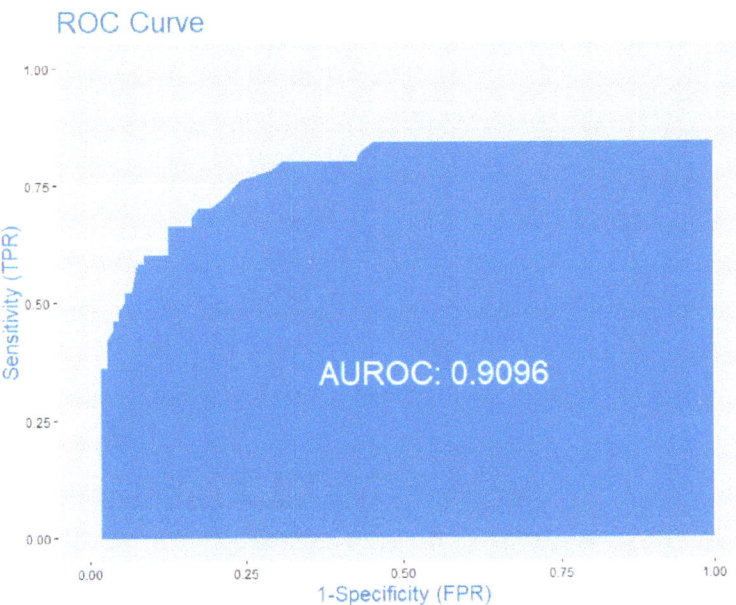

Figure 1. ROC-AUC report the high accuracy of the model in distinguishing the diagnosis of COVID-19 between the two groups.

4. Discussion

In this study, we were able to prove that a composite measure that includes increased blood levels of Reactive C-Protein, the evidence of suggestive CT-scan alterations and the presence of dyspnea and respiratory failure in addition to the NPS are highly predictive of SARS-CoV-2 infection. The current gold standard to make a diagnosis of active COVID-19 infection should remain the positive detection of viral RNA in respiratory specimens. The use of RT-PCR assay to detect SARS-CoV-2 RNA from the nasopharyngeal tract should remain the preferred initial diagnostic test, although it should be implemented with other evaluations to avoid uncertainties [16]. It has been proven that negative test results do not necessarily rule out the possibility of COVID-19 infection and other complementary measurements, such as bronchoalveolar lavage, should be performed in case of high suspicion of disease [17–22]. In such a manner, the diagnostic confirmation of COVID-19 infection can require some days, causing difficulties in terms of management of hospital beds and patients' follow-up in dedicated units. Suspected SARS-CoV-2 patients generally can stand for days in the "grey areas" of the Emergency Care Unit, receiving assistance while they are waiting for the test results. Therefore, there is the need to implement complementary tools for the decision-making process to accelerate the diagnosis of COVID-19 and facilitate the management of suspected COVID-19 patients. To our knowledge, this is the first study that evaluated, in the real-life scenario of two Italian regions with high and low COVID-19 prevalence, the importance of clinical, radiological and laboratory parameters to implement the diagnosis of COVID-19 and accelerate the decision-making.

As previously demonstrated, CT scan plays a fundamental role in the diagnosis and management of subjects with COVID-19 disease, and it can also be essential in detecting the disease at an early stage [23,24]. In line with these findings, we were also able to demonstrate that imaging could help to detect SARS-CoV-2-infected patients. Specifically, we found that a positive chest CT scan can increase the risk of the presence of SARS-CoV-2 infection, whereas the presence of pleural effusion reduces it. A recent study highlighted the high diagnostic sensitivity of chest CT at certain stages after viral infection [23]. In a study by Xie et al., it was found that all patients presented characteristic CT features of

COVID-19 at an early stage, which was confirmed by a positive RT-PCR assay during the isolation period [25]. Similar results were obtained by Ai et al. in a study that evaluated the consistency of chest CT scans in the diagnosis of COVID-19 [26]. CT imaging features of COVID-19 can differ at various disease stages [27,28]. The most frequent CT abnormalities observed in patients with COVID-19 are ground-glass opacities (GGO), usually with multiple and bilateral focal lesions in the posterior and peripheral lung segments, "crazy paving" pattern and less commonly at early stages, pure consolidations [27,29–32]. In the current study, we were also able to demonstrate that the presence of pleural effusion is indicative of a lower risk of COVID-19 diagnosis. This is in line with the study of Woon et al. [33], who showed that the reported incidence of pleural effusions in COVID-19 pneumonia is low (7.3%). Pleural effusions may occur several days after the onset of symptoms, more likely resembling advanced stages of COVID-19 pneumonia [33]. Therefore, pleural effusion in COVID-19 patients could more likely be considered a more severe radiological evolution of COVID-19 pneumonia [14,34–36]. Surely, a chest CT-scan alone is not sufficient to exclude or confirm the diagnosis of COVID-19. Indeed, chest CT-scans should be combined with other relevant clinical information. We proved that patients that reported dyspnea with respiratory failure had an increased risk to be infected by SARS-CoV-2. This is of great importance, given that SARS-CoV-2 infection may result in hypoxemia [37] and the occurrence of respiratory failure increases mortality [38].

In addition to the radiological and clinical findings, we explored other markers able to support the RT-PCR NPS and accelerate the diagnosis of SARS-CoV-2 infection. In this regard, our analysis indicated that increased serum levels of C-reactive protein (CPR) could enhance the risk of SARS-CoV-2 diagnosis. As shown in other studies, the levels of CRP would optimally be rechecked on days 3, 5 and 7 after admission [3,39].

5. Conclusions

In conclusion, our findings suggest that NPS tests should be combined with chest CT-scans, clinical symptoms and blood CPR evaluation, to increase the accuracy of the diagnosis of COVID-19 in suspected patients with respiratory symptoms.

Supplementary Materials: The following supporting information can be downloaded at: https://www.mdpi.com/article/10.3390/jcm11112993/s1, Table S1: Logistic regression model with symptoms and physiological features. OR: Odd ratio; CI(95%): Confidence interval at 95%; Table S2: Logistic regression model with radiological findings. OR: Odd ratio; CI(95%): Confidence interval at 95%. CT: Chest-Tomography; Table S3: Logistic regression model with laboratory findings. OR: Odd ratio; CI(95%): Confidence interval at 95%. CPR: C-Reactive Protein; LDH: Lactic dehydrogenase.

Author Contributions: Conceptualization, S.P., N.S., A.G.C. and A.G.; methodology, S.P., N.S., A.G.C. and S.B.; software, S.P., S.B., F.A. and A.G.; validation, S.P., A.G., A.B., F.A., S.B., E.G., M.A., I.P., A.G.C. and N.S.; formal analysis, S.P., S.B. and E.G.; investigation, S.P., A.B. and A.G.; resources S.P., A.G., N.S., A.G.C., M.A., I.P., F.A. and E.G.; data curation S.P., A.B., N.S., A.G., A.G.C. and S.B.; writing—original draft preparation, S.P., N.S., A.G.C., M.A. and I.P.; writing—review and editing S.P., A.G., A.B., F.A., S.B., E.G., M.A., I.P., A.G.C. and N.S. Visualization, S.P., A.G., A.B., F.A., S.B. and E.G.; supervision, A.B., N.S. and A.G.C.; project administration, N.S., A.G.C., S.P. and A.G. All authors have read and agreed to the published version of the manuscript.

Funding: This research received no external funding.

Institutional Review Board Statement: The study was conducted in accordance with the Declaration of Helsinki, and approved by the Institutional Review Board (or Ethics Committee) of the Fondazione IRCCS Policlinico San Matteo, University of Pavia (protocol code P-20200052973 of the 12/06/2020) and AOUP Policlinico Paolo Giaccone, University of Palermo (protocol code 5/2020 of the 20/05/2020.

Informed Consent Statement: Not applicable.

Data Availability Statement: The data presented in this study are available on request from the corresponding author. The data are no publicly available due to privacy.

Conflicts of Interest: The authors declare no conflict of interest.

References

1. Zhu, N.; Zhang, D.; Wang, W.; Li, X.; Yang, B.; Song, J.; Zhao, X.; Huang, B.; Shi, W.; Lu, R.; et al. A Novel Coronavirus from Patients with Pneumonia in China, 2019. *N. Engl. J. Med.* **2020**, *382*, 727–733. [CrossRef] [PubMed]
2. WHO/Europe | Coronavirus Disease (COVID-19) Outbreak. Available online: https://www.euro.who.int/en/health-topics/health-emergencies/coronavirus-covid-19 (accessed on 26 April 2022).
3. Huang, C.; Wang, Y.; Li, X.; Ren, L.; Zhao, J.; Hu, Y.; Zhang, L.; Fan, G.; Xu, J.; Gu, X.; et al. Clinical Features of Patients Infected with 2019 Novel Coronavirus in Wuhan, China. *Lancet* **2020**, *395*, 497–506. [CrossRef]
4. Zhou, P.; Yang, X.L.; Wang, X.G.; Hu, B.; Zhang, L.; Zhang, W.; Si, H.R.; Zhu, Y.; Li, B.; Huang, C.L.; et al. A Pneumonia Outbreak Associated with a New Coronavirus of Probable Bat Origin. *Nature* **2020**, *579*, 270–273. [CrossRef] [PubMed]
5. Dramé, M.; Tabue Teguo, M.; Proye, E.; Hequet, F.; Hentzien, M.; Kanagaratnam, L.; Godaert, L. Should RT-PCR Be Considered a Gold Standard in the Diagnosis of COVID-19? *J. Med. Virol.* **2020**, *92*, 2312–2313. [CrossRef] [PubMed]
6. Xiang, F.; Wang, X.; He, X.; Peng, Z.; Yang, B.; Zhang, J.; Zhou, Q.; Ye, H.; Ma, Y.; Li, H.; et al. Antibody Detection and Dynamic Characteristics in Patients with Coronavirus Disease 2019. *Clin. Infect. Dis.* **2020**, *71*, 1930–1934. [CrossRef]
7. Mouliou, D.S.; Gourgoulianis, K.I. False-Positive and False-Negative COVID-19 Cases: Respiratory Prevention and Management Strategies, Vaccination, and Further Perspectives. *Expert Rev. Respir. Med.* **2021**, *15*, 993–1002. [CrossRef] [PubMed]
8. Arevalo-Rodriguez, I.; Buitrago-Garcia, D.; Simancas-Racines, D.; Zambrano-Achig, P.; Del Campo, R.; Ciapponi, A.; Sued, O.; Martinez-García, L.; Rutjes, A.W.; Low, N.; et al. False-Negative Results of Initial RT-PCR Assays for COVID-19: A Systematic Review. *PLoS ONE* **2020**, *15*, e0242958. [CrossRef]
9. Sartor, G.; Del Riccio, M.; Dal Poz, I.; Bonanni, P.; Bonaccorsi, G. COVID-19 in Italy: Considerations on Official Data. *Int. J. Infect. Dis.* **2020**, *98*, 188–190. [CrossRef]
10. POLITICO–European Politics, Policy, Government News. Available online: https://www.politico.eu/ (accessed on 26 April 2022).
11. Scichilone, N.; Basile, L.; Battaglia, S.; Benfante, A.; Fonte, R.; Gambino, F.; Marino, S.; Messina, R.; Poma, S.; Principe, S.; et al. Management of Suspected COVID-19 Patients in a Low Prevalence Region. *Chron. Respir. Dis.* **2020**, *17*, 1479973120961843. [CrossRef]
12. Hua, W.; Xiaofeng, L.; Zhenqiang, B.; Jun, R.; Ban, W.; Liming, L. The Epidemiological Characteristics of an Outbreak of 2019 Novel Coronavirus Diseases (COVID-19) in China. *Zhonghua Liu Xing Bing Xue Za Zhi* **2020**, *41*, 297–300. [CrossRef]
13. Sverzellati, N.; Ryerson, C.J.; Milanese, G.; Renzoni, E.A.; Volpi, A.; Spagnolo, P.; Bonella, F.; Comelli, I.; Affanni, P.; Veronesi, L.; et al. Chest Radiography or Computed Tomography for COVID-19 Pneumonia? Comparative Study in a Simulated Triage Setting. *Eur. Respir. J.* **2021**, *58*, 745. [CrossRef] [PubMed]
14. Shi, H.; Han, X.; Jiang, N.; Cao, Y.; Alwalid, O.; Gu, J.; Fan, Y.; Zheng, C. Radiological Findings from 81 Patients with COVID-19 Pneumonia in Wuhan, China: A Descriptive Study. *Lancet Infect. Dis.* **2020**, *20*, 425–434. [CrossRef]
15. Baudouin, S.; Turner, L.; Blumenthal, S.; Cooper, B.; Davidson, C.; Davison, A.; Elliott, M.; Kinnear, W.; Paton, R.; Sawicka, E. Non-Invasive Ventilation in Acute Respiratory Failure. *Thorax* **2002**, *57*, 192–211. [CrossRef]
16. Patel, A.; Jernigan, D.B. 2019-nCoV CDC Response Team Initial Public Health Response and Interim Clinical Guidance for the 2019 Novel Coronavirus Outbreak-United States, 31 December 2019–4 February 2020. *Am. J. Transplant* **2020**, *20*, 889–895. [CrossRef] [PubMed]
17. Li, Y.; Yao, L.; Li, J.; Chen, L.; Song, Y.; Cai, Z.; Yang, C. Stability Issues of RT-PCR Testing of SARS-CoV-2 for Hospitalized Patients Clinically Diagnosed with COVID-19. *J. Med. Virol.* **2020**, *92*, 903–908. [CrossRef]
18. Kucirka, L.M.; Lauer, S.A.; Laeyendecker, O.; Boon, D.; Lessler, J. Variation in False-Negative Rate of Reverse Transcriptase Polymerase Chain Reaction–Based SARS-CoV-2 Tests by Time Since Exposure. *Ann. Intern. Med.* **2020**, *173*, 262–268. [CrossRef]
19. Winichakoon, P.; Chaiwarith, R.; Liwsrisakun, C.; Salee, P.; Goonn, A.; Limsukon, A.; Kaewpoowat, Q. Negative Nasopharyngeal and Oropharyngeal Swabs Do Not Rule Out COVID-19. *J. Clin. Microbiol.* **2020**, *58*, e00297-20. [CrossRef]
20. Xiao, A.T.; Tong, Y.X.; Zhang, S. False Negative of RT-PCR and Prolonged Nucleic Acid Conversion in COVID-19: Rather than Recurrence. *J. Med. Virol.* **2020**, *92*, 1755–1756. [CrossRef]
21. Young, B.E.; Ong, S.W.X.; Kalimuddin, S.; Low, J.G.; Tan, S.Y.; Loh, J.; Ng, O.T.; Marimuthu, K.; Ang, L.W.; Mak, T.M.; et al. Epidemiologic Features and Clinical Course of Patients Infected With SARS-CoV-2 in Singapore. *JAMA* **2020**, *323*, 1488–1494. [CrossRef]
22. Zou, L.; Ruan, F.; Huang, M.; Liang, L.; Huang, H.; Hong, Z.; Yu, J.; Kang, M.; Song, Y.; Xia, J.; et al. SARS-CoV-2 Viral Load in Upper Respiratory Specimens of Infected Patients. *N. Engl. J. Med.* **2020**, *9*, 1177–1179. [CrossRef]
23. Fang, Y.; Zhang, H.; Xie, J.; Lin, M.; Ying, L.; Pang, P.; Ji, W. Sensitivity of Chest CT for COVID-19: Comparison to RT-PCR. *Radiology* **2020**, *296*, E115–E117. [CrossRef] [PubMed]
24. Wang, S.; Kang, B.; Ma, J.; Zeng, X.; Xiao, M.; Guo, J.; Cai, M.; Yang, J.; Li, Y.; Meng, X.; et al. A Deep Learning Algorithm Using CT Images to Screen for Corona Virus Disease (COVID-19). *Eur. Radiol.* **2021**, *31*, 6096–6104. [CrossRef] [PubMed]
25. Xie, X.; Zhong, Z.; Zhao, W.; Zheng, C.; Wang, F.; Liu, J. Chest CT for Typical 2019-NCoV Pneumonia: Relationship to Negative RT-PCR Testing. *Radiology* **2020**, *296*, E41–E45. [CrossRef] [PubMed]

26. Ai, T.; Yang, Z.; Hou, H.; Zhan, C.; Chen, C.; Lv, W.; Tao, Q.; Sun, Z.; Xia, L. Correlation of Chest CT and RT-PCR Testing in Coronavirus Disease 2019 (COVID-19) in China: A Report of 1014 Cases. *Radiology* **2020**, *296*, E32–E40. [CrossRef] [PubMed]
27. Wu, J.; Wu, X.; Zeng, W.; Guo, D.; Fang, Z.; Chen, L.; Huang, H.; Li, C. Chest CT Findings in Patients with Coronavirus Disease 2019 and Its Relationship With Clinical Features. *Investig. Radiol.* **2020**, *55*, 257. [CrossRef]
28. Franquet, T. Imaging of Pulmonary Viral Pneumonia. *Radiology* **2011**, *260*, 18–39. [CrossRef]
29. Song, F.; Shi, N.; Shan, F.; Zhang, Z.; Shen, J.; Lu, H.; Ling, Y.; Jiang, Y.; Shi, Y. Emerging 2019 Novel Coronavirus (2019-NCoV) Pneumonia. *Radiology* **2020**, *295*, 210–217. [CrossRef]
30. Ng, M.Y.; Lee, E.Y.P.; Yang, J.; Yang, F.; Li, X.; Wang, H.; Lui, M.M.S.; Lo, C.S.Y.; Leung, B.; Khong, P.L.; et al. Imaging Profile of the COVID-19 Infection: Radiologic Findings and Literature Review. *Radiol. Cardiothorac. Imaging* **2020**, *2*, e200034. [CrossRef]
31. Zu, Z.Y.; Di Jiang, M.; Xu, P.P.; Chen, W.; Ni, Q.Q.; Lu, G.M.; Zhang, L.J. Coronavirus Disease 2019 (COVID-19): A Perspective from China. *Radiology* **2020**, *296*, E15–E25. [CrossRef]
32. Pan, F.; Ye, T.; Sun, P.; Gui, S.; Liang, B.; Li, L.; Zheng, D.; Wang, J.; Hesketh, R.L.; Yang, L.; et al. Time Course of Lung Changes at Chest CT during Recovery from Coronavirus Disease 2019 (COVID-19). *Radiology* **2020**, *295*, 715–721. [CrossRef]
33. Chong, W.H.; Saha, B.K.; Conuel, E.; Chopra, A. The Incidence of Pleural Effusion in COVID-19 Pneumonia: State-of-the-Art Review. *Hear. Lung* **2021**, *50*, 481. [CrossRef] [PubMed]
34. Bernheim, A.; Mei, X.; Huang, M.; Yang, Y.; Fayad, Z.A.; Zhang, N.; Diao, K.; Lin, B.; Zhu, X.; Li, K.; et al. Chest CT Findings in Coronavirus Disease-19 (COVID-19): Relationship to Duration of Infection. *Radiology* **2020**, *295*, 685–691. [CrossRef] [PubMed]
35. Xiong, Y.; Sun, D.; Liu, Y.; Fan, Y.; Zhao, L.; Li, X.; Zhu, W. Clinical and High-Resolution CT Features of the COVID-19 Infection: Comparison of the Initial and Follow-up Changes. *Investig. Radiol.* **2020**, *55*, 332–339. [CrossRef] [PubMed]
36. Guan, C.S.; Lv, Z.B.; Yan, S.; Du, Y.N.; Chen, H.; Wei, L.G.; Xie, R.M.; Chen, B.D. Imaging Features of Coronavirus Disease 2019 (COVID-19): Evaluation on Thin-Section CT. *Acad. Radiol.* **2020**, *27*, 609. [CrossRef] [PubMed]
37. Yi, Y.; Lagniton, P.N.P.; Ye, S.; Li, E.; Xu, R.H. COVID-19: What Has Been Learned and to Be Learned about the Novel Coronavirus Disease. *Int. J. Biol. Sci.* **2020**, *16*, 1753. [CrossRef] [PubMed]
38. Haimovich, A.D.; Ravindra, N.G.; Stoytchev, S.; Young, H.P.; Wilson, F.P.; van Dijk, D.; Schulz, W.L.; Taylor, R.A. Development and Validation of the Quick COVID-19 Severity Index: A Prognostic Tool for Early Clinical Decompensation. *Ann. Emerg. Med.* **2020**, *76*, 442. [CrossRef]
39. Chen, L.D.; Zhang, Z.Y.; Wei, X.J.; Cai, Y.Q.; Yao, W.Z.; Wang, M.H.; Huang, Q.F.; Zhang, X. Bin Association between Cytokine Profiles and Lung Injury in COVID-19 Pneumonia. *Respir. Res.* **2020**, *21*, 201. [CrossRef]

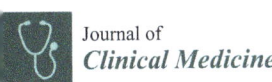

Article

Does the Serum Concentration of Angiotensin II Type 1 Receptor Have an Effect on the Severity of COVID-19? A Prospective Preliminary Observational Study among Healthcare Professionals

Jarosław Janc [1,*], Michał Suchański [1], Magdalena Mierzchała-Pasierb [2], Ewa Woźnica-Niesobska [3], Lidia Łysenko [3] and Patrycja Leśnik [1]

1. Department of Anaesthesiology and Intensive Therapy, 4th Military Clinical Hospital, 50-981 Wroclaw, Poland; michal.suchanski@icloud.com (M.S.); patrycja.lesnik@gmail.com (P.L.)
2. Department of Medical Biochemistry, Wroclaw Medical University, 50-369 Wroclaw, Poland; magdalena.mierzchala-pasierb@umw.edu.pl
3. Department of Anaesthesiology and Intensive Therapy, Wroclaw Medical University, 50-556 Wroclaw, Poland; ewa.anna.woznica@gmail.com (E.W.-N.); lidia.lysenko@umw.edu.pl (L.Ł.)
* Correspondence: jjanc@4wsk.pl; Tel.: +48-71-712-89-39

Citation: Janc, J.; Suchański, M.; Mierzchała-Pasierb, M.; Woźnica-Niesobska, E.; Łysenko, L.; Leśnik, P. Does the Serum Concentration of Angiotensin II Type 1 Receptor Have an Effect on the Severity of COVID-19? A Prospective Preliminary Observational Study among Healthcare Professionals. *J. Clin. Med.* **2022**, *11*, 1769. https://doi.org/10.3390/jcm11071769

Academic Editors: Robert Flisiak and Jan Jelrik Oosterheert

Received: 18 February 2022
Accepted: 21 March 2022
Published: 23 March 2022

Publisher's Note: MDPI stays neutral with regard to jurisdictional claims in published maps and institutional affiliations.

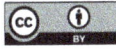

Copyright: © 2022 by the authors. Licensee MDPI, Basel, Switzerland. This article is an open access article distributed under the terms and conditions of the Creative Commons Attribution (CC BY) license (https://creativecommons.org/licenses/by/4.0/).

Abstract: SARS-CoV-2 is a virus that causes severe respiratory distress syndrome. The pathophysiology of COVID-19 is related to the renin–angiotensin system (RAS). SARS-CoV-2, a vector of COVID-19, uses angiotensin-converting enzyme 2 (ACE-2), which is highly expressed in human lung tissue, nasal cavity, and oral mucosa, to gain access into human cells. After entering the cell, SARS-CoV-2 inhibits ACE-2, thus favouring the ACE/Ang II/angiotensin II type 1 receptor (AT1R) axis, which plays a role in the development of acute lung injury (ALI). This study aimed to analyse the influence of angiotensin 1 receptor (AT1R) levels in the serum on the course of the severity of symptoms in healthcare professionals who had a SARS-CoV-2 infection. This prospective observational study was conducted on a group of 82 participants. The study group included physicians and nurses who had a COVID-19 infection confirmed by real-time reverse transcription-polymerase chain reaction (RT-PCR) test for SARS-CoV-2. The control group consisted of healthy medical professionals who had not had a SARS-CoV-2 infection or who had no symptoms of COVID-19 and who tested negative for SARS-CoV-2 on the day of examination. We analysed the correlation between AT1R concentration and the severity of COVID-19, as well as with sex, age, blood group, and comorbidities. There were no statistically significant differences in the mean values of AT1R concentration in the recovered individuals and the non-COVID-19 subjects (3.29 vs. 3.76 ng/mL; $p = 0.32$). The ROC curve for the AT1R assay showed an optimal cut-off point of 1.33 (AUC = 0.44; 95% CI = 0.32–0.57; $p = 0.37$). There was also no correlation between AT1R concentration and the severity of symptoms associated with COVID-19. Blood type analysis showed statistically significantly lower levels of AT1R in COVID-19-recovered participants with blood group A than in those with blood group O. In conclusion, AT1R concentration does not affect the severity of symptoms associated with COVID-19 among healthcare professionals.

Keywords: SARS-CoV-2; COVID-19; angiotensin 1 receptor (AT1R); AT1R concentration; angiotensin II; symptoms' severity

1. Introduction

Coronavirus Disease 2019 (COVID-19) was declared a world pandemic by the World Health Organization (WHO) on 11 March 2020 [1]. Since then, the understanding of COVID-19 pathophysiology and therapeutic options has evolved. The incubation period of COVID-19 is estimated to be 14 days from exposure, with a median time of 4–5 days [2], and the severity of the disease may range from asymptomatic to severe pneumonia with acute respiratory distress syndrome (ARDS). The symptoms of coronavirus type 2 (SARS-CoV-2) infection and the severity of COVID-19 are evaluated according to the illness categories described in the Clinical Spectrum of SARS-CoV-2 Infection section of the COVID-19 Treatment Guidelines developed by the National Institutes of Health (NIH) [3].

An asymptomatic or presymptomatic infection is described in individuals with a positive virologic test for SARS-CoV-2 but without symptoms consistent with COVID-19. Symptoms such as fever, cough, sore throat, muscle pain, diarrhoea, loss of smell and taste, malaise, and fatigue are classified as mild illness [3]. Patients with lower respiratory disease with a saturation of oxygen (SpO_2) $\geq$ 94% in room air at sea level are classified as having a moderate illness, and those with SpO_2 < 94% and PaO_2/FiO_2 < 300 mmHg as having a severe illness. A critical illness is described in individuals with respiratory failure, septic shock, and/or multiple organ dysfunction [3].

The pathophysiology of COVID-19 is related to the renin–angiotensin system (RAS). SARS-CoV-2, a vector of COVID-19, uses angiotensin-converting enzyme 2 (ACE-2), which is highly expressed in human lung tissue, nasal cavity, and oral mucosa, to gain access into human cells [4].

The substrate of the RAS pathway, angiotensinogen, is released into the circulation by the liver, where it is cleaved by an enzyme, renin, into angiotensin I (AngI) [5]. AngI is converted into angiotensin II (AngII) by ACE upon entering the ACE/AngII/AT1R axis of RAS. AngI and AngII are converted by ACE-2 into Ang1–9 and Ang1–7, respectively, which are the molecules of the ACE-2/AT2R axis. AngII, by interacting with its receptor– AngII receptor type 1 (AT1R), causes vasoconstriction, cell proliferation, hypertrophy, fibrosis, and inflammation [6]. By contrast, its interaction with AT2R is responsible for counterbalancing the effects of AT1R activation [7]. After entering the cell, SARS-CoV-2 inhibits ACE-2, thus favouring the ACE/AngII/AT1R axis, which plays a role in the development of acute lung injury (ALI) [8]. Elevated AngII levels have been determined in ALI and correlated with the severity and mortality of the disease (Figure 1) [9,10].

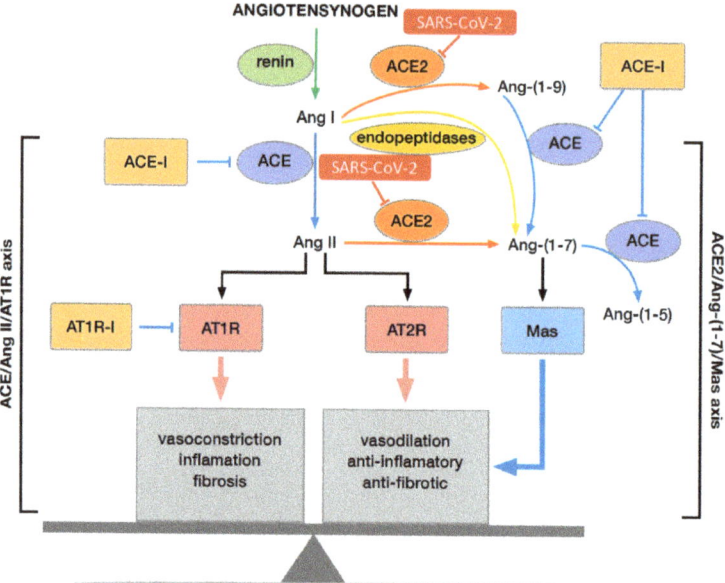

Figure 1. Influence of SARS-CoV-2 on RAS pathway.

AngII/AT1R activation leads to endothelial dysfunction and the activation of the coagulation cascade. AngII/AT1R acts by increasing reactive oxidative species (ROS) and promoting inflammation, inter alia leading to an increase in C-reactive protein (CRP) and interleukin-6 (IL-6) levels; such changes are observed in COVID-19 infection and are considered predictors of disease severity [11]. The formation of ROS results in the production of inflammatory factors, such as tumour necrosis factor-alpha (TNF-α), monocyte chemoattractant protein-1 (MCP-1), tissue factor (TF), nuclear factor kappa B (NF-κB), IL-6, CRP, and plasminogen activator inhibitor-1 (PAI-1), which may add to the state of overwhelming systemic inflammation, and hypercoagulability [12]. Further, increased aldosterone release, mediated by AngII/AT1R, may be associated with thrombotic events [13]. It should be emphasised that AngII and aldosterone increase the expression of PAI-1, a major inhibitor of fibrinolysis in vivo, in vascular smooth muscle and endothelial cells [14]. Aldosterone release, stimulated by AngII/AT1R activation, also upregulates protein-C receptors in the human vascular endothelium [15] and is strongly associated with a prothrombotic state [16].

This study aimed to determine the correlation between AT1R serum concentration and the severity of SARS-CoV-2 in healthcare professionals who work with patients with COVID-19.

2. Materials and Methods

2.1. Design and Settings

The single-centre prospective observational study was conducted in January 2021 at the Department of Anaesthesiology and Intensive Therapy of the 4th Military Clinical Hospital in Wroclaw, Poland. The study was prospectively registered in the Australian New Zealand Clinical Trials Registry (ANZCTR), with registration no. ACTRN 12621000013864. The Strengthening the Reporting of Observational Studies in Epidemiology (STROBE) standards were followed, and the relevant checklist for enrolment and allocation of participants was used [17]. Written informed consent was obtained from all eligible participants prior to the study.

2.2. Ethics

The study protocol was approved by the Bioethics Committee of the Wroclaw Medical University, Poland (approval no. KB–815/2020). The study was carried out according to the Declaration of Helsinki and Good Clinical Practice guidelines. Written informed consent was obtained from all the participants prior to the study.

2.3. Participants

The study was carried out on 82 participants, including 47 physicians and 35 nurses. Two study groups were identified. The first group (study group, $n = 40$) included healthcare professionals who had a symptomatic COVID-19 infection with a confirmed real-time reverse transcription-polymerase chain reaction (RT-PCR) test for SARS-CoV-2. The second group (control group, $n = 42$) included medical staff who, until the study, had always obtained a negative result (every 14 days) of the RT-PCR test for SARS-CoV-2. The primary study outcome was to assess serum AT1R levels relative to COVID severity. We also analysed demographic data (age, sex, blood group, and body mass index (BMI)) and collected information on chronic diseases (diabetes, hypertension, nicotinism, and kidney failure) and medications. None of the study participants took AT1R blockers or ACE inhibitors.

2.4. Outcomes

2.4.1. AT1R Serum Concentration

On the day of the examination, one sample of blood (2.7 mL) was taken from each patient to determine the AT1R levels. After collection, the blood samples were left at room temperature to clot (about 30 min). They were then centrifuged at 3000 rpm for 10 min. The resulting serum was frozen and stored at $-70\ °C$ until the determination was performed. A 96-well plate coated with an anti-human AT1R antibody was used for test purposes. For analysis, 100 μL of the standard solution at 0, 0.156, 0.312, 0.625, 1.25, 2.5, 5, and 10 ng/mL, was added in duplicate. The remaining wells were filled with 100 μL of patient/control sera, added in duplicate. After 2 h of incubation at 37 °C, the liquid from each well was removed. Then, 100 μL of detection reagent A was added to each well and left for 1 h at 37 °C temperature. After 1 h of incubation, the wells were washed three times with 350 μL of a wash buffer. Subsequently, 100 μL of detection reagent B was added to each well and left for 1 h at 37 °C temperature. After the next washing step (five times with 350 μL of the wash buffer), 90 μL of 3,3′,5,5′-tetramethylbenzidine (TMB) was added to each well. After 10 min of incubation at 37 °C temperature, the reaction was stopped with a stop solution. Absorbance was read using a microplate reader Tecan Infinite 200 (Tecan Austria GmbH, Grödig, Austria) at 450 nm. Serum level of AT1R was determined in accordance with the recommendations of the manufacturer Biomatik (Kitchener, Ontario, Canada) no. EKU02409 AT1R ELISA Kit. According to the manufacturer's description, the detection range is 0.156–10 ng/mL. The minimum detectable dose of AT1R is typically less than 0.055 ng/mL. The sensitivity of this assay, or Lower Limit of Detection (LLD) was defined as the lowest protein concentration that could be differentiated from zero. It was determined by subtracting two standard deviations to the mean optical density value of 20 zero-standard replicates and calculating the corresponding concentration. This assay has high sensitivity and excellent specificity for detection of AT1R. No significant cross-reactivity or interference between AT1R and analogues was observed.

2.4.2. COVID Severity

In the COVID-19-recovered individuals, SARS-CoV-2 infection symptoms and the severity of COVID-19 were additionally evaluated according to the illness categories described in the Clinical Spectrum of SARS-CoV-2 Infection section of the COVID-19 Treatment Guidelines developed by the NIH [3]:

1. Asymptomatic or Presymptomatic Infection: Individuals who tested positive for SARS-CoV-2 using a virologic test (i.e., a nucleic acid amplification test or an antigen test) but had no symptoms that were consistent with COVID-19;
2. Mild Illness: Individuals who had any of the various signs and symptoms of COVID-19 (e.g., fever, cough, sore throat, malaise, headache, muscle pain, nausea, vomiting, diarrhoea, loss of taste and smell) but who did not have shortness of breath, dyspnoea, or abnormal chest imaging;
3. Moderate Illness: Individuals who showed lower respiratory disease evidence during clinical assessment or imaging and had a saturation of oxygen (SpO_2) $\geq$ 94% on room air at sea level;
4. Severe Illness: Individuals who had SpO_2 < 94% on room air at sea level, a ratio of the arterial partial pressure of oxygen to fraction of inspired oxygen (PaO_2/FiO_2) < 300 mmHg, a respiratory rate > 30 breaths per minute, or lung infiltrates >50%;
5. Critical Illness: Individuals who had respiratory failure, septic shock, and/or multiple organ dysfunction.

2.5. Sample Size

Sample size analysis was performed using Statistica 13 (TIBCO Software Inc., Palo Alto, CA, USA). The difference in the serum AT1R level (ng/mL) between the groups of COVID-19-recovered subjects ($n = 6$) and healthy subjects ($n = 6$) was evaluated based on the available preliminary results of the study conducted at our centre (pilot study, $n = 12$). The sample size estimation analysis used the mean scores and standard deviations of the AT1R level (ng/mL) in both groups: the mean score in the COVID-19-recovered group was 3.02 ng/mL (SD = 1.71 ng/mL); the mean score in the group of health subjects was 4.10 ng/mL (SD = 1.79 ng/mL). The estimated sample size was calculated with a two-sample t-test for means (t-test for independent samples). The α level was set at 0.05, and the power of the test was 0.8. We assumed that there was no correlation between the evaluated variables, and a two-sided null hypothesis was adopted. The final sample size was set at $n = 40$ in each group.

2.6. Statistical Analysis

The statistical analysis was performed using Statistica 13 (TIBCO Software Inc., Palo Alto, CA, USA). For measurable variables, arithmetic means, medians, quartiles, standard deviations, and the range of variability (extreme values) were calculated. The frequency of the occurrence (percentage) of the qualitative variables was calculated. All the measured quantitative variables were tested with the Shapiro–Wilk test to determine the type of distribution. Qualitative variables were compared between the groups using the chi-square test (χ^2). The comparison of the results of quantitative variables between the groups was performed using the Student's t-test for independent samples or the Mann–Whitney U test, depending on the fulfilment of the test assumptions. The receiver operating characteristic (ROC) curve analysis (with Youden's index) was performed to determine the optimal cut-off level for AT1R to detect the occurrence of COVID-19. Univariable logistic regression was used to evaluate the influence of individual predictor variables in predicting COVID-19 disease. The results were considered statistically significant when the *p*-value was lower than 0.05.

3. Results

A group of 82 participants enrolled in the study, including healthy individuals who never had a positive RT-PCR test for COVID-19 (control group, $n = 42$), and individuals who had recovered from COVID-19 (study group, $n = 40$). Women represented 59.75% ($n = 49$) and men 40.25% ($n = 33$). The mean age of the participants was 39.9 years (SD = 9.8 years). Table 1 shows the detailed characteristics of the group together with a comparison of these characteristics between the COVID-19 recovered subjects and the control group. The groups were homogeneous regarding the selected characteristics (Table 1).

Table 1. Characteristics of study participants.

	All $n = 82$	COVID-19 Recovered $n = 40$	Non-COVID-19 $n = 42$	*p*
Age (years)				0.58 *
M ± SD	39.9 ± 9.8	39.3 ± 10.7	39.9 ± 9.8	
Me (Q1–Q3)	38.0 (31.0–47.0)	36.0 (29.5–48.0)	38.0 (31.0–47.0)	
Min–Max	25.0–64.0	25.0–64.0	25.0–64.0	
Weight (kg)				0.62 *
M ± SD	77.9 ± 16.8	78.9 ± 18.6	77.0 ± 15.1	
Me (Q1–Q3)	77.5 (67.0–87.0)	79.0 (66.0–89.5)	76.5 (67.0–82.0)	
Min–Max	45.0–135.0	45.0–135.0	50.0–116.0	
Height (cm)				0.43 *
M ± SD	171.5 ± 8.9	172.4 ± 10.0	170.8 ± 7.8	
Me (Q1–Q3)	173.0 (164.0–180.0)	173.0 (163.5–180.5)	172.5 (164.0–176.0)	
Min–Max	155.0–189.0	157.0–189.0	155.0–184.0	
BMI (kg/m^2)				0.92 *
M ± SD	26.4 ± 4.7	26.4 ± 5.2	26.3 ± 4.3	
Me (Q1–Q3)	26.3 (22.8–29.4)	26.2 (22.8–29.7)	26.3 (23.3–29.0)	
Min–Max	17.4–37.8	17.4–37.8	18.9–36.3	
Sex (female) *n* (%)	49 (60%)	23 (58%)	26 (62%)	0.68 **
Blood group *n* (%)				0.36 **
O	17 (23%)	5 (14%)	12 (31%)	
AB	8 (11%)	5 (14%)	3 (8%)	

Table 1. Cont.

	All n = 82	COVID-19 Recovered n = 40	Non-COVID-19 n = 42	p
A	33 (44%)	17 (49%)	16 (41%)	
B	6 (22%)	8 (23%)	11 (20%)	
Rh factor n (%)				0.12 **
Rh −	14 (19%)	4 (11%)	10 (26%)	
Rh +	60 (81%)	31 (89%)	29 (74%)	
Chronic disease n (%)				
Hypertension (Yes)	8 (10%)	5 (13%)	3 (7%)	0.41 **
Diabetes (Yes)	2 (2%)	1 (3%)	1 (2%)	0.97 **
Thyroid disease (Yes)	7 (9%)	4 (10%)	4 (7%)	0.64 **

Abbreviations: n, number of participants; M, mean; Me, median; Min, minimum value; Max, maximum value; Q1, lower quartile; Q3, upper quartile; SD, standard deviation; p, level of statistical significance. Notes: * t-test for independent samples; ** χ^2 test.

3.1. Analysis of AT1R Serum Concentration and Selected Values in Both Groups

There were no statistically significant differences in the mean values of AT1R serum concentration in the recovered individuals and the non-COVID-19 subjects (control group) (3.29 vs. 3.76 ng/mL; $p = 0.32$) (Figure 2). The ROC curve for the AT1R assay revealed that the optimal cut-off point was 1.33 (area under the curve, 0.44; 95% confidence interval, 0.32–0.57; $p = 0.37$) (Figure 3). The relationship between the selected variables and AT1R levels was assessed in all subjects. The analysis of the unifactorial logistic regression model did not show a significant statistical relationship between the variables (age, sex, body weight, height, BMI, blood group, Rh factor, hypertension, diabetes, thyroid disease, and COVID-19) and the level of AT1R (Table 2).

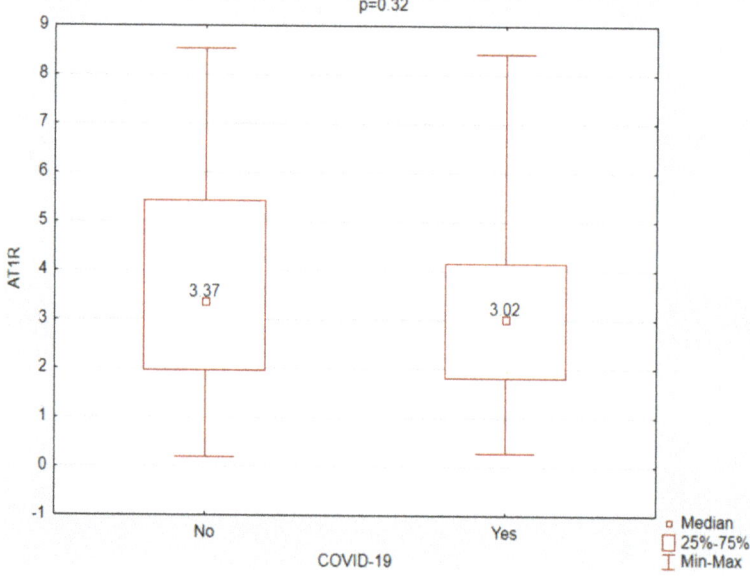

Figure 2. AT1R concentration in the non-COVID-19 and the COVID-19 recovered individuals. Abbreviations: AT1R, angiotensin II type 1 receptor.

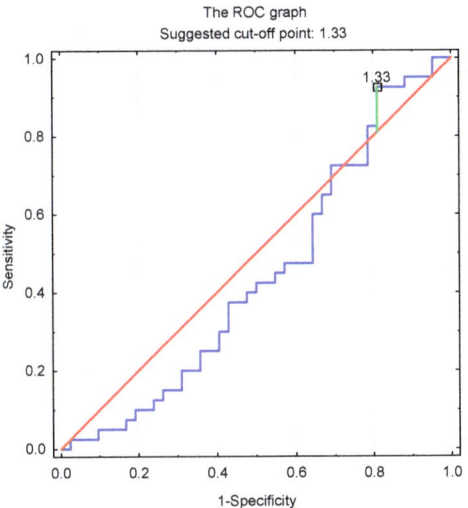

Figure 3. ROC curve for AT1R serum concentration in the non-COVID-19 and the COVID-19 recovered individuals. Abbreviations: ROC, receiver operating characteristic curve.

Table 2. Linear regression analysis between AT1R serum concentration and selected variables in all subjects.

AT1R Level—Linear Regression						
Variables		B	SE	t	p-Value	ß
Age		−0.01	0.02	−0.63	0.53	−0.07
Body height		0.01	0.03	0.26	0.79	0.03
Body weight		−0.02	0.01	−1.11	0.27	−0.12
BMI		−0.07	0.05	−1.43	0.16	−0.16
Sex	F	Ref.				
	M	−0.33	0.23	−1.41	0.16	−0.16
Blood group	O	Ref.				
	A	0.22	0.38	0.57	0.57	0.08
	B	−0.18	0.46	−0.39	0.70	−0.06
	AB	0.03	0.60	0.05	0.96	0.01
Rh factor	−	Ref.				
	+	0.18	0.31	0.58	0.57	0.07
COVID-19	No	Ref				
	Yes	−0.23	0.23	−1.01	0.32	−0.11
Hypertension	No	Ref.				
	Yes	−0.16	0.39	−0.42	0.67	−0.05
Diabetes	No	Ref.				
	Yes	0.84	0.75	1.12	0.27	0.12
Thyroid disease	No	Ref.				
	Yes	0.28	0.48	0.58	0.57	0.09

Abbreviations: B, unstandardized regression coefficient B; SE, standard error; t: B/standard error; ß, standardized regression coefficient ß; F, female; M, male.

3.2. Analysis of AT1R Serum Concentration and Selected Variables in the COVID-19 Recovered

An attempt was also made to compare intragroup and intergroup AT1R levels with stratification according to the aforementioned variables. No statistically significant differences were found in the inter- and intra-group comparisons (Table 3). The relationship between the selected variables and the AT1R level in the COVID-19-recovered group was assessed. The univariate logistic regression model showed a statistically significantly lower levels of AT1R in volunteers with blood group A than in those with blood group O. The other variables did not have a statistically significant influence on the level of AT1R (Table 4). Further, in the COVID-19-recovered group, the effect of AT1R serum concentration on the severity of the course was assessed according to the NIH guidelines. There was no statistically significant effect of AT1R serum levels on the severity of SARS-CoV-2 infection (Table 5).

Table 3. Comparison of AT1R serum concentration between the groups depending on the selected variables.

Variable		\multicolumn{7}{c}{AT1R Concentration}								p *
		COVID-19 Recovered (n = 40)							Non-COVID-19 (n = 42)						
		M	Me	Min	Max	Q1	Q3	SD	M	Me	Min	Max	Q1	Q3	SD	
Sex	M	3.03	2.99	0.28	7.19	1.48	4.32	2.03	3.25	2.74	0.20	6.71	1.52	5.36	2.26	0.63
	F	3.49	3.05	1.35	8.43	2.48	3.95	1.64	4.07	3.44	0.20	8.53	2.86	5.44	2.35	0.30
p-value *					0.48							0.37				
Blood group	O	4.02	3.98	1.82	5.55	3.43	5.31	1.52	3.19	3.13	0.49	6.55	1.17	5.45	2.21	1.00
	AB	4.41	3.95	1.33	8.43	2.48	5.88	2.82	2.06	1.96	0.20	4.02	0.20	4.02	1.91	1.00
	A	2.59	2.87	0.88	5.04	1.78	3.05	1.02	4.91	4.90	1.15	8.53	2.68	7.14	2.52	0.08
	B	3.91	3.76	1.35	7.19	2.92	4.69	1.74	2.73	3.35	0.20	3.89	1.95	3.57	1.40	0.96
p-value **					0.72							0.42				
Rh	−	3.57	2.88	1.35	7.19	1.56	5.59	2.67	3.13	3.35	0.49	8.13	1.13	3.89	2.30	0.62
	+	3.33	3.05	0.88	8.43	2.34	3.95	1.61	3.91	3.32	0.20	8.53	2.06	5.79	2.39	0.34
p-value *					0.98							0.41				
Hypertension	No	3.23	2.99	0.28	8.43	1.80	3.98	1.77	3.86	3.42	0.20	8.53	1.98	5.44	2.28	0.23
	Yes	3.71	3.43	1.78	7.19	1.82	4.33	2.23	2.44	1.13	0.20	5.99	0.20	5.99	3.11	0.37
p-value *					0.59							0.31				
Diabetes	No	3.27	2.99	0.28	8.43	1.80	3.98	1.82	3.70	3.32	0.20	8.53	1.96	5.23	2.33	0.41
	Yes	4.33	4.33	4.33	4.33	4.33	4.33	-	5.99	5.99	5.99	5.99	5.99	5.99	-	-
p-value *					-							-				
Thyroid disease	No	3.24	2.98	0.28	8.43	1.79	4.15	1.86	3.67	3.42	0.20	8.53	1.91	5.44	2.30	0.42
	Yes	3.79	3.19	2.91	5.88	2.95	4.63	1.41	4.84	3.28	3.11	8.13	3.11	8.13	2.85	0.60
p-value *					0.43							0.56				

Abbreviations: n, number of participants; M, mean; Me, median; Min, minimum value; Max, maximum value; Q1, lower quartile; Q3, upper quartile; SD, standard deviation; AT1R, angiotensin II type 1 receptor; M, male; F, female; p, level of statistical significance. Notes: * Mann–Whitney U test; ** Kruskal–Wallis test; Bonferroni correction was used for all comparisons.

Table 4. Results of the logistic regression for COVID-19 recovered group.

AT1R Level—Linear Regression						
Variables		B	SE	t	p-Value	ß
Age		0.00	0.03	0.17	0.86	0.03
Body height		0.01	0.03	0.41	0.69	0.07
Body weight		0.00	0.02	−0.01	0.99	0.00
BMI		−0.01	0.06	−0.22	0.83	−0.04
Sex	F	Ref.				
	M	−0.23	0.29	−0.78	0.44	−0.13
Blood group	0	Ref.				
	A	−1.14	0.41	−2.78	0.009	−0.48
	B	0.18	0.50	0.35	0.73	0.06
	AB	0.68	0.59	1.15	0.26	0.22
Rh factor	−	Ref.				
	+	−0.12	0.46	−0.26	0.79	−0.05
Symptoms	1–2	Ref				
	2–3	−0.15	0.30	−0.49	0.63	−0.08
Hypertension	No	Ref.				
	Yes	0.24	0.44	0.55	0.59	0.09
Diabetes	No	Ref.				
	Yes	0.53	0.92	0.58	0.57	0.09
Thyroid disease	No	Ref.				
	Yes	0.28	0.48	0.58	0.57	0.09

Abbreviations: BMI, body mass index; AT1R, angiotensin II type 1 receptor; M, male; F, female; B, unstandardized regression coefficient; SE, standard error; t: B/standard error; ß, standardized regression coefficient ß.

Table 5. Comparison of AT1R serum concentration with illness category according to NIH Treatment Guidelines in COVID-19 recovered individuals.

NIH Illness Category	n	AT1R Serum Concentration in COVID-19 Recovered Group (n = 40)							p
		M	Me	Min	Max	Q1	Q3	SD	
1	1	7.19	7.19	7.19	7.19	7.19	7.19	-	
2	25	3.24	2.99	1.35	6.34	2.46	3.95	1.30	0.21 *
3	10	3.24	3.28	0.28	5.55	1.71	5.04	1.72	
4	4	2.75	1.11	0.35	8.43	0.62	4.88	3.81	
1–2	26	3.40	3.02	1.35	7.19	2.46	3.98	1.49	0.45 **
3–4	14	3.10	3.01	0.28	8.43	1.33	5.04	2.33	

Abbreviations: NIH, National Institutes of Health; n, number of participants; M, mean; Me, median; Min, minimum value; Max, maximum value; Q1, lower quartile; Q3, upper quartile; SD, standard deviation; AT1R, angiotensin II type 1 receptor; p, level of statistical significance. Notes: * Kruskal–Wallis test; ** Mann–Whitney U test.

4. Discussion

In our study, we found no statistical relationship between AT1R serum levels and the severity of infection based on the NIH COVID-19 Treatment Guidelines [3]. There were no statistically significant differences in the mean AT1R serum levels in the recovered individuals and the non-COVID-19 subjects. There was no statistical relationship between AT1R serum concentration in subjects with comorbidities such as hypertension, type II diabetes, and thyroid disease, or with COVID-19 severity.

The methodology assumes that although the AT1R is a membrane GPCR receptor occurring mainly in the vascular endothelium, part of it may be in the blood, which will allow its detection and quantification. To date, no soluble version of this receptor has been described, however, the available test for the determination of AT1R has been validated for determination in blood serum. Especially in the COVID-19 recovered group due to the significant stimulation of AT1R by AngII, it was assumed that its amount may be higher compared to the non-COVID-19 group. The results did not confirm an increase in receptor concentration in the COVID-19 group. Studies of AT1R concentration were also carried out in other body fluids.

Hu et al. [18] in 2009 determined the concentration of AT1R in the urine of Sugar Rats using immunoblotting method, comparing the results with the number of receptors in renal biopsies. The work does not explain in detail the mechanism of the presence of receptors in the urine but suggest that AT1R can be expressed in vascular tissues throughout the body and may be filtered to some extent through the glomerulus. On the other hand, in the study by Bansal et al. [19], the concentration of the AT1R receptor in serum exosomes was determined by Western blot and densitometry analysis.

Knowing the nature of the AT1R receptor, we are not able describe the mechanism of the appearance of this receptor in the sera we studied. We would point out that the presence of the receptor was determined in both groups: recovered from COVID-19 and patients who did not undergo this disease, and none of the results showed the absence of the receptor in serum.

The RAS system plays a crucial role in SARS-CoV-2 infection. One component of this system, ACE2, functions as a receptor for the virus. In their study, Guzzi et al. [20] indicated that a decrease in ACE2 expression following COVID-19 infection leads to excessive AT1R activation by AngII. Increased AT1R activation exerts proinflammatory, prothrombotic, and pro-apoptotic effects [21]. Inflammation following a cytokine storm is one of the major causes of mortality in SARS-CoV-2 infection. The severity of inflammation is further exacerbated by AT1R activation by AngII [22].

Currently, there are many ongoing studies on the effect of angiotensin receptor blockers (ARBs) on the course of SARS-CoV-2 infection. Several authors have shown that this type of drug has dual-phase effects with possible antagonistic outcomes [23,24]. Dublin et al. [25] suggested that ARBs may be effective in SARS-CoV-2 infection, modifying disease progression. Further, ARBs possess inverse agonist properties that give them an additional pharmacological effect and improve drug efficacy [26]. Given the hypothesis that the severity of inflammation in COVID-19 depends on AT1 receptor stimulation by AngII, drugs that act on AT1R have been proposed as a treatment for COVID-19 [27]. Zhang et al. [28] found that among COVID-19 patients hospitalised with hypertension, patient treatment with ACEI/ARB was related to a lower risk of all-cause mortality.

At present, the use of ARBs in preventing excessive proinflammatory effects of AngII in COVID-19 is quite controversial. The present study did not show a correlation between AT1R levels and the severity of the symptoms associated with COVID-19, which is a consequence of the dynamics of the inflammatory state. Rothlin et al. [29] demonstrated that the use of ARBs in the treatment of COVID-19 should be considered, depending on the stage and severity of disease, rather than as a component of the continuation of antihypertensive treatment in the group of patients with COVID-19.

Notably, our analysis showed a relationship between the blood group and AT1R serum levels in the COVID-19-recovered group. The univariate logistic regression model showed a statistically significantly lower level of AT1R in volunteers with blood group A than in those with blood group O. Studies published so far have shown a protective effect of anti-A antibodies against the intracellular uptake of SARS-CoV-2 [30,31]. Four studies showed a correlation between blood group and severity of COVID-19; five studies did not find any correlation [32–40]. Ray et al. [36] published a study on a cohort of 7031 patients with positive tests for SARS-CoV-2. The authors found that individuals with type O blood were less likely to contract SARS-CoV-2 compared to non-type O blood groups. In our study, we found that participants with type A blood had higher levels of AT1R than those with type O blood among patients who had a SARS-CoV-2 infection; however, there was no correlation between AT1R levels and the severity of infection. An updated meta-analysis published in 2021 by Bhattacharjee et al. [41] showed no significant differences in unadjusted mortality or severity outcomes related to COVID-19 illness in patients with blood groups A/AB compared to those with B/O blood groups.

Although the role of the RAS has been extensively studied in COVID-19 patients, there are, unquestionably, information gaps concerning this topic, especially regarding the role of AT1-inverse agonists and their mechanism action in SARS-CoV-2 infection.

Study Limitations

This study has some potential methodological limitations that need to be mentioned. A foremost limitation is the single-centre nature of the study. In our opinion, thorough multicentre research is needed on the topic. The number of patients enrolled was relatively small, which calls for future studies with a larger population size.

5. Conclusions

The serum levels of AT1R did not correlate with the severity of the course of COVID-19 in the healthcare professional sampled in this study. No statistically significant difference in AT1R serum concentration was found between the recovered individuals and the non-COVID-19 subjects. Our univariate logistic regression model showed a statistically significantly lower level of serum AT1R in volunteers with blood group A than in participants with blood group O. Thus, further studies on the influence of the virus on the RAS system and the effect of AT1R-blocking drugs on the disease course are necessary.

Author Contributions: Conceptualization, J.J., M.S., L.Ł. and P.L.; methodology, J.J., M.S., L.Ł. and P.L.; software, J.J., M.M.-P. and E.W.-N.; validation, J.J., M.S., M.M.-P. and E.W.-N.; formal analysis, J.J., M.S., L.Ł. and P.L.; investigation, J.J., M.S., L.Ł. and P.L.; resources, J.J., M.M.-P. and E.W.-N.; data curation, J.J., M.S., E.W.-N., L.Ł. and P.L.; writing—original draft preparation, J.J., M.S., E.W.-N. and P.L.; writing—review and editing, J.J., M.M.-P. and L.Ł.; visualization, J.J., M.S. and M.M.-P.; supervision, J.J., L.Ł. and P.L.; project administration, J.J. and P.L.; funding acquisition, J.J. and L.Ł. All authors have read and agreed to the published version of the manuscript.

Funding: This research was partially supported by the Ministry of Health subventions according to number of SUB.A040.19.016 from the IT Simple system of the Wroclaw Medical University.

Institutional Review Board Statement: The study was conducted in accordance with the Declaration of Helsinki, and approved by the Bioethics Committee of the Wroclaw Medical University, Poland (approval no. KB–815/2020).

Informed Consent Statement: Informed consent was obtained from all subjects involved in the study.

Data Availability Statement: The data presented in this study are available on request from the corresponding author.

Conflicts of Interest: The authors declare no conflict of interest.

References

1. Cucinotta, D.; Vanelli, M. WHO Declares COVID-19 a Pandemic. *Acta Bio-Med. Atenei Parm.* **2020**, *91*, 157–160. [CrossRef]
2. Guan, W.-J.; Ni, Z.-Y.; Hu, Y.; Liang, W.-H.; Ou, C.-Q.; He, J.-X.; Liu, L.; Shan, H.; Lei, C.-L.; Hui, D.S.C.; et al. Clinical Characteristics of Coronavirus Disease 2019 in China. *N. Engl. J. Med.* **2020**, *382*, 1708–1720. [CrossRef] [PubMed]
3. COVID-19 Treatment Guidelines Panel. *Coronavirus Disease (COVID-19) Treatment Guidelines: Clinical Spectrum of SARS-CoV-2 Infection*; National Institutes of Health: Bethesda, MA, USA, 2021.
4. Hamming, I.; Timens, W.; Bulthuis, M.L.C.; Lely, A.T.; Navis, G.J.; van Goor, H. Tissue Distribution of ACE2 Protein, the Functional Receptor for SARS Coronavirus. A First Step in Understanding SARS Pathogenesis. *J. Pathol.* **2004**, *203*, 631–637. [CrossRef] [PubMed]
5. Sparks, M.A.; Crowley, S.D.; Gurley, S.B.; Mirotsou, M.; Coffman, T.M. Classical Renin-Angiotensin System in Kidney Physiology. *Compr. Physiol.* **2014**, *4*, 1201–1228. [CrossRef]

6. Bernard, A.; Broeckaert, F.; De Poorter, G.; De Cock, A.; Hermans, C.; Saegerman, C.; Houins, G. The Belgian PCB/Dioxin Incident: Analysis of the Food Chain Contamination and Health Risk Evaluation. *Environ. Res.* **2002**, *88*, 1–18. [CrossRef] [PubMed]
7. Guang, C.; Phillips, R.D.; Jiang, B.; Milani, F. Three Key Proteases–Angiotensin-I-Converting Enzyme (ACE), ACE2 and Renin–within and beyond the Renin-Angiotensin System. *Arch. Cardiovasc. Dis.* **2012**, *105*, 373–385. [CrossRef] [PubMed]
8. D'Ardes, D.; Boccatonda, A.; Rossi, I.; Guagnano, M.T.; Santilli, F.; Cipollone, F.; Bucci, M. COVID-19 and RAS: Unravelling an Unclear Relationship. *Int. J. Mol. Sci.* **2020**, *21*, 3003. [CrossRef]
9. Khan, A.; Benthin, C.; Zeno, B.; Albertson, T.E.; Boyd, J.; Christie, J.D.; Hall, R.; Poirier, G.; Ronco, J.J.; Tidswell, M.; et al. A Pilot Clinical Trial of Recombinant Human Angiotensin-Converting Enzyme 2 in Acute Respiratory Distress Syndrome. *Crit. Care Lond. Engl.* **2017**, *21*, 234. [CrossRef]
10. Lundström, A.; Ziegler, L.; Havervall, S.; Rudberg, A.-S.; von Meijenfeldt, F.; Lisman, T.; Mackman, N.; Sandén, P.; Thålin, C. Soluble Angiotensin-Converting Enzyme 2 Is Transiently Elevated in COVID-19 and Correlates with Specific Inflammatory and Endothelial Markers. *J. Med. Virol.* **2021**, *93*, 5908–5916. [CrossRef]
11. Liu, F.; Li, L.; Xu, M.; Wu, J.; Luo, D.; Zhu, Y.; Li, B.; Song, X.; Zhou, X. Prognostic Value of Interleukin-6, C-Reactive Protein, and Procalcitonin in Patients with COVID-19. *J. Clin. Virol.* **2020**, *127*, 104370. [CrossRef]
12. Dandona, P.; Dhindsa, S.; Ghanim, H.; Chaudhuri, A. Angiotensin II and Inflammation: The Effect of Angiotensin-Converting Enzyme Inhibition and Angiotensin II Receptor Blockade. *J. Hum. Hypertens.* **2007**, *21*, 20–27. [CrossRef]
13. Gromotowicz-Poplawska, A.; Stankiewicz, A.; Kramkowski, K.; Gradzka, A.; Wojewodzka-Zeleznikowicz, M.; Dzieciol, J.; Szemraj, J.; Chabielska, E. The Acute Prothrombotic Effect of Aldosterone in Rats Is Partially Mediated via Angiotensin II Receptor Type 1. *Thromb. Res.* **2016**, *138*, 114–120. [CrossRef] [PubMed]
14. Sawathiparnich, P.; Murphey, L.J.; Kumar, S.; Vaughan, D.E.; Brown, N.J. Effect of Combined AT1 Receptor and Aldosterone Receptor Antagonism on Plasminogen Activator Inhibitor-1. *J. Clin. Endocrinol. Metab.* **2003**, *88*, 3867–3873. [CrossRef] [PubMed]
15. Ducros, E.; Berthaut, A.; Mirshahi, S.S.; Faussat, A.M.; Soria, J.; Agarwal, M.K.; Mirshahi, M. Aldosterone Modifies Hemostasis via Upregulation of the Protein-C Receptor in Human Vascular Endothelium. *Biochem. Biophys. Res. Commun.* **2008**, *373*, 192–196. [CrossRef] [PubMed]
16. Remková, A.; Remko, M. The Role of Renin-Angiotensin System in Prothrombotic State in Essential Hypertension. *Physiol. Res.* **2010**, *59*, 13–23. [CrossRef]
17. von Elm, E.; Altman, D.G.; Egger, M.; Pocock, S.J.; Gøtzsche, P.C.; Vandenbroucke, J.P. STROBE Initiative The Strengthening the Reporting of Observational Studies in Epidemiology (STROBE) Statement: Guidelines for Reporting Observational Studies. *J. Clin. Epidemiol.* **2008**, *61*, 344–349. [CrossRef]
18. Hu, J.; Tiwari, S.; Riazi, S.; Hu, X.; Wang, X.; Ecelbarger, C.M. Regulation of Angiotensin II Type I Receptor (AT1R) Protein Levels in the Obese Zucker Rat Kidney and Urine. *Clin. Exp. Hypertens.* **2009**, *31*, 49–63. [CrossRef]
19. Bansal, S.; Tokman, S.; Fleming, T.; Maine, G.N.; Sanborn, K.; Hachem, R.; Bharat, A.; Smith, M.A.; Bremner, R.M.; Mohanakumar, T. SARS-CoV-2 Infection in Lung Transplant Recipients Induces Circulating Exosomes with SARS-CoV-2 Spike Protein S2. *Clin. Transl. Med.* **2021**, *11*, e576. [CrossRef]
20. Guzzi, P.H.; Mercatelli, D.; Ceraolo, C.; Giorgi, F.M. Master Regulator Analysis of the SARS-CoV-2/Human Interactome. *J. Clin. Med.* **2020**, *9*, 982. [CrossRef]
21. Speth, R.C. Angiotensin II Administration to COVID-19 Patients Is Not Advisable. *Crit. Care Lond. Engl.* **2020**, *24*, 296. [CrossRef]
22. Forrester, S.J.; Booz, G.W.; Sigmund, C.D.; Coffman, T.M.; Kawai, T.; Rizzo, V.; Scalia, R.; Eguchi, S. Angiotensin II Signal Transduction: An Update on Mechanisms of Physiology and Pathophysiology. *Physiol. Rev.* **2018**, *98*, 1627–1738. [CrossRef] [PubMed]
23. Dworakowska, D.; Grossman, A.B. Renin-Angiotensin System Inhibitors in Management of Hypertension during the COVID-19 Pandemic. *J. Physiol. Pharmacol.* **2020**, *71*. [CrossRef]
24. Mehta, P.; McAuley, D.F.; Brown, M.; Sanchez, E.; Tattersall, R.S.; Manson, J.J. HLH Across Speciality Collaboration, UK COVID-19: Consider Cytokine Storm Syndromes and Immunosuppression. *Lancet Lond. Engl.* **2020**, *395*, 1033–1034. [CrossRef]
25. Dublin, S.; Walker, R.; Floyd, J.S.; Shortreed, S.M.; Fuller, S.; Albertson-Junkans, L.; Harrington, L.B.; Greenwood-Hickman, M.A.; Green, B.B.; Psaty, B.M. Renin-Angiotensin-Aldosterone System Inhibitors and COVID-19 Infection or Hospitalization: A Cohort Study. *medRxiv* **2020**. [CrossRef] [PubMed]
26. Akazawa, H.; Yasuda, N.; Komuro, I. Mechanisms and Functions of Agonist-Independent Activation in the Angiotensin II Type 1 Receptor. *Mol. Cell. Endocrinol.* **2009**, *302*, 140–147. [CrossRef]
27. Gurwitz, D. Angiotensin Receptor Blockers as Tentative SARS-CoV-2 Therapeutics. *Drug Dev. Res.* **2020**, *81*, 537–540. [CrossRef]
28. Zhang, P.; Zhu, L.; Cai, J.; Lei, F.; Qin, J.-J.; Xie, J.; Liu, Y.-M.; Zhao, Y.-C.; Huang, X.; Lin, L.; et al. Association of Inpatient Use of Angiotensin-Converting Enzyme Inhibitors and Angiotensin II Receptor Blockers with Mortality Among Patients With Hypertension Hospitalized With COVID-19. *Circ. Res.* **2020**, *126*, 1671–1681. [CrossRef]
29. Rothlin, R.P.; Duarte, M.; Pelorosso, F.G.; Nicolosi, L.; Salgado, M.V.; Vetulli, H.M.; Spitzer, E. Angiotensin Receptor Blockers for COVID-19: Pathophysiological and Pharmacological Considerations About Ongoing and Future Prospective Clinical Trials. *Front. Pharmacol.* **2021**, *12*, 603736. [CrossRef]
30. Guillon, P.; Clément, M.; Sébille, V.; Rivain, J.-G.; Chou, C.-F.; Ruvoën-Clouet, N.; Le Pendu, J. Inhibition of the Interaction between the SARS-CoV Spike Protein and Its Cellular Receptor by Anti-Histo-Blood Group Antibodies. *Glycobiology* **2008**, *18*, 1085–1093. [CrossRef]

31. Ritchie, G.; Harvey, D.J.; Feldmann, F.; Stroeher, U.; Feldmann, H.; Royle, L.; Dwek, R.A.; Rudd, P.M. Identification of N-Linked Carbohydrates from Severe Acute Respiratory Syndrome (SARS) Spike Glycoprotein. *Virology* **2010**, *399*, 257–269. [CrossRef]
32. Hoiland, R.L.; Fergusson, N.A.; Mitra, A.R.; Griesdale, D.E.G.; Devine, D.V.; Stukas, S.; Cooper, J.; Thiara, S.; Foster, D.; Chen, L.Y.C.; et al. The Association of ABO Blood Group with Indices of Disease Severity and Multiorgan Dysfunction in COVID-19. *Blood Adv.* **2020**, *4*, 4981–4989. [CrossRef] [PubMed]
33. Latz, C.A.; DeCarlo, C.; Boitano, L.; Png, C.Y.M.; Patell, R.; Conrad, M.F.; Eagleton, M.; Dua, A. Blood Type and Outcomes in Patients with COVID-19. *Ann. Hematol.* **2020**, *99*, 2113–2118. [CrossRef]
34. Leaf, R.K.; Al-Samkari, H.; Brenner, S.K.; Gupta, S.; Leaf, D.E. ABO Phenotype and Death in Critically Ill Patients with COVID-19. *Br. J. Haematol.* **2020**, *190*, e204–e208. [CrossRef] [PubMed]
35. Li, J.; Wang, X.; Chen, J.; Cai, Y.; Deng, A.; Yang, M. Association between ABO Blood Groups and Risk of SARS-CoV-2 Pneumonia. *Br. J. Haematol.* **2020**, *190*, 24–27. [CrossRef] [PubMed]
36. Ray, J.G.; Schull, M.J.; Vermeulen, M.J.; Park, A.L. Association Between ABO and Rh Blood Groups and SARS-CoV-2 Infection or Severe COVID-19 Illness: A Population-Based Cohort Study. *Ann. Intern. Med.* **2021**, *174*, 308–315. [CrossRef]
37. Zhao, J.; Yang, Y.; Huang, H.; Li, D.; Gu, D.; Lu, X.; Zhang, Z.; Liu, L.; Liu, T.; Liu, Y.; et al. Relationship between the ABO Blood Group and the COVID-19 Susceptibility. *Clin. Infect. Dis.* **2021**, *73*, 328–331. [CrossRef]
38. Zietz, M.; Zucker, J.; Tatonetti, N.P. Testing the Association between Blood Type and COVID-19 Infection, Intubation, and Death. *medRxiv* **2020**. [CrossRef]
39. Boudin, L.; Janvier, F.; Bylicki, O.; Dutasta, F. ABO Blood Groups Are Not Associated with Risk of Acquiring the SARS-CoV-2 Infection in Young Adults. *Haematologica* **2020**, *105*, 2841–2843. [CrossRef]
40. Barnkob, M.B.; Pottegård, A.; Støvring, H.; Haunstrup, T.M.; Homburg, K.; Larsen, R.; Hansen, M.B.; Titlestad, K.; Aagaard, B.; Møller, B.K.; et al. Reduced Prevalence of SARS-CoV-2 Infection in ABO Blood Group O. *Blood Adv.* **2020**, *4*, 4990–4993. [CrossRef]
41. Bhattacharjee, S.; Banerjee, M.; Pal, R. ABO Blood Groups and Severe Outcomes in COVID-19: A Meta-Analysis. *Postgrad. Med. J.* **2020**. [CrossRef]

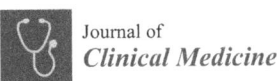

Journal of
Clinical Medicine

Article

Demographic and Clinical Overview of Hospitalized COVID-19 Patients during the First 17 Months of the Pandemic in Poland

Robert Flisiak [1,*,†], Piotr Rzymski [2,3,*,†], Dorota Zarębska-Michaluk [4,*,†], Magdalena Rogalska [1], Marta Rorat [5,6], Piotr Czupryna [7], Beata Lorenc [8], Przemysław Ciechanowski [9], Dorota Kozielewicz [10], Anna Piekarska [11], Maria Pokorska-Śpiewak [12], Katarzyna Sikorska [13], Magdalena Tudrujek [14], Beata Bolewska [15], Grzegorz Angielski [16], Justyna Kowalska [17], Regina Podlasin [18], Włodzimierz Mazur [19], Barbara Oczko-Grzesik [20], Izabela Zaleska [21], Aleksandra Szymczak [22], Paulina Frańczak-Chmura [23], Małgorzata Sobolewska-Pilarczyk [10], Krzysztof Kłos [24], Magdalena Figlerowicz [25], Piotr Leszczyński [26], Izabela Kucharek [27] and Hubert Grabowski [28]

1. Department of Infectious Diseases and Hepatology, Medical University of Białystok, 15-089 Bialystok, Poland; pmagdar@gmail.com
2. Department of Environmental Medicine, Poznan University of Medical Sciences, 60-806 Poznan, Poland
3. Integrated Science Association (ISA), Universal Scientific Education and Research Network (USERN), 60-806 Poznan, Poland
4. Department of Infectious Diseases, Jan Kochanowski University, 25-369 Kielce, Poland
5. Department of Forensic Medicine, Wrocław Medical University, 50-367 Wrocław, Poland; marta.rorat@gmail.com
6. First Infectious Diseases Ward, Gromkowski Regional Specialist Hospital in Wrocław, 51-149 Wroclaw, Poland
7. Department of Infectious Diseases and Neuroinfections, Medical University of Białystok, 15-089 Bialystok, Poland; piotr.czupryna@umb.edu.pl
8. Pomeranian Center of Infectious Diseases, Department of Infectious Diseases, 80-210 Gdansk, Poland; lormar@gumed.edu.pl
9. Department of Paediatrics and Infectious Diseases, Regional Hospital in Szczecin, 71-455 Szczecin, Poland; przciechanowski@spwsz.szczecin.pl
10. Department of Infectious Diseases and Hepatology, Faculty of Medicine, Collegium Medicum in Bydgoszcz, Nicolaus Copernicus University, 87-100 Torun, Poland; d.kozielewicz@wsoz.pl (D.K.); m.pilarczyk@wsoz.pl (M.S.-P.)
11. Department of Infectious Diseases, Medical University of Łódź, 90-549 Lodz, Poland; annapiekar@gmail.com
12. Department of Children's Infectious Diseases, Medical University of Warsaw, 01-201 Warsaw, Poland; mpspiewak@gmail.com
13. Department of Tropical Medicine and Epidemiology, Medical University of Gdańsk, 80-210 Gdańsk, Poland; ksikorska@gumed.edu.pl
14. Department of Infectious Diseases and Hepatology, Medical University of Lublin, 20-059 Lublin, Poland; magdalena.tudrujek@gmail.com
15. Department of Infectious Diseases, Poznan University of Medical Sciences, 61-701 Poznan, Poland; bbolewska@ump.edu.pl
16. 7th Navy Hospital, 80-305 Gdansk, Poland; grzegorzangielski1@gmail.com
17. Department of Adults' Infectious Diseases, Medical University of Warsaw, 02-091 Warsaw, Poland; jdkowalska@gmail.com
18. Regional Hospital of Infectious Diseases in Warsaw, 01-301 Warsaw, Poland; podlasin@zakazny.pl
19. Clinical Department of Infectious Diseases in Chorzów, Medical University of Silesia, 41-500 Katowice, Poland; wlodek.maz@gmail.com
20. Department of Infectious Diseases and Hepatology, Medical University of Silesia, 40-055 Katowice, Poland; bgrzesik@hoga.pl
21. Department of Paediatrics and Infectious Diseases, Wroclaw Medical University, 50-367 Wroclaw, Poland; izabela.zaleska9@gmail.com
22. Department of Infectious Diseases, Liver Diseases and Acquired Immune Deficiencies, Wroclaw Medical University, 51-149 Wroclaw, Poland; ola.szymczak@gmail.com
23. Department of Children's Infectious Diseases, Provincial Jan Boży Hospital, 20-089 Lublin, Poland; franczak_paulina@wp.pl
24. Department of Infectious Diseases and Allergology, Military Institute of Medicine, 04-141 Warsaw, Poland; kklos@wim.mil.pl
25. Department of Infectious Diseases and Child Neurology, Poznan University of Medical Sciences, 60-572 Poznan, Poland; mfiglerowicz@gmail.com
26. Department of Rheumatology, Rehabilitation and Internal Medicine, Poznan University of Medical Sciences, 61-701 Poznan, Poland; piotr_leszczynski@wp.pl

Citation: Flisiak, R.; Rzymski, P.; Zarębska-Michaluk, D.; Rogalska, M.; Rorat, M.; Czupryna, P.; Lorenc, B.; Ciechanowski, P.; Kozielewicz, D.; Piekarska, A.; et al. Demographic and Clinical Overview of Hospitalized COVID-19 Patients during the First 17 Months of the Pandemic in Poland. *J. Clin. Med.* **2022**, *11*, 117. https://doi.org/10.3390/jcm11010117

Academic Editors: Kaio Kitazato and Jan Jelrik Oosterheert

Received: 24 November 2021
Accepted: 23 December 2021
Published: 26 December 2021

Publisher's Note: MDPI stays neutral with regard to jurisdictional claims in published maps and institutional affiliations.

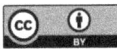

Copyright: © 2021 by the authors. Licensee MDPI, Basel, Switzerland. This article is an open access article distributed under the terms and conditions of the Creative Commons Attribution (CC BY) license (https://creativecommons.org/licenses/by/4.0/).

[27] 2nd Department of Paediatrics, Centre of Postgraduate Medical Education, 02-507 Warsaw, Poland; izaqcharek@gmail.com
[28] General, Endocrine and Transplant Surgery Department, Medical University of Gdańsk, 80-214 Gdansk, Poland; hubert1grabowski@gmail.com
* Correspondence: robert.flisiak1@gmail.com (R.F.); rzymskipiotr@ump.edu.pl (P.R.); dorota1010@tlen.pl (D.Z.-M.)
† These authors contributed equally to this work.

Abstract: Long-term analyses of demographical and clinical characteristics of COVID-19 patients can provide a better overview of the clinical course of the disease. They can also help understand whether changes in infection symptomatology, disease severity, and outcome occur over time. We aimed to analyze the demographics, early symptoms of infection, laboratory parameters, and clinical manifestation of COVID-19 patients hospitalized during the first 17 months of the pandemic in Poland (March 2020–June 2021). The patients' demographical and clinical data ($n = 5199$) were extracted from the national SARSTer database encompassing 30 medical centers in Poland and statistically assessed. Patients aged 50–64 were most commonly hospitalized due to COVID-19 regardless of the pandemic period. There was no shift in the age of admitted patients and patients who died throughout the studied period. Men had higher C-reactive protein and interleukin-6 levels and required oxygenation and mechanical ventilation more often. No gender difference in fatality rate was seen, although the age of males who died was significantly lower. A share of patients with baseline $SpO_2 < 91\%$, presenting respiratory, systemic and gastrointestinal symptoms was higher in the later phase of a pandemic than in the first three months. Cough, dyspnea and fever were more often presented in men, while women had a higher frequency of anosmia, diarrhea, nausea and vomiting. This study shows some shifts in SARS-CoV-2 pathogenicity between March 2020 and July 2021 in the Polish cohort of hospitalized patients and documents various gender-differences in this regard. The results represent a reference point for further analyses conducted under the dominance of different SARS-CoV-2 variants.

Keywords: epidemiology; SARS-CoV-2; clinical outcome; symptomatology; pandemic

1. Introduction

The outbreak of coronavirus disease (COVID-19) caused by severe acute respiratory syndrome coronavirus 2 (SARS-CoV-2) in late December 2019 in China quickly became an emerging, continuously evolving situation, spreading inevitably outside the Asian continent. It was declared a Public Health Emergency of International Concern at the end of January 2020 and a pandemic in March 2020 by the World Health Organization (WHO) [1]. Globally, nearly 84 million cases and 1.9 million deaths due to COVID-19 were reported by the end of 2020; both figures increased more than twofold in the following half-year. Although SARS-CoV-2 infections remain predominantly asymptomatic or mild, the clinical spectrum of COVID-19 is vast and includes severe progressive pneumonia and acute respiratory distress syndrome, both of which can be accompanied by cytokine storm, thrombosis, and multiple organ dysfunction [2,3]. The risk of severe COVID-19 is associated with increased age, obesity, male sex, and selected pre-existing medical conditions [4].

Since the publication of the first whole-genome sequence in January 2020, SARS-CoV-2 has been evolving, with numerous variants identified through genomic surveillance. In late 2020 and at the beginning of 2021, the emergence of variants posing higher public health risks, classified as variants of interest (VOIs) and variants of concern (VOCs), were observed. Two main evolutionary trajectories of SARS-CoV-2 include an increase in transmissibility (e.g., B.1.1.7 and B.1.617.2 variants) and evading host immune response (e.g., B.1.351 and others bearing E484K mutation) [5]. This has raised questions of whether these adaptive changes may be associated with increased vulnerability of different groups (e.g., younger, healthier subjects) to severe disease or influence the clinical presentation and outcome of COVID-19. It has been suggested that selected nonsynonymous mutations may be associated with more severe disease and inferior outcomes [6]. In vivo data indicated that infection with VOCs such as B.1.1.7 and B.1.351 reveal significant differences in pathogenicity with increased clinical progression and lower survival [7]. However, this has not been confirmed in the observational studies of hospitalized patients [8]. There has also been a discussion of whether shifts in the dominant SARS-CoV-2 variants in circulation may lead to changes in symptomatology [9].

Analyzing the long-term characteristics and trends of demographical and clinical data of patients hospitalized throughout a pandemic in a selected region can help assess whether there is a change in disease manifestation, severity and outcome, and understand the potential responsible factors. The present study summarized such data for COVID-19 patients hospitalized in 30 clinical centers in Poland between March 2020 and June 2021 and assessed whether there was any significant change in demographics (age, gender), early symptoms of infection, laboratory parameters, clinical manifestation, severity and outcome of the disease.

2. Materials and Methods

2.1. Data Collection

The data for this study was extracted from the SARSTer national database—an ongoing project led by the Polish Association of Epidemiologists and Infectiologists and supported by the Medical Research Agency (grant number 2020/ABM/COVID19/PTEILCHZ), collecting data on clinical characteristics of COVID-19 and treatment. Data for all COVID-19 patients hospitalized in 30 Polish centers between early March 2020 and mid-July 2021 were used in the analysis. Patients were diagnosed and treated with respect to applicable national recommendations for the management of COVID-19 [10–13].

The extracted demographical data included age, gender, body mass index (BMI) and comorbidities. Laboratory analysis data at admission included C-reactive protein (CRP), interleukin-6 (IL-6), procalcitonin (PCT), d-dimer, alanine aminotransferase (ALT), white blood cell count (WBC), absolute lymphocyte count (ALC), absolute neutrophil count (ANC) and platelet count (PLT). Early symptoms of infection before the treatment and oxygen saturation (SpO_2) upon admission were also included. The clinical course of the disease was assessed with the ordinal scale based on the WHO recommendation, although modified to an 8-score version to fit the specificity of the Polish healthcare system and used in previous SARSTer studies [14,15]. The scores were given at baseline and after 7, 14, 21 and 28 days of hospitalization and were defined as follows: (1) not hospitalized, no activity restrictions; (2) not hospitalized, no activity restrictions and/or requiring oxygen supplementation at home; (3) hospitalized, does not require oxygen supplementation and does not require medical care; (4) hospitalized, requiring no oxygen supplementation, but requiring medical care; (5) hospitalized, requiring normal oxygen supplementation; (6) hospitalized, on non-invasive ventilation with high-flow oxygen equipment; (7) hospitalized, for invasive mechanical ventilation or extracorporeal membrane oxygenation; (8) death. Improvement in the clinical course of COVID-19 was defined as a reduction in the score of at least 2 points.

The demographical and clinical characteristics of patients were divided into five groups depending on the date of hospitalization: (i) early March 2020 to 30 June 2020, (ii) 1 July to 30 September 2020, (iii) 1 October to 31 December 2020, (iv) 1 January to 31 March 2021, and (v) 1 April to 15 July 2021. Two main pandemic phases were used for comparisons: early-phase (March to 30 September 2020) and late-phase (October 2020–July 2021). The former had a lower national number of identified infections (91,515), but shortages in equipment and medicine and a lower level of knowledge on COVID-19 among healthcare workers. The latter phase was characterized by high infection numbers (2,789,636) and an overwhelmed healthcare system, but the supplies of medicines (e.g., remdesivir) and oxygen, and experience in COVID-19 clinical course were much improved, while Polish recommendations of management of SARS-CoV-2 infections were already effectively implemented [10–13].

2.2. Statistical Analyses

The data analysis was done with Statistica v.13.1 (StatSoft, Tulsa, OK, USA). For continuous variables (age, BMI, length of hospitalization), differences were tested with a Student's t test. For nominal categorical variables, differences in frequencies were tested with Pearson's χ^2 test. Trends in patient's age and length of hospitalization were analyzed with a linear regression function and the coefficient of determination (R^2). To evaluate associations between early symptoms of infection and the need for oxygen therapy, mechanical ventilation and death, the classical odds ratios (ORs) with a confidence interval were calculated according to the formulas given by Bland and Altman using MedCalc (MedCalc, Ostend, Belgium). To account for alpha inflation and limit the probability of type 1 error, Bonferroni corrections were applied in all multiple comparisons. A p-value < 0.05 was considered statistically significant.

3. Results

3.1. Demographic Characteristics

Overall, 5199 patients were included in this analysis, of whom 21.8% ($n = 1133$) were hospitalized between 6 March 2020 and 30 June 2020, 19.5% ($n = 1012$) between 1 July and 30 September 2020, 30.4% ($n = 1581$) between 1 October and 31 December 2020, 20.9% ($n = 1087$) between 1 January and 31 March 2021, and 7.4% ($n = 386$) between 1 April and 15 July 2021. Women constituted 45.7% of all patients; their share in considered periods fluctuated from 50.5% (till June 2020), 47.0% (July–September 2020), 42.0% (October–December 2020), 45.2% (January–March 2021) to 44.8% (April–July 2021). Fatality rates did not differ between women and men, although the age of male patients who died was significantly lower. The demographic breakdown of the studied population is presented in Table 1.

Table 1. Demographic characteristics of COVID-19 patients hospitalized between 1 March 2020 and 15 July 2021, and differences in parameters between women and men measured with χ^2 test or Student's t-test.

	All ($n = 5199$)	Female ($n = 2376$)	Male ($n = 2823$)	p-Value
Age (years), mean ± SD (min–max)	53.4 ± 24.5 (0–100)	55.3 ± 25.4 (0–100)	51.9 ± 23.6 (0–97)	**$p < 0.001$**
BMI (kg/m^2), mean ± SD (min–max)	26.7 ± 6.4 (7.4–58.8)	26.1 ± 6.6 (7.4–56.9)	27.1 ± 6.3 (9.6–58.8)	**$p < 0.001$**
Obese adults, % (n)	23.2 (1207)	22.4 (532)	23.9 (675)	$p > 0.05$
Comorbidities, % (n)	67.0 (3481)	68.6 (1629)	65.6 (1852)	**$p = 0.02$**
Need for oxygenation, % (n)	44.9 (2333)	40.1 (952)	48.9 (1381)	**$p < 0.001$**
Need for mechanical ventilation, % (n)	4.5 (233)	3.5 (84)	5.3 (149)	**$p = 0.003$**
Time of hospitalization (days), mean ± SD	11.9 ± 8.9	11.9 ± 9.0	11.9 ± 8.8	$p > 0.05$
Fatality, % (n)	9.2 (479)	8.8 (208)	9.6 (271)	$p > 0.05$
Age of patients who died (years), mean ± SD (min–max)	75.9 ± 12.0	77.9 ± 11.7	74.3 ± 12.0	**$p < 0.001$**

BMI: body mass index; COVID-19: coronavirus disease 2019. Statistically significant p-values are highlighted in bold.

The majority of hospitalized patients had at least one comorbidity and were aged ≥ 50 years (64.4%), with the highest share of individuals aged 50–64 (24–28%) regardless of the pandemic period (Figure 1A). There was no linear trend between patient's age and month of hospitalization (y = 0.021x + 6.84; $R^2 = 0.018$), also when analyzed separately for women (y = 0.022x + 6.56; $R^2 = 0.021$) and men (y = 0.016x + 10.12; $R^2 = 0.0024$). However, the age of hospitalized patients was lower in the early phase than the late phase of the pandemic (mean ± SD 48.2 ± 25.5 vs. 57.1 ± 23.1 years, $p < 0.001$) (Figure 1B).

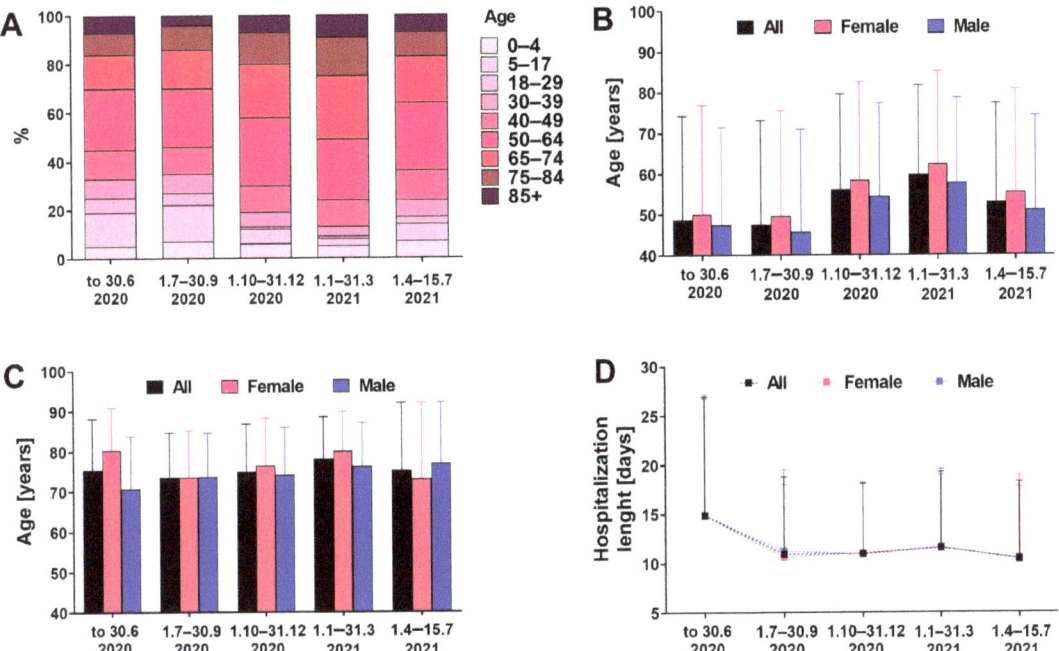

Figure 1. Structure of age (**A**) and mean ± SD age (**B**) of patients hospitalized in different periods of pandemic ($n = 5199$). (**C**) Age of patients who died in different periods of the pandemic. (**D**) Time of hospitalization (mean ± SD) in different periods of the pandemic.

The age of patients who died was similar across different periods (Figure 1C) and no linear trend was seen for the total population ($y = 0.024x + 6.98$; $R^2 = 0.0063$), women ($y = 0.0162x + 10.12$; $R^2 = 0.0024$) and men ($y = 0.054x + 4.79$; $R^2 = 0.034$). The age of patients who died was similar in the early and late phases of the pandemic (mean ± SD 74.7 ± 12.2 vs. 76.3 ± 11.9 years, $p > 0.05$). The hospitalization length was the highest in March–June 2020 period (mean ± SD 14.9 ± 12.1 days) and then decreased to the 10–11 days range (Figure 1D). There was no linear trend between length and month of hospitalization for total population ($y = 0.34x + 14.6$; $R^2 = 0.021$), group of women ($y = 0.062x + 8.49$; $R^2 = 0.021$) and men ($y = 0.063x + 8.86$; $R^2 = 0.022$). However, in general, the hospitalization stay was longer in the early pandemic phase compared to the late phase (mean ± SD 13.0 ± 10.5 vs. 11.1 ± 7.5 days).

3.2. Early Symptoms of Infection

Fever (69.6%), cough (60.4%), and dyspnea (43.6%) were the most common early COVID-19 symptoms, followed by fatigue (33.0%), anosmia (13.9%), diarrhea (11.2%) and headaches (10.9%), while nausea (5.6%) and vomiting (5.3%) were the least commonly observed. Fluctuations in the frequency of early symptoms was observed in different periods of the pandemic. There was a steady increase of diarrhea reporting from 9.2% (March–June 2020) to 14.8% (April–July 2021). Compared to the early months of the pandemic, the frequencies of cough, fever, dyspnea and fatigue were also higher in subsequent months (Figure 2).

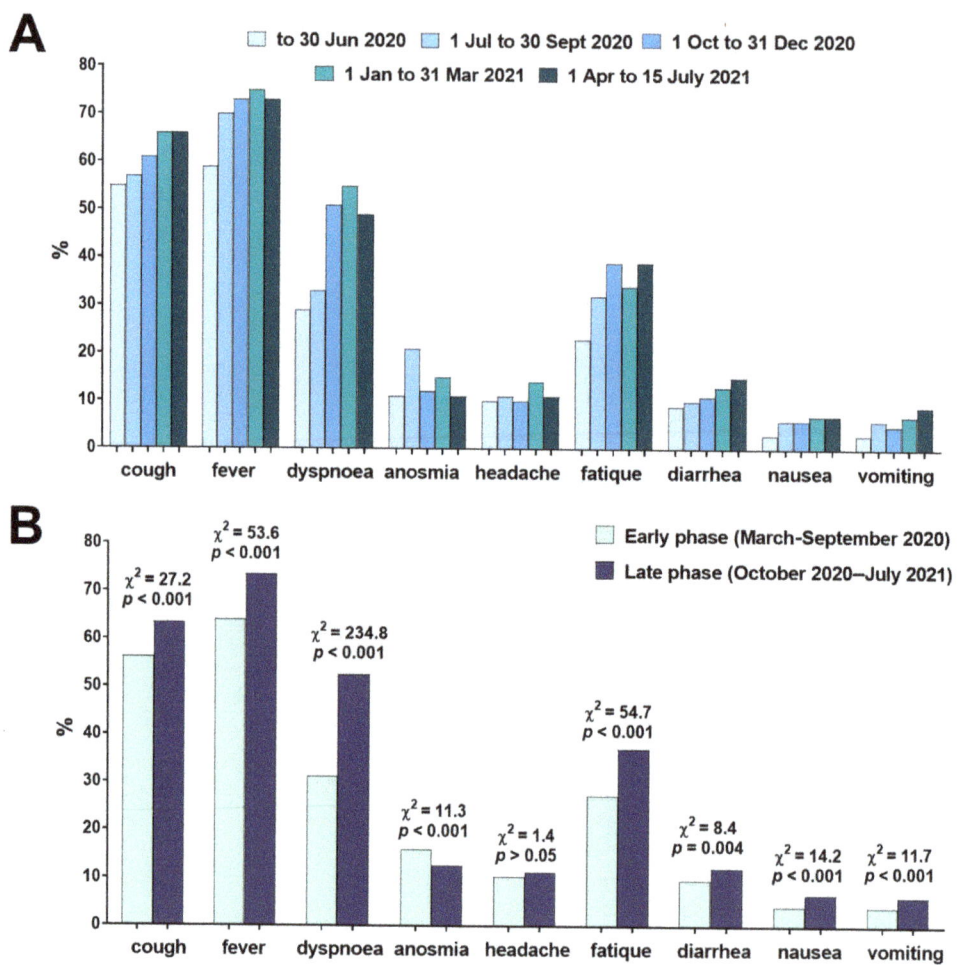

Figure 2. (**A**) Frequency of early COVID-19 symptoms presented by patients hospitalized in different periods of the pandemic (n = 5199) and (**B**) comparison in symptoms frequency between the early and late phase of the pandemic.

Significant gender differences in early symptoms were found. Compared to men, women had a lower frequency of cough (57.4 vs. 62.9%; $\chi^2 = 16.3$, $p < 0.001$), fever (64.0 vs. 74.4%; $\chi^2 = 65.2$, $p < 0.001$) and dyspnea (40.3 vs 46.4%; $\chi^2 = 19.9$, $p < 0.001$), but higher frequency of anosmia (15.3 vs. 12.8%; $\chi^2 = 7.1$, $p = 0.007$), headache (17.2 vs. 9.4%; $\chi^2 = 20$, $p < 0.001$), diarrhea (13.0 vs. 9.6%; $\chi^2 = 15.1$, $p < 0.001$), nausea (7.0 vs. 4.4%, $\chi^2 = 17.5$, $p < 0.001$) and vomiting (7.4 vs. 3.6%, $\chi^2 = 36.0$, $p < 0.001$). The presence of cough and dyspnea increased the odds of requiring oxygen therapy, mechanical ventilation and death in both women and men. Fever was associated with higher odds for oxygen therapy in women and men, and mechanical ventilation in men. Women presenting anosmia had lower odds for oxygen therapy and fatal outcome. Headache was associated with increased odds for oxygen therapy in women. Men and women presenting fatigue had higher odds for oxygen therapy. Gastrointestinal manifestations (diarrhea, nausea and vomiting) were not related to change in odds of the analyzed events (Table 2).

Table 2. The odds ratio (95% confidence interval) for mechanical ventilation and death in relation to different early COVID-19 symptoms presented by hospitalized patients.

Symptom	Outcome	All (n = 5199)	Female (n = 2376)	Male (n = 2823)
Cough	Oxygen therapy	2.0 (1.7–2.2) $p < 0.001$	1.8 (1.5–2.1) $p < 0.001$	2.1 (1.8–2.4) $p < 0.001$
	Mechanical ventilation	1.9 (1.4–2.5) $p < 0.001$	2.2 (1.3–3.5) $p = 0.003$	1.0 (0.8–1.4) $p > 0.05$
	Death	0.8 (0.6–0.9) $p = 0.01$	0.8 (0.6–1.1) $p > 0.05$	0.7 (0.6–1.0) $p = 0.02$
Dyspnea	Oxygen therapy	6.3 (5.6–7.2) $p < 0.001$	5.3 (4.7–6.4) $p < 0.001$	7.2 (6.1–8.5) $p < 0.001$
	Mechanical ventilation	6.0 (4.3–8.3) $p < 0.001$	7.9 (4.4–14.1) $p < 0.001$	4.9 (3.3–7.4) $p < 0.001$
	Death	3.7 (3.0–4.5) $p < 0.001$	3.5 (2.6–4.7) $p < 0.001$	3.8 (2.9–5.1) $p < 0.001$
Fever	Oxygen therapy	2.0 (1.7–2.3) $p < 0.001$	1.7 (1.4–2.0) $p < 0.001$	2.2 (1.9–2.6) $p < 0.001$
	Mechanical ventilation	2.2 (1.6–3.2) $p < 0.001$	1.6 (1.0–2.6) $p > 0.05$	2.8 (1.7–4.7) $p < 0.001$
	Death	0.9 (0.7–1.1) $p > 0.05$	0.8 (0.6–1.1) $p > 0.05$	0.9 (0.7–1.2) $p > 0.05$
Anosmia	Oxygen therapy	0.8 (0.7–0.9) $p = 0.003$	0.7 (0.6–0.9) $p = 0.005$	0.9 (0.7–1.1) $p > 0.05$
	Mechanical ventilation	0.7 (0.5–1.1) $p > 0.05$	0.5 (0.2–1.1) $p > 0.05$	0.9 (0.5–1.5) $p > 0.05$
	Death	0.4 (0.3–0.6) $p < 0.001$	0.3 (0.2–0.6) $p < 0.001$	0.5 (0.3–0.8) $p = 0.004$
Headache	Oxygen therapy	0.7 (0.6–0.9) $p = 0.003$	0.6 (0.4–0.8) $p < 0.001$	0.9 (0.7–1.2) $p > 0.05$
	Mechanical ventilation	1.1 (0.7–1.6) $p > 0.05$	0.6 (0.3–1.4) $p > 0.05$	1.5 (0.9–2.5) $p > 0.05$
	Death	0.7 (0.5–1.0) $p > 0.05$	0.7 (0.4–1.2) $p > 0.05$	0.7 (0.4–1.1) $p > 0.05$
Fatigue	Oxygen therapy	1.6 (1.5–1.8) $p < 0.001$	1.4 (1.2–1.7) $p < 0.001$	1.9 (1.6–2.2) $p < 0.001$
	Mechanical ventilation	1.4 (1.1–1.8) $p = 0.02$	1.2 (0.7–1.8) $p > 0.05$	1.6 (1.1–2.2) $p = 0.007$
	Death	1.2 (0.9–1.5) $p > 0.05$	1.0 (0.8–1.4) $p > 0.05$	1.1 (0.7–2.0) $p > 0.05$
Diarrhea	Oxygen therapy	1.1 (0.9–1.3) $p > 0.05$	1.2 (0.9–1.5) $p > 0.05$	1.1 (0.9–1.5) $p > 0.05$
	Mechanical ventilation	1.1 (0.7–1.6) $p > 0.05$	1.0 (0.5–1.9) $p > 0.05$	1.1 (0.7–1.9) $p > 0.05$
	Death	1.1 (0.8–1.5) $p > 0.05$	1.0 (0.7–1.5) $p > 0.05$	1.2 (0.8–1.8) $p > 0.05$
Nausea	Oxygen therapy	1.0 (0.8–1.2) $p > 0.05$	1.0 (0.7–1.4) $p > 0.05$	1.0 (0.7–1.5) $p > 0.05$
	Mechanical ventilation	0.8 (0.4–1.5) $p > 0.05$	0.7 (0.2–1.8) $p > 0.05$	0.9 (0.4–2.2) $p > 0.05$
	Death	0.8 (0.5–1.3) $p > 0.05$	1.0 (0.6–1.8) $p > 0.05$	0.6 (0.3–1.2) $p > 0.05$
Vomiting	Oxygen therapy	0.9 (0.7–1.2) $p > 0.05$	1.0 (0.7–1.4) $p > 0.05$	0.9 (0.6–1.6) $p > 0.05$
	Mechanical ventilation	0.7 (0.4–1.4) $p > 0.05$	0.8 (0.3–2.0) $p > 0.05$	0.7 (0.3–2.0) $p > 0.05$
	Death	0.8 (0.5–1.2) $p > 0.05$	0.8 (0.4–1.4) $p > 0.05$	0.8 (0.4–1.7) $p > 0.05$

Statistically significant p-values are highlighted in bold.

3.3. Laboratory and Clinical Characteristics

The summary of laboratory parameters at admission is provided in Table 3. Male patients were characterized by significantly higher inflammatory markers (CRP and IL-6), ALT, higher neutrophil count, and lower platelet count. Significant differences in the majority of considered parameters between patients hospitalized in the early and late phases of the COVID-19 pandemic were observed. The latter group had higher concentrations of CRP, IL-6, d-dimer and ALT, higher counts of WBC and neutrophils, but lower counts of lymphocytes and platelets (Table 3).

Table 3. Laboratory parameters (mean ± SD) of hospitalized patients and differences between women and men, and early and late phase of the COVID-19 pandemic evaluated with Student's t-test.

	All (n = 5199)	Female (n = 2376)	Male (n = 2823)	p-Value	Early Phase (n = 2145)	Late Phase (n = 3054)	p-Value
CRP, mg/L	70.2 ± 76.1	57.0 ± 68.9	81.3 ± 80.2	<0.001	50.4 ± 68.0	83.8 ± 78.5	<0.001
PCT, ng/mL	0.5 ± 3.5	0.4 ± 2.9	0.6 ± 3.9	>0.05	0.5 ± 4.7	0.5 ± 2.6	>0.05
IL-6, pg/mL	67.7 ± 175.2	58.9 ± 200.3	75.2 ± 150.3	<0.001	44.5 ± 150.1	80.1 ± 186.1	<0.001
d-dimer, ng/mL	1964.0 ± 6153.7	1865.5 ± 5309.3	2046.4 ± 6779.5	>0.05	1331.6 ± 4345.1	2361.7 ± 7029.2	<0.001
ALT, IU/L	40.6 ± 56.2	34.0 ± 50.1	46.2 ± 60.3	<0.001	34.9 ± 54.6	44.6 ± 56.9	<0.001
WBC, $\times 10^3/\mu L$	7.0 ± 4.4	6.7 ± 3.8	7.2 ± 4.7	<0.001	6.6 ± 4.2	7.3 ± 4.4	<0.001
Lymphocytes, $\times 10^3/\mu L$	1.4 ± 1.8	1.5 ± 1.4	1.4 ± 2.0	>0.05	1.6 ± 2.0	1.4 ± 1.6	<0.001
Neutrophils, $\times 10^3/\mu L$	4.9 ± 3.7	4.6 ± 3.2	5.1 ± 4.2	<0.001	4.2 ± 2.8	5.3 ± 4.2	<0.001
Platelets, $\times 10^3/\mu L$	227.2 ± 102.4	235.2 ± 98.7	220.5 ± 104.9	0.003	231.3 ± 98.0	224.8 ± 105.2	0.04

ALT: alanine aminotransferase; COVID-19: coronavirus disease 2019; CRP: C-reactive protein; IL-6: Interleukin-6; PCT: procalcitonin; SD: standard deviation; WBC: white blood cell. Statistically significant p-values are highlighted in bold.

Considering that the odds for oxygen therapy and death were significantly lowered in subjects with anosmia (Table 2), the comparison of laboratory parameters between patients displaying or not displaying this symptom was performed. As shown, the former were characterized by significantly lower values of inflammatory markers: CRP (64.3 ± 70.7 mg/L vs. 71.2 ± 77.0 mg/L, $p = 0.03$), IL-6 (45.2 ± 76.5 pg/mL vs. 72.0 ± 187.8 pg/mL, $p < 0.001$) and PCT (0.2 ± 1.0 ng/mL vs. 0.5 ± 3.8 ng/mL, $p < 0.001$), and lower counts of WBC (6.4 ± 3.1 × $10^3/\mu L$ vs. 7.1 ± 4.5 × $10^3/\mu L$) and neutrophils (4.5 ± 2.7 × $10^3/\mu L$ vs. 4.9 ± 3.9 × $10^3/\mu L$).

During the entire studied period, the share of patients with $SpO_2 < 91\%$ at admission and requiring oxygen therapy was 32.5 and 46.1%, respectively, although their share increased since 1 October 2020 (Figure 3A). Compared to the late pandemic phase, the early phase of the pandemic had a significantly lower percentage of patients with $SpO_2 < 91\%$ at admission requiring oxygen therapy. The overall percentage of patients requiring mechanical ventilation was 4.5%, with no difference between the early and late phases of the pandemic. The fatality rate in the studied period was 9.2% and increased significantly from 5.8% in the early pandemic phase to 11.6% in the late phase (Figure 3B). Men had higher odds for $SpO_2 < 91\%$ (OR (95%CI) = 1.5 (1.3–1.6), $p < 0.001$), oxygen therapy (OR (95%CI) = 1.4 (1.3–1.6), $p < 0.001$) and mechanical ventilation (OR (95%CI) = 1.5 (1.2–2.0), $p = 0.003$), but not higher odds of death (OR (95%CI) = 1.1 (0.9–1.4, $p > 0.05$)). Clinical improvement, defined by a reduction in the score of at least 2 points on the ordinal scale, was less frequently recorded in the first period of the pandemic (March–July 2020), especially in the seven days and 14 days follow-ups (Figure 3C,D).

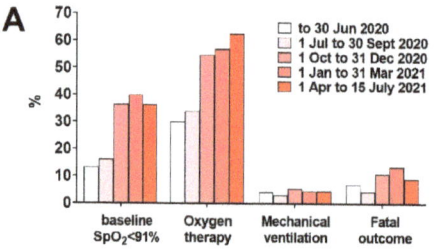 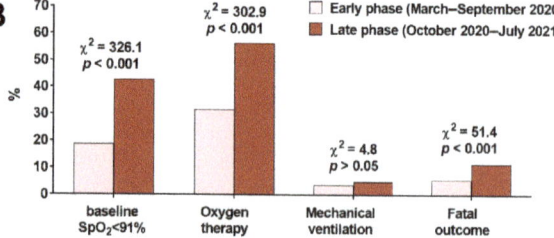

Figure 3. Cont.

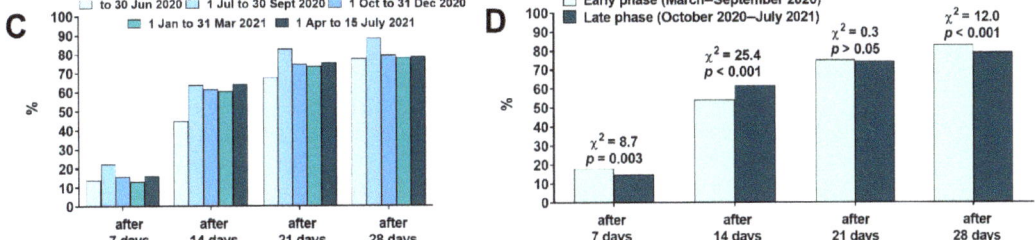

Figure 3. (**A**) The frequency of patients with baseline SpO$_2$ < 91%, requiring oxygen therapy and mechanical ventilation, and with fatal outcome in different periods of the pandemic (n = 5199) and (**B**) comparison of these events between the early and late phase of the pandemic. (**C**) Percentage of patients with improvement in the clinical course of COVID-19 defined as a reduction in the score of at least 2 points on the ordinal 8-score scale (see Material & Methods for a detailed explanation of each score) in different periods of the pandemic and (**D**) comparison of these percentages between the early and late phase of the pandemic.

4. Discussion

This study provides a comprehensive overview of the COVID-19 patients hospitalized in Poland over the first 17 months of the pandemic and a reference point for further epidemiological analyses and comparisons. Consistent with various other observations, the investigated cohort was characterized mainly by elderly subjects suffering from at least one comorbidity, slightly more frequently represented by men.

The conducted analysis indicates some potential changes in pathogenicity of SARS-CoV-2 after September 2020, manifested by an increased share of patients with SpO$_2$ < 91% and requiring oxygen therapy. The frequency of cough, fever, dyspnea also increased in later pandemic phases compared to the first three months. In general, the frequency of all considered symptoms except headache was higher in the late phase of the pandemic (October 2020–July 2021). Moreover, this phase was also characterized by patients exhibiting significantly increased levels of inflammatory markers, including IL-6, as well as differences in blood morphology: higher WBC and neutrophils counts but lower counts of lymphocytes and platelets. This may be due to the increase of the G superclade frequency in SARS-CoV-2 variants circulating in Poland in 2020 [16]. Its hallmark D614G substitution in spike protein was associated with increased transmissibility and higher viral loads [17]. Although the general human mortality was not found to be affected by D614G mutation, the animal studies demonstrated a modest increase in virulence—this slight increase may also be reflected in our observations [17,18].

According to some studies, infections with the B.1.1.7 (alpha) variant could be associated with higher mortality, although this was contradicted by other observations [18,19]. There have been some concerns, magnified by media reports, that the B.1.1.7 (alpha) variant may have a larger impact on the younger population by leading to a more severe clinical course of COVID-19 [20]. According to the national genomic surveillance, B.1.1.7 was steadily increasing in circulation in the Polish population since January 2021 to become dominant by mid-February and constitute over 80% of infections throughout March and April (>80% of infections). In this period, most hospitalizations were constituted by individuals >50 years, while a share of the younger population decreased between January and March 2021.

Furthermore, the age of patients who died did not differ throughout the considered 17 months. This observation contradicts various media reports, often based on the short-term experience of a single-center, claiming a gradual rise in COVID-19 deaths in younger individuals in the studied period. This is despite the worsening epidemiological situation in the late pandemic phase (October 2020–July 2021) in Poland compared to the early phase (March–September 2020) and the fact that COVID-19 vaccine rollout in the country was initiated on 27 December 2020 and 17.6 million people (46.5% of the population) had received at least one dose by 15 July 2021, while the elderly constituted a priority group in the national vaccination campaign. As shown previously, deaths from COVID-19 occurred very rarely in the fully vaccinated group and mostly concerned the immunocompromised, vaccine non-responders and individuals > 70 years with comorbidities [15].

At the same time, the length of hospital stay was the highest in the first months of the pandemic and decreased in the late pandemic phase. This should not be associated with any shifts in SARS-CoV-2 pathogenicity, as it was mostly due to epidemiological regulations enforced in Poland at the beginning of the pandemic (requirement to hospitalize patients for at least 14 days and obtaining two negative results for SARS-CoV-2 by PCR), as well as due to better experience in managing COVID-19 patients and increased availability of oxygen supply and treatment options. It is also likely that these aspects have also influenced the observed slight differences in the share of patients with clinical improvement rates between the early and late phases of the pandemic.

This study reports that gender differences in early COVID-19 symptoms were found. Respiratory symptoms (cough and dyspnea) and fever were more frequently observed in men, while women reported anosmia and gastrointestinal symptoms more often. This likely mirrors the differences in the immune response to the SARS-CoV-2 infection as indicated by significantly lower inflammatory markers (CRP and IL-6) in women. Previous research has shown that women reveal a more robust antiviral interferon response and increased adaptive immune response toward viral antigens, ultimately resulting in better viral control and lower disease severity [21]. Here, men also required oxygenation and mechanical ventilation more frequently, although it must be stressed that no gender disparity in fatality ratio was seen.

Although the previous research suggested that diarrhea may be related to worse COVID-19 outcomes, this was not seen in the present cohort [22]. The presence of gastrointestinal symptoms (diarrhea, nausea or vomiting) did not increase odds for oxygen therapy, mechanical ventilation and death, regardless of gender. In turn, patients with anosmia had lower odds for oxygen therapy and death. This is in line with previous findings linking smell loss with lower COVID-19 severity and better prognosis [23,24]. The mechanism behind these observations remains to be elucidated, although it could be hypothesized that the local inflammation of the olfactory bulb correlates with a more appropriate antiviral response. As shown in the present study, hospitalized subjects experiencing anosmia were characterized by significantly lower inflammatory markers at admission (IL-6, CRP and procalcitonin), confirming that the presence of this symptom is somewhat related to better control of the immune response to viral infection.

Although men were also characterized by higher mean levels of inflammatory markers (CRP and IL-6) and required oxygenation and mechanical ventilation more frequently, their hospitalization length and fatality rate were not increased compared to women. Male sex has been previously established as a risk factor for severe COVID-19 with the higher odds for death, as indicated by a meta-analysis of the global cases [21]. However, epidemiological reports from different U.S. states, Iran, Pakistan, and Finland, show no sex bias in mortality odds ratio [21]. The basis of these exceptional findings requires further research, although it may not solely be related to biological factors but also to socio-cultural and behavioral differences, as well as local healthcare capacities. In our study, women had comorbidities more often than men, and this may partially account for the lack of gender difference in survival.

It should be stressed that this study only included hospitalized COVID-19 patients. Thus, its observations, e.g., regarding changes in early symptoms of infection, may not necessarily translate to milder cases. Moreover, no genomic surveillance of SARS-CoV-2 was conducted for the studied cohort of patients; therefore, relationships between demographic and clinical characteristics and particular variants must be formulated with caution. However, the observations of this study do not translate to the B.1.617.2 (delta) variant that was first detected in Poland in May 2021 but became dominant in July 2021. Further studies are required to understand whether infections with B.1.617.2 are associated with different severity and outcomes in the Polish population.

5. Conclusions

In this study, we demonstrated shifts in SARS-CoV-2 pathogenicity that occurred between March 2020 and July 2021 in the Polish cohort of hospitalized patients and documented various gender differences in this regard. The clinical course of the disease did change, but it could have been caused, at least partially, by the varying burden on the health care system in different periods of the pandemic. This view is supported by the constant mean age of patients with a fatal outcome of the disease. The results represent a reference point for further analyses conducted under the dominance of different SARS-CoV-2 variants.

Author Contributions: Conceptualization, R.F.; methodology, R.F., P.R. and D.Z.-M.; investigation, R.F., P.R., D.Z.-M., M.R. (Magdalena Rogalska), M.R. (Marta Rorat), P.C. (Piotr Czupryna), B.L., P.C. (Przemysław Ciechanowski), D.K., A.P., M.P.-Ś., K.S., M.T., B.B., G.A., J.K., R.P., W.M., B.O.-G., I.Z., A.S., P.F.-C., M.S.-P., K.K., M.F., P.L., I.K. and H.G.; writing—original draft preparation, R.F., P.R. and D.Z.-M.; P.R.; supervision, R.F.; project administration, R.F.; funding acquisition, R.F. All authors have read and agreed to the published version of the manuscript.

Funding: This research was funded by Medical Research Agency, grant number 2020/ABM/COVID19/PTEILCHZ and Polish Association of Epidemiologists and Infectiologists.

Institutional Review Board Statement: This study was retrospective, non-interventional and based on data collected in the national SARSTer database. Therefore it does not require approval of the Ethics Committee. Due to the retrospective nature of the presented study, written consent by participants was not necessary. The patients' data was protected according to the European Union General Data Protection Regulation.

Informed Consent Statement: Not applicable.

Data Availability Statement: The datasets used and analyzed during the current study are available from the corresponding author upon reasonable request.

Conflicts of Interest: The authors declare no conflict of interest.

References

1. Cucinotta, D.; Vanelli, M. WHO Declares COVID-19 a Pandemic. *Acta Bio-Med. Atenei Parm.* **2020**, *91*, 157–160. [CrossRef]
2. Gu, S.X.; Tyagi, T.; Jain, K.; Gu, V.W.; Lee, S.H.; Hwa, J.M.; Kwan, J.M.; Krause, D.S.; Lee, A.I.; Halene, S.; et al. Thrombocytopathy and endotheliopathy: Crucial contributors to COVID-19 thromboinflammation. *Nat. Rev. Cardiol.* **2021**, *18*, 194–209. [CrossRef] [PubMed]
3. Robba, C.; Battaglini, D.; Pelosi, P.; Rocco, P.R.M. Multiple organ dysfunction in SARS-CoV-2: MODS-CoV-2. *Expert Rev. Respir. Med.* **2020**, *14*, 865–868. [CrossRef] [PubMed]
4. Li, J.; Huang, D.Q.; Zou, B.; Yang, H.; Hui, W.Z.; Rui, F.; Yee, N.T.S.; Liu, C.; Nerurkar, S.N.; Kai, J.C.Y.; et al. Epidemiology of COVID-19: A systematic review and meta-analysis of clinical characteristics, risk factors, and outcomes. *J. Med. Virol.* **2021**, *93*, 1449–1458. [CrossRef] [PubMed]
5. Rochman, N.D.; Wolf, Y.I.; Faure, G.; Mutz, P.; Zhang, F.; Koonin, E.V. Ongoing global and regional adaptive evolution of SARS-CoV-2. *Proc. Natl. Acad. Sci. USA* **2021**, *118*, e2104241118. [CrossRef] [PubMed]
6. Nagy, Á.; Pongor, S.; Győrffy, B. Different mutations in SARS-CoV-2 associate with severe and mild outcome. *Int. J. Antimicrob. Agents* **2021**, *57*, 106272. [CrossRef]
7. Horspool, A.M.; Ye, C.; Wong, T.Y.; Russ, B.P.; Lee, K.S.; Winters, M.T.; Bevere, J.R.; Kieffer, T.; Martinez, I.; Sourimant, J.; et al. SARS-CoV-2 B.1.1.7 and B.1.351 variants of concern induce lethal disease in K18-hACE2 transgenic mice despite convalescent plasma therapy. *bioRxiv* **2021**. [CrossRef]
8. Frampton, D.; Rampling, T.; Cross, A.; Bailey, H.; Heaney, J.; Byott, M.; Scott, R.; Sconza, R.; Price, J.; Margaritis, M.; et al. Genomic characteristics and clinical effect of the emergent SARS-CoV-2 B.1.1.7 lineage in London, UK: A whole-genome sequencing and hospital-based cohort study. *Lancet Infect. Dis.* **2021**, *21*, 1246–1256. [CrossRef]
9. Graham, M.S.; Sudre, C.H.; May, A.; Antonelli, M.; Murray, B.; Varsavsky, T.; Kläser, K.; Canas, L.S.; Molteni, E.; Modat, M.; et al. Changes in symptomatology, reinfection, and transmissibility associated with the SARS-CoV-2 variant B.1.1.7: An ecological study. *Lancet Public Health* **2021**, *6*, e335–e345. [CrossRef]

10. Flisiak, R.; Horban, A.; Jaroszewicz, J.; Kozielewicz, D.; Pawłowska, M.; Parczewski, M.; Piekarska, A.; Simon, K.; Tomasiewicz, K.; Zarębska-Michaluk, D. Management of SARS-CoV-2 infection: Recommendations of the Polish Association of Epidemiologists and Infectiologists as of 31 March 2020. *Pol. Arch. Intern. Med.* **2020**, *130*, 352–357. [CrossRef]
11. Flisiak, R.; Horban, A.; Jaroszewicz, J.; Kozielewicz, D.; Pawłowska, M.; Parczewski, M.; Piekarska, A.; Simon, K.; Tomasiewicz, K.; Zarębska-Michaluk, D. Management of SARS-CoV-2 infection: Recommendations of the Polish Association of Epidemiologists and Infectiologists. Annex no. 1 as of 8 June 2020. *Pol. Arch. Intern. Med.* **2020**, *130*, 557–558. [CrossRef] [PubMed]
12. Flisiak, R.; Parczewski, M.; Horban, A.; Jaroszewicz, J.; Kozielewicz, D.; Pawłowska, M.; Piekarska, A.; Simon, K.; Tomasiewicz, K.; Zarębska-Michaluk, D. Management of SARS-CoV-2 infection: Recommendations of the Polish Association of Epidemiologists and Infectiologists. Annex no. 2 as of 13 October 2020. *Pol. Arch. Intern. Med.* **2020**, *130*, 915–918. [CrossRef] [PubMed]
13. Flisiak, R.; Horban, A.; Jaroszewicz, J.; Kozielewicz, D.; Mastalerz-Migas, A.; Owczuk, R.; Parczewski, M.; Pawłowska, M.; Piekarska, A.; Simon, K.; et al. Management of SARS-CoV-2 infection: Recommendations of the Polish Association of Epidemiologists and Infectiologists as of 26 2April 021. *Pol. Arch. Intern. Med.* **2021**, *131*, 487–496. [CrossRef]
14. Flisiak, R.; Jaroszewicz, J.; Rogalska, M.; Łapiński, T.; Berkan-Kawińska, A.; Bolewska, B.; Tudrujek-Zdunek, M.; Kozielewicz, D.; Rorat, M.; Leszczyński, P.; et al. Tocilizumab Improves the Prognosis of COVID-19 in Patients with High IL-6. *J. Clin. Med.* **2021**, *10*, 1583. [CrossRef] [PubMed]
15. Rzymski, P.; Pazgan-Simon, M.; Simon, K.; Łapiński, T.; Zarębska-Michaluk, D.; Szczepańska, B.; Chojnicki, M.; Mozer-Lisewska, I.; Flisiak, R. Clinical Characteristics of Hospitalized COVID-19 Patients Who Received at Least One Dose of COVID-19 Vaccine. *Vaccines* **2021**, *9*, 781. [CrossRef] [PubMed]
16. Hryhorowicz, S.; Ustaszewski, A.; Kaczmarek-Ryś, M.; Lis, E.; Witt, M.; Pławski, A.; Ziętkiewicz, E. European context of the diversity and phylogenetic position of SARS-CoV-2 sequences from Polish COVID-19 patients. *J. Appl. Genet.* **2021**, *62*, 327–337. [CrossRef] [PubMed]
17. Volz, E.; Hill, V.; McCrone, J.T.; Price, A.; Jorgensen, D.; O'Toole, Á.; Southgate, J.; Johnson, R.; Jackson, B.; Nascimento, F.F.; et al. Evaluating the Effects of SARS-CoV-2 Spike Mutation D614G on Transmissibility and Pathogenicity. *Cell* **2021**, *184*, 64–75. [CrossRef]
18. Hou, Y.J.; Chiba, S.; Halfmann, P.; Ehre, C.; Kuroda, M.; Dinnon, K.H., 3rd; Leist, S.R.; Schäfer, A.; Nakajima, N.; Takahashi, K.; et al. SARS-CoV-2 D614G variant exhibits efficient replication ex vivo and transmission in vivo. *Science* **2020**, *370*, 1464–1468. [CrossRef]
19. Davies, N.G.; Jarvis, C.I.; van Zandvoort, K.; Clifford, S.; Sun, F.Y.; Funk, S.; Medley, G.; Jafari, Y.; Meakin, S.R.; Lowe, R.; et al. Increased mortality in community-tested cases of SARS-CoV-2 lineage B.1.1.7. *Nature* **2021**, *593*, 270–274. [CrossRef]
20. Brookman, S.; Cook, J.; Zucherman, M.; Broughton, S.; Harman, K.; Gupta, A. Effect of the new SARS-CoV-2 variant B.1.1.7 on children and young people. *Lancet Child Adolesc Health* **2021**, *5*, e9–e10. [CrossRef]
21. Peckham, H.; de Gruijter, N.M.; Raine, C.; Radziszewska, A.; Ciurtin, C.; Wedderburn, L.R.; Rosser, E.C.; Webb, K.; Deakin, C.T. Male sex identified by global COVID-19 meta-analysis as a risk factor for death and ITU admission. *Nat. Commun.* **2020**, *11*, 6317. [CrossRef]
22. Ghimire, S.; Sharma, S.; Patel, A.; Budhathoki, R.; Chakinala, R.; Khan, H.; Lincoln, M.; Georgeston, M. Diarrhea Is Associated with Increased Severity of Disease in COVID-19: Systemic Review and Metaanalysis. *SN Compr. Clin. Med.* **2021**, *3*, 28–35. [CrossRef] [PubMed]
23. Talavera, B.; García-Azorín, D.; Martínez-Pías, E.; Trigo, J.; Hernández-Pérez, I.; Valle-Peñacoba, G.; Simón-Campo, P.; de Lera, M.; Chavarría-Miranda, A.; López-Sanz, C.; et al. Anosmia is associated with lower in-hospital mortality in COVID-19. *J. Neurol. Sci.* **2020**, *419*, 117163. [CrossRef] [PubMed]
24. Foster, K.J.; Jauregui, E.; Tajudeen, B.; Bishehsari, F.; Mahdavinia, M. Smell loss is a prognostic factor for lower severity of coronavirus disease 2019. *Ann. Allergy Asthma Immunol.* **2020**, *125*, 481–483. [CrossRef] [PubMed]

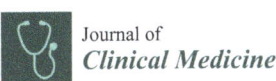

Article

Clinical and Epidemiological Characteristics of 1283 Pediatric Patients with Coronavirus Disease 2019 during the First and Second Waves of the Pandemic—Results of the Pediatric Part of a Multicenter Polish Register SARSTer

Maria Pokorska-Śpiewak [1,†], Ewa Talarek [1,*,†], Anna Mania [2], Małgorzata Pawłowska [3], Jolanta Popielska [1], Konrad Zawadka [1], Magdalena Figlerowicz [2], Katarzyna Mazur-Melewska [2], Kamil Faltin [2], Przemysław Ciechanowski [4], Joanna Łasecka-Zadrożna [4], Józef Rudnicki [4], Barbara Hasiec [5], Martyna Stani [5], Paulina Frańczak-Chmura [5], Izabela Zaleska [6], Leszek Szenborn [6], Kacper Toczyłowski [7], Artur Sulik [7], Barbara Szczepańska [8], Ilona Pałyga-Bysiecka [8], Izabela Kucharek [9], Adam Sybilski [9], Małgorzata Sobolewska-Pilarczyk [3], Urszula Dryja [10], Ewa Majda-Stanisławska [10], Sławomira Niedźwiecka [11], Ernest Kuchar [12], Bolesław Kalicki [13], Anna Gorczyca [14] and Magdalena Marczyńska [1]

Citation: Pokorska-Śpiewak, M.; Talarek, E.; Mania, A.; Pawłowska, M.; Popielska, J.; Zawadka, K.; Figlerowicz, M.; Mazur-Melewska, K.; Faltin, K.; Ciechanowski, P.; et al. Clinical and Epidemiological Characteristics of 1283 Pediatric Patients with Coronavirus Disease 2019 during the First and Second Waves of the Pandemic—Results of the Pediatric Part of a Multicenter Polish Register SARSTer. *J. Clin. Med.* **2021**, *10*, 5098. https://doi.org/10.3390/jcm10215098

Academic Editors: Robert Flisiak and Marco Sebastiani

Received: 16 August 2021
Accepted: 27 October 2021
Published: 30 October 2021

Publisher's Note: MDPI stays neutral with regard to jurisdictional claims in published maps and institutional affiliations.

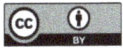

Copyright: © 2021 by the authors. Licensee MDPI, Basel, Switzerland. This article is an open access article distributed under the terms and conditions of the Creative Commons Attribution (CC BY) license (https://creativecommons.org/licenses/by/4.0/).

[1] Department of Children's Infectious Diseases, Regional Hospital of Infectious Diseases in Warsaw, Medical University of Warsaw, 01-201 Warsaw, Poland; mpspiewak@gmail.com (M.P.-Ś.); jolanta.popielska@wum.edu.pl (J.P.); konrad.zawadka@wum.edu.pl (K.Z.); magdalena.marczynska@wum.edu.pl (M.M.)
[2] Department of Infectious Diseases and Child Neurology, Poznan University of Medical Sciences, 60-572 Poznan, Poland; amania@ump.edu.pl (A.M.); mfiglerowicz@gmail.com (M.F.); katarzynamelewska@ump.edu.pl (K.M.-M.); faltinkamil@interia.pl (K.F.)
[3] Department of Infectious Diseases and Hepatology, Faculty of Medicine, Collegium Medicum, Nicolaus Copernicus University, 85-030 Bydgoszcz, Poland; mpawlowska@cm.umk.pl (M.P.); m.pilarczyk@wsoz.pl (M.S.-P.)
[4] Department of Paediatrics and Infectious Diseases, Regional Hospital in Szczecin, 71-455 Szczecin, Poland; przciechanowski@spwsz.szczecin.pl (P.C.); zadrozna@spwsz.szczecin.pl (J.Ł.-Z.); rudnicki@spwsz.szczecin.pl (J.R.)
[5] Department of Children's Infectious Diseases, Provincial Jan Boży Hospital in Lublin, 20-089 Lublin, Poland; bhasiec@wp.pl (B.H.); martyna.stani@janbozy.pl (M.S.); paulina.franczak@janbozy.pl (P.F.-C.)
[6] Department of Paediatrics and Infectious Diseases, Wroclaw Medical University, 50-368 Wroclaw, Poland; izabela.zaleska@gmail.com (I.Z.); leszek.szenborn@umed.wroclaw.pl (L.S.)
[7] Department of Pediatric Infectious Diseases, Medical University of Bialystok, 15-274 Bialystok, Poland; kacper.toczylowski@umb.edu.pl (K.T.); artur.sulik@umb.edu.pl (A.S.)
[8] 1st Department of Pediatrics, Collegium Medicum Jan Kochanowski University, 25-317 Kielce, Poland; g.b.szczepanski@onet.eu (B.S.); bysiecka@gmail.com (I.P.-B.)
[9] 2nd Department of Paediatrics, Centre of Postgraduate Medical Education, Department of Paediatrics and Neonatology with Allergology Center, Central Clinical Hospital of the Ministry of the Interior, 02-507 Warsaw, Poland; iza.orlinska@gmail.com (I.K.); adam.sybilski@cskmswia.pl (A.S.)
[10] Department of Paediatric Infectious Diseases, Medical University of Lodz, 91-347 Lodz, Poland; urszuladryja@gmail.com (U.D.); emajda@lodz.home.pl (E.M.-S.)
[11] Department of Paediatric Infectious Diseases, Pomeranian Center of Infectious Diseases and Tuberculosis in Gdansk, 80-214 Gdansk, Poland; sniedzwiecka@szpitalepomorskie.eu
[12] Department of Paediatrics with Clinical Assessment Unit, Medical University of Warsaw, 02-091 Warsaw, Poland; ekuchar@wum.edu.pl
[13] Department of Paediatrics, Paediatric Nephrology and Allergology, Military Institute of Medicine, 04-349 Warsaw, Poland; kalicki@wim.mil.pl
[14] The Ward of Pediatric Infectious Diseases and Hepatology, The John Paul II Hospital in Krakow, 31-202 Krakow, Poland; agorczyc@szpitaljp2.krakow.pl
* Correspondence: ewa.talarek@wum.edu.pl; Tel.: +48-22-33-55-250; Fax: +48-22-33-55-379
† Equal contribution.

Abstract: This prospective multicenter cohort study aimed to analyze the epidemiological and clinical characteristics of coronavirus disease 2019 (COVID-19) in children. The study, based on the pediatric part of the Polish SARSTer register, included 1283 children (0 to 18 years) who were diagnosed with COVID-19 between 1 March 2020 and 31 December 2020. Household contact was reported in 56% of cases, more frequently in younger children. Fever was the most common symptom (46%). The youngest children (0–5 years) more frequently presented with fever, rhinitis and diarrhea. Teenagers more often complained of headache, sore throat, anosmia/ageusia and weakness. One fifth of patients were reported to be asymptomatic. Pneumonia was diagnosed in 12% of patients, more frequently in younger children. During the second wave patients were younger than during the first wave (median age 53 vs. 102 months, $p < 0.0001$) and required longer hospitalization ($p < 0.0001$). Significantly fewer asymptomatic patients were noted and pneumonia as well as gastrointestinal symptoms were more common. The epidemiological characteristics of pediatric patients and the clinical presentation of COVID-19 are age-related. Younger children were more frequently infected by close relatives, more often suffered from pneumonia and gastrointestinal symptoms and required hospitalization. Clinical courses differed significantly during the first two waves of the pandemic.

Keywords: children; clinical presentation; coronavirus disease 2019 (COVID-19); epidemiology; severe acute respiratory syndrome coronavirus 2 (SARS-CoV-2)

1. Introduction

Due to the rapid spread and enormous burden of coronavirus disease 2019 (COVID-19), the World Health Organization declared it a pandemic in March 2020 [1]. By 31 December 2020, almost 1,295,000 cases of COVID-19 had been diagnosed in Poland. The proportion of pediatric patients remains unknown. However, according to available data from the first two months of the pandemic, children constituted 6.68% of cases ($n = 1191$) in Poland, with an infection rate of 15.49/100,000 children, which increased with age (10.79/100,000 in children below 4 years of age to 21.59/100,000 in patients between 15 and 19 years old) [2]. From the beginning of the pandemic, available observations suggested that pediatric populations are less affected than adults, with a lower incidence and milder clinical course of the disease [3–6]. Many reports, including both observational studies [7–12] and systematic reviews [13–16], address the epidemiological and clinical characteristics of pediatric patients with COVID-19, most of which were published in the first months of the pandemic, providing valuable information about the novel disease in children. As the pandemic continues, the number of pediatric cases grows, and answering some critical questions should become easier, e.g., which children are more vulnerable to severe acute respiratory syndrome coronavirus 2 (SARS-CoV-2) infection, whether any factors can predict a more severe clinical course and whether the disease remained the same and had the same clinical picture during subsequent waves of the pandemic.

This study aimed to analyze the clinical and epidemiological characteristics of COVID-19 in children. In particular, we investigated differences in disease course according to patient age and wave of the pandemic (the first vs. the second). In addition, predictors of COVID-19-related pneumonia and gastrointestinal symptoms were analyzed.

2. Material and Methods

2.1. Study Design and Setting

This multicenter prospective cohort study based on the pediatric part of the SARSTer register (SARSTer-PED) included children (0 to 18 years) who were diagnosed with COVID-19 between 1 March 2020, and 31 December 2020. Fourteen Polish inpatient centers dedicated to pediatric patients with COVID-19 reported their cases using an electronic questionnaire addressing epidemiological and clinical data. Any patient younger than 18 years with confirmed SARS-CoV-2 infection was eligible for inclusion.

2.2. SARS-CoV-2 Testing

COVID-19 was diagnosed by a positive real-time polymerase chain reaction (RT-PCR) on a nasopharyngeal swab performed in certified molecular diagnostics laboratories using certified RT-PCR testing methods for SARS-CoV-2 infection. After validation and approval of second-generation antigen testing for SARS-CoV-2 infection as a reliable method for the diagnosis of COVID-19 (30 October 2020), cases confirmed by this method were also included.

2.3. Data Collection and Study Definitions

Demographic data included age and sex. Epidemiologic data included known exposure to a person with confirmed SARS-CoV-2 infection (in the household or otherwise), history of international travel in the 14 days before disease onset, the duration of symptoms before presentation and any comorbidity, including bronchial asthma, cardiovascular disease, immunodeficiency, obesity, diabetes and arterial hypertension. Immunodeficiency was defined as congenital or acquired immunodeficiency or as the concurrent use of an immunosuppressive agent. Obesity was defined as body mass index $\geq$ the 95th percentile for age/sex. All symptoms at the time of admission and during hospitalization (if applicable) were documented. Fever was defined as a body surface temperature $\geq 38.5\ °C$. Laboratory testing and imaging results (if performed due to clinical indications) were recorded. Diagnosis of pneumonia was based on clinical signs, auscultation findings and/or chest X-ray abnormalities. Criteria for hospitalization varied across the study period. In the first several weeks, due to limited availability of PCR testing and scarce experience with pediatric COVID-19, most patients were admitted to the hospital for confirmation of SARS-CoV-2 infection and clinical assessment. Later, indications for hospital admission were clinical. For the purpose of this study, two waves of the pandemic were defined: the first wave lasted from March to August 2020 and the second wave lasted from September to December 2020, reflecting the two waves of the pandemic observed in Poland.

2.4. Statistical Analysis

Statistical analysis was performed using MedCalc Statistical Software version 19.2.1 (MedCalc, Ostend, Belgium, https://www.medcalc.org, accessed on 7 October 2021). Categorical variables were compared using the chi-square test. Continuous variables are presented as medians with interquartile ranges (IQRs) and were compared using the Mann–Whitney U test. A two-sided p value < 0.05 was considered significant. In addition, logistic regression analysis was performed. Parameters with a significant difference were included in the univariate analysis, and parameters significant in the univariate analysis were included in the multivariate analysis. The results were presented as odds ratios (ORs) and 95% confidence intervals (95% CIs). Results with a CI not including 1.0 were considered significant.

2.5. Ethical Statement

The study was performed in accordance with the ethical standards in the 1964 Declaration of Helsinki and its later amendments. The local ethics committee of the Regional Medical Chamber in Warsaw approved this study (No KB/1270/20; date of approval: 3 April 2020).

3. Results

3.1. Study Group

Between 1 March 2020 and 31 December 2020, 1283 patients with COVID-19 were reported: 465 during the first wave of the pandemic (March to August) and 818 during the second wave (September to December, Figure 1), including 650 boys and 633 girls aged 5 days to 18 years, with a median age of 6 (1; 13) years. Among the 1283 patients, 1008 (78%) were hospitalized: 349 (35%) patients were hospitalized for no longer than 24 h and the remaining 659 (65%) patients were hospitalized for longer than 24 h, with a median hospital stay of 5 (3; 8) days. Twenty-five (2%) of the patients required oxygen therapy but none of them needed mechanical ventilation. The median duration of clinical symptoms before admission was 2 (1; 4) days. Two hundred fifty-one patients (20%) suffered from chronic comorbidities, including those potentially related to a high risk of severe COVID-19, e.g., bronchial asthma (26 patients), cardiovascular disease (22), immunodeficiency (19), obesity (8), diabetes (5) and arterial hypertension (4). Comorbidities were significantly more frequently reported in teenagers (26%) than in younger children ($p < 0.0001$) (Table 1). Three patients required admission to the intensive care unit (ICU). No fatal outcomes were reported.

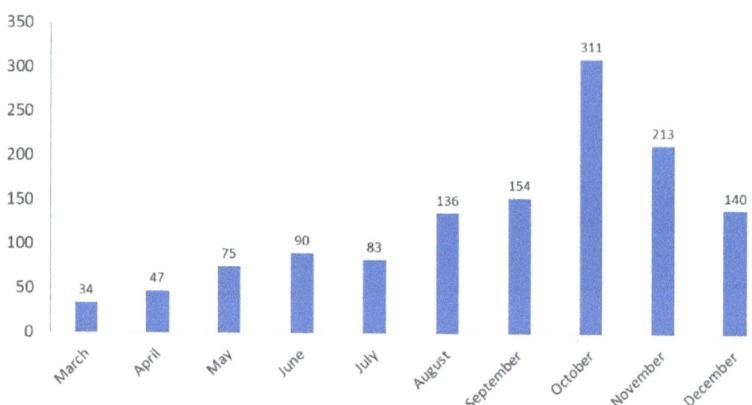

Figure 1. The number of COVID-19 cases in pediatric patients reported in the SARSTer-PED register throughout 2020.

Epidemiological features in the three age groups (0–5; >5–10; and >10–18 years) are presented in Table 1. Household contact with a relative infected with SARS-CoV-2 was reported in 716 (56%) cases, more frequently in younger children. Among 606 patients for whom COVID-19 was confirmed in a family member, in 260 (43%) cases, the diagnosis had been established in relatives before the children; in 281 (46%) cases, the diagnoses were established simultaneously; and in 65 (11%) cases, relatives were diagnosed after the children. Exposure other than household contact was confirmed in 83 (6%) patients, significantly more frequently in teenagers (12%), $p < 0.0001$. Forty-three (3%) patients had a history of international travel 14 days before disease onset.

3.2. Clinical Presentation

Fever was the most frequent symptom of COVID-19, with a prevalence of 46%. In an additional 14% of patients, low-grade fever (up to 38.5°C) was observed. The frequencies of clinical symptoms in the study group are presented in Table 1 and Figure 2. Anosmia and/or ageusia, the most specific symptoms of COVID-19, were reported in 8% of patients, including 20% of teenagers, but not in any children up to 5 years old. The youngest children (0–5 years old) more frequently presented with fever, rhinitis, diarrhea, loss of appetite and rash than teenagers, who more often complained of weakness, headache, sore throat, anosmia, muscle pain and chest pain (Table 1). In addition, dyspnea was significantly more frequently observed in teenagers (9%) than in younger children (4% in children aged 0–5 years and 3% in children aged 5–10 years, $p = 0.0002$). Two hundred seventy-one patients (21%) were reported to be asymptomatic (they were admitted for epidemiological reasons, mainly during the first weeks of the pandemic).

Table 1. Clinical presentation and epidemiological characteristics of COVID-19 in the study group and in different age groups.

Characteristics	Total N = 1283	Age (Years)			p *
		0–5 N = 589	>5–10 N = 225	>10 N = 469	
	n (%)	n (%)	n (%)	n (%)	
Epidemiological:					
Household contact with an infected family member	716 (56)	348 (59)	149 (66)	219 (47)	<0.0001
Confirmed other contact	83 (6)	11 (2)	18 (8)	54 (12)	<0.0001
History of international travel (during 14 days before disease onset)	43 (3)	9 (2)	4 (2)	30 (6)	<0.0001
Comorbidities	251 (20)	84 (14)	43 (19)	124 (26)	
Bronchial asthma	26 (2)	5 (0.8)	7 (3)	14 (3)	
Cardiovascular disease	22 (1.7)	8 (1)	2 (1)	12 (3)	<0.0001
Immunodeficiency	19 (1.5)	5 (0.8)	8 (4)	5 (1)	
Obesity	8 (0.6)	0	0	8 (2)	0.005
Diabetes	5 (0.4)	0	0	5 (1)	
Arterial hypertension	4 (0.3)	0	0	4 (1)	
Number of patients during 1st/2nd waves of the pandemic	465 (36)/ 818 (64)	155 (26)/ 434 (74)	116 (52)/109 (48)	194 (41)/275 (59)	<0.0001
Clinical Presentation					
Fever	597 (46)	351 (60)	91 (40)	155 (33)	<0.0001
Cough	417 (33)	209 (35)	46 (20)	162 (35)	0.0001
Rhinitis	339 (26)	190 (32)	36 (16)	113 (24)	<0.0001
Weakness	305 (24)	120 (20)	53 (19)	142 (30)	0.0002
Diarrhea	191 (15)	128 (22)	20 (9)	43 (9)	<0.0001
Headache	139 (11)	6 (1)	34 (15)	101 (22)	<0.0001
Sore throat	114 (9)	19 (3)	18 (8)	129 (28)	<0.0001
Abdominal pain	118 (9)	42 (7)	36 (16)	40 (9)	<0.0001
Vomiting	111 (9)	59 (10)	23 (10)	29 (6)	0.05
Anosmia/ageusia	104 (8)	0 (0)	11 (5)	92 (20)	<0.0001
Muscle pain	96 (7)	9 (2)	12 (5)	75 (16)	<0.0001
Loss of appetite	93 (7)	78 (13)	9 (4)	6 (1)	<0.0001
Dyspnea	76 (6)	26 (4)	6 (3)	44 (9)	0.0002
Rash	70 (5)	47 (8)	9 (4)	14 (3)	0.001
Chest pain	47 (4)	1 (<1)	3 (1)	43 (9)	<0.0001
Seizures	24 (2)	13 (2)	4 (2)	5 (1)	0.36
Pneumonia related to COVID-19	156 (12)	112 (19)	13 (6)	31 (7)	<0.0001
Gastrointestinal symptoms	295 (23)	175 (30)	47 (21)	73 (16)	<0.0001
Asymptomatic course	271 (21)	97 (16)	69 (31)	105 (22)	<0.0001
Hospitalization	1008 (79)	500 (85)	165 (73)	343 (73)	<0.0001

Data are presented as a number (%); * p values were calculated for the three age groups (0–5 vs. > 5–10 vs. > 10 years). 3.2. Epidemiological Characteristics

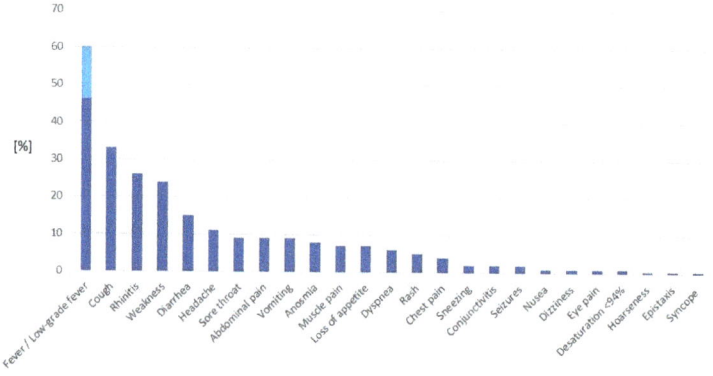

Figure 2. Clinical symptoms of COVID-19 in 1283 children. Data are presented as the frequency of the symptoms (%).

3.3. COVID-19-Related Pneumonia

Based on the clinical presentation and chest X-ray (CXR) results, pneumonia associated with COVID-19 was diagnosed in 156 (12%) patients. Typical CXR findings included bilateral patchy consolidation and ground-glass opacities with a peripheral and lower lung predominance, which were often bilateral. In our study group, children with pneumonia were younger: their median age was 18.0 (6.0; 84.5) months compared to 86.0 (20.0; 160.0) months in children without pneumonia ($p < 0.0001$). They also more frequently presented with fever, cough and gastrointestinal symptoms (Table 2). On laboratory testing, children with pneumonia had higher leukocyte counts and C-reactive protein (CRP), D-dimer, interleukin-6 (Il-6) and alanine as well as aspartate aminotransferase (ALT and AST) levels than patients without pneumonia. Interestingly, the presence of comorbidities did not cause a higher risk of COVID-19-related pneumonia (Table 2).

Table 2. Clinical factors associated with COVID-19-related pneumonia.

Factor	Pneumonia		p	OR (95% CI)
	With Pneumonia (n = 156)	Without Pneumonia (n = 1127)		
Age (months)	18.0 (6.0; 84.5)	86.0 (20.0; 160.0)	<0.0001	0.99 (0.98–0.99)
Sex	M: 89 (57) F: 67 (43)	M: 561 (50) F: 566 (50)	0.08	-
Fever (>38.5 °C)	103 (66)	494 (44)	<0.0001	1.48 (1.17–1.88)
Cough	79 (51)	338 (30)	<0.0001	2.06 (1.47–2.88)
Gastrointestinal symptoms	46 (29)	249 (22)	0.04	1.47 (1.01–2.14)
Leukocyte count ($10^3/\mu L$)	8.9 (6.4; 12.6)	7.4 (5.3; 10.9)	0.0005	-
CRP (mg/L)	6.0 (2.4; 27.8)	3.0 (0.7; 10.6)	<0.0001	1.01 (1.01–1.01)
Interleukin-6 (pg/mL)	8.9 (2.8; 43.6)	4.5 (2.2; 9.9)	0.02	-
D-dimer (ng/mL)	451.0 (230.0; 980.0)	311.0 (205.0; 486.2)	0.0004	-
ALT (IU/L)	22.0 (15.3; 34.7)	17.0 (13.0; 25.0)	<0.0001	-
AST (IU/L)	41.0 (30.0; 53.0)	32.0 (24.0; 42.0)	<0.0001	-
Comorbidities *	36 (23)	232 (21)	0.47	-

Data are presented as the median (IQR) or n (%), as appropriate. ALT—alanine aminotransferase; AST—aspartate aminotransferase; CI—confidence interval; CRP—C-reactive protein; and OR—odds ratio. * Comorbidities included: bronchial asthma, cardiovascular disease, immunodeficiency, obesity, diabetes, arterial hypertension and other.

3.4. Gastrointestinal (GI) Symptoms

A total of 295 (23%) patients presented with at least one GI symptom (abdominal pain, diarrhea or vomiting). These children were younger than the remaining group without GI presentation (median age 36 vs. 87 months, $p < 0.0001$), and presented more frequently with fever and higher CRP, D-dimer and AST levels. No difference in the GI symptom incidence was noted between patients with comorbidities and otherwise healthy children (Table 3).

Table 3. Clinical factors associated with gastrointestinal symptoms in the course of COVID-19.

Factor	Gastrointestinal (GI) Symptoms (Abdominal Pain, Diarrhea or Vomiting)		p	OR (95% CI)
	Patients with GI Symptoms ($n = 295$)	Patients without GI Symptoms ($n = 988$)		
Age (months)	36 (9; 120)	87 (20; 164)	<0.0001	0.99 (0.99–0.99)
Sex	M: 153 (52) F: 142 (48)	M: 497 (50) F: 491 (50)	0.63	-
Fever (> 38.5 °C)	192 (65)	405 (41)	<0.0001	2.58 (1.96–3.38)
Leukocyte count ($10^3/\mu L$)	8.8 (6.1; 12.8)	7.3 (5.3; 10.6)	<0.0001	-
CRP (mg/L)	5.2 (1.3; 21.0)	3.0 (0.6; 9.8)	0.0002	-
Interleukin-6 (pg/mL)	4.2 (2.1; 18.5)	4.8 (2.6; 10.6)	0.97	-
D-dimer (ng/mL)	443.5 (266.3; 739.7)	290.9 (194.3; 481.8)	<0.0001	-
ALT (IU/L)	17 (13; 26)	17 (13; 26)	0.69	-
AST (IU/L)	35 (27; 46)	32 (24; 44)	0.02	-
Comorbidities	64 (21)	204 (21)	0.69	-

Data are presented as the median (IQR) or n (%), as appropriate. ALT—alanine aminotransferase; AST—aspartate aminotransferase; CI—confidence interval; CRP—C-reactive protein; and OR—odds ratio.

3.5. Comparison of the Clinical Presentation of COVID-19 between the First and Second Pandemic Waves

We found significant differences in the course of COVID-19 and epidemiological features among patients reported during the second wave of the pandemic compared to the patients from the first wave (Table 4). Children diagnosed during the second wave were younger, with a median age of 53 vs. 102 months ($p < 0.0001$) and required significantly longer hospitalization ($p < 0.0001$). Household exposure to SARS-CoV-2 was reported less frequently ($p < 0.0001$), whereas another source of exposure was confirmed more often. Significantly fewer asymptomatic patients were noted, whereas COVID-19-related pneumonia, GI symptoms and most other clinical symptoms were more common (Table 4).

Table 4. Comparison of the clinical presentation of COVID-19 in children between the 1st and 2nd waves of the pandemic.

Clinical Factor	Patients Diagnosed between March and August 2020 N = 465	Patients Diagnosed between September and December 2020 N = 818	p	OR (95% CI)
Age (months) Median (IQR)	102.0 (44.0; 154.7)	53.0 (9.0; 156.0)	<0.0001	0.99 (0.99–0.99)
Sex (male/female)	223 (48)/242 (52)	427 (52)/391 (48)	0.14	-
Hospitalized	321 (69)	687 (84)	<0.0001	2.29 (1.74–3.01)
Duration of hospitalization (days), median (IQR)	1 (1; 3)	3 (1; 6)	<0.0001	1.07 (1.04–1.11)

Table 4. Cont.

Clinical Factor	Patients Diagnosed between March and August 2020 N = 465	Patients Diagnosed between September and December 2020 N = 818	p	OR (95% CI)
Household contact with an infected family member	360 (78)	355 (43)	<0.0001	0.39 (0.31–0.49)
Confirmed other contact	5 (1)	43 (5)	0.0001	-
International travel during the 14 days before symptom onset	31 (7)	12 (1)	<0.0001	0.20 (0.10–0.40)
Comorbidities	70 (15)	198 (24)	0.0001	1.72 (1.27–2.31)
CLINICAL PRESENTATION				
Asymptomatic disease course	167 (36)	104 (13)	<0.0001	0.26 (0.19–0.34)
Pneumonia related to COVID-19	42 (9)	114 (14)	0.009	1.63 (1.12–2.38)
Gastrointestinal symptoms	58 (12)	237 (29)	<0.0001	2.87 (2.10–3.94)
Fever	152 (33)	445 (54)	<0.0001	2.30 (1.81–2.93)
Cough	109 (23)	308 (38)	<0.0001	1.86 (1.43–2.41)
Rhinitis	79 (17)	260 (32)	<0.0001	2.17 (1.63–2.89)
Weakness	68 (15)	237 (29)	<0.0001	2.25 (1.66–3.03)
Diarrhea	40 (9)	151 (18)	<0.0001	2.27 (1.57–3.29)
Headache	39 (8)	102 (12)	0.02	1.48 (1.01–2.19)
Sore throat	41 (9)	73 (9)	0.94	-
Anosmia	45 (10)	59 (7)	0.12	-
Vomiting	19 (4)	92 (11)	<0.0001	2.74 (1.66–4.52)
Abdominal pain	18 (4)	100 (12)	<0.0001	3.16 (1.91-5.25)
Loss of appetite	9 (2)	84 (10)	<0.0001	6.51 (3.24-13.09)
Muscle pain	26 (6)	70 (9)	0.05	-
Dyspnea	19 (4)	57 (7)	0.03	-
Rash	20 (4)	50 (6)	0.17	-
Chest pain	13 (3)	34 (4)	0.21	-
Conjunctivitis	7 (2)	18 (2)	0.38	-
Seizures	3 (1)	21 (3)	0.01	-

Data are presented as a number (%) unless otherwise indicated. CI—confidence interval and OR—odds ratio.

4. Discussion

This study presents our experience with COVID-19 in 1283 patients from 14 pediatric hospital settings in Poland. Children aged 0–5 years accounted for a high proportion of our patients (45%), similarly to preliminary data from Italy [9], but other authors reported a higher prevalence among older children [8,11,16]. Both sexes were equally affected, whereas in a number of studies a slight male predominance has been reported [5,7,10,11,14,17]. Almost 80% of patients were hospitalized. This proportion was significantly higher during the second wave than during the first wave (84% vs. 69%, respectively, $p < 0.0001$). The difference might be caused by the fact that testing for SARS-CoV-2 during the first weeks/months of the pandemic was available in Poland mainly in hospital settings; thus, some children with suspected SARS-CoV-2 infection were referred to the hospital for confirmation of the infection. Later, access to testing was easy in primary care; thus, children with confirmed SARS-CoV-2 infection were referred to the hospital for clinical indications, which may also explain the higher proportion of asymptomatic patients during the first pandemic wave than during the second wave (36% vs. 13%, respectively, $p < 0.0001$). Young children (5 days–5 years old) were also admitted to the hospital more frequently than those older than 5 years. The possible explanation may be a higher tendency for parents to seek medical care for younger children and/or a higher tendency for clinicians to admit them to the hospital. Younger age is recognized as a risk factor of a more severe course of some infections, e.g., influenza. In this age group of our cohort pneumonia and gastrointestinal symptoms were significantly more frequent, which may suggest need of supportive treatment, even if it does mean a severe clinical course. Hospitalization rates were reported only in a limited number of previous studies, which varied from 11% to 74% during the first few months of the pandemic [4,5,7,10,11,18]. Most hospitalizations were short, which is consistent with other observations [7,10], although some systematic reviews reported a mean LoHS exceeding 10 days [14,16]. The need for a stay longer than 7 days was reported in 17% of our inpatients; these children were significantly younger (median age 52 vs. 78.5 months, respectively, $p = 0.001$) and more commonly had comorbidities (38% vs. 18%, respectively, $p < 0.0001$). According to other studies, 1 to 18% of pediatric patients required admission to the intensive care unit (ICU) [4,11,14,17]. In our cohort, only three children (< 1%) were hospitalized in the ICU.

Most children were infected in the household, and exposure to a family member with SARS-CoV-2 infection, mainly a parent, was confirmed in 52–76% of pediatric patients [3,9–11,14]. Our results support these observations for the first pandemic wave, when 78% of patients had a history of household exposure compared with 46% during the second wave ($p < 0.0001$). Analysis of age groups revealed that household exposure was less common in children >10–18 years old, which may be explained by the greater mobility of teenagers, even in lockdown conditions when schools were closed. Although predominant community exposure (60%) was reported in South America by Antunez-Montes et al., they explained that this result was due to the lack of a strict lockdown [19].

The pediatric population is not commonly affected by comorbidities compared to adults, but children with chronic underlying conditions were reported in all studies. At least one comorbidity was reported in 20 to 45% of pediatric patients with COVID-19 [4,7,9,11,14]. The most common condition was chronic pulmonary disease, including bronchial asthma. In the present cohort, the prevalence of comorbidities was 20%, with bronchial asthma as the most commonly reported condition. Comorbidities were significantly more widely reported among patients during the second wave (24% vs. 15%, respectively, $p < 0.0001$). Some authors found that comorbidities (e.g., pulmonary, endocrine, neurologic and immunocompromising conditions) increase both the odds of hospitalization and the need for respiratory support [7,11], but these observations are not confirmed by others [10] or our results. It seems that comorbidity in a patient with SARS-CoV-2 infection may be a cause for referral to the hospital rather than a cause of a more severe clinical course of the disease, since COVID-19-related pneumonia was not more frequent than among patients with no underlying conditions.

An asymptomatic course of SARS-CoV-2 infection was observed in 2.5–19% of patients [7,9,11,12,14,16]; in this study, an asymptomatic course was found in 21% of the whole cohort, with a significant difference between the first and second waves of the pandemic (36% vs. 13%, respectively, $p < 0.0001$). Different diagnostic approaches may explain this result during the first months of the pandemic when testing for SARS-CoV-2 infection was partially performed for epidemiologic purposes regardless of the clinical presentation. In the second wave, as the number of COVID-19 cases significantly increased, patients were tested mainly because of clinical suspicion of the disease. The proportion of asymptomatic cases was age-related, with approximately one third in children > 5–10 years old. Among symptomatic patients, the most commonly reported signs were fever (46%), followed by a cough (33%), rhinitis (26%) and weakness (24%); these same symptoms were the most common in a systemic review including 7780 pediatric patients conducted by Hoang et al., although their proportions varied (59%, 56%, 20% and 19%, respectively) [14]. When comparing the prevalence of these symptoms in different age groups, we found that fever and rhinitis were significantly more common in children aged 0–5 years and weakness in those aged > 10–18 years. The relationship between age and the prevalence of symptoms was demonstrated in a UK pediatric study [17] and a multinational study with both pediatric and adult populations [20]. In contrast to others, Badal et al. reported headache as the most common symptom, which was present in 60–74% of pediatric patients [16]. In our whole cohort and in the >10–18 years group the prevalence rates of headache were 11% and 22%, respectively. GI symptoms, e.g., the presence of at least one of the following: vomiting, diarrhea or abdominal pain, were observed in 23% of patients, which is similar to data reported by others (22–24%) [9,11]. GI symptoms had the highest prevalence (30%) in children aged 5 days–5 years. Patients with GI symptoms were significantly younger (36 vs. 87 months, respectively, $p < 0.0001$) and more commonly presented with fever and higher levels of inflammatory markers: leukocyte count, CRP and D-dimer. Comorbidities were not a predictor of a GI presentation. When comparing the two pandemic waves, GI symptoms were approximately 2.5 times more frequent during the second wave. At that time, Polish pediatricians (and parents) were more aware of both COVID-19 and pediatric inflammatory multisystem syndrome temporally associated with SARS-CoV-2 (PIMS); thus, children with abdominal pain and diarrhea (especially accompanied by fever), were tested for SARS-CoV-2 infection due to the suspicion of PIMS.

Pneumonia is a relatively common clinical feature in children with COVID-19, which is reported in 25–65% of pediatric patients [21]. Due to the heterogeneity of the data, including the basis of diagnosis (clinical symptoms vs. chest imaging), comparisons are difficult. According to studies published early in the pandemic, chest imaging (mainly CXR) was also performed in asymptomatic children. Patients with mild clinical symptoms and abnormalities were found in some proportions of these studies [3,12]. As knowledge about the presentation and evolution of COVID-19-related pneumonia in pediatric patients increased, indications for chest imaging were limited [22]. In our cohort, pneumonia was diagnosed in a relatively low proportion of patients (12%). Of note, patients with comorbidities were not at a greater risk in contrast to children presenting GI symptoms during the clinical course. Pneumonia was more frequent during the second wave of the pandemic than during the first wave.

Loss of smell and/or taste, which appeared in the first months of the pandemic as a specific and common symptom of SARS-CoV-2 infection in adults [23,24], was also observed in children [18,25]. In one American cohort study, loss of smell was reported in 6% of pediatric patients, but in others, anosmia or ageusia was not listed among clinical presentations. The prevalence of these symptoms was 8% in our cohort, which reached 20% in the oldest age group (> 10–18 years old). The prevalence also seemed higher during the first vs. the second wave of the pandemic, although without statistical significance (10% vs. 7%, respectively, $p = 0.12$).

The differences in the clinical course of COVID-19 between the two waves of the pandemic suggest the probable influence of new variants of SARS-CoV-2 on disease presentation. However, as the first cases of infection caused by SARS-CoV-2 variants were reported in Poland in January and February 2021, we are not able to analyze the possible influence of different mutations on the clinical course of COVID-19 in the described period of 2020.

This study has limitations. It was conducted in hospital settings, and the spectrum of pediatric COVID-19 may have been affected by the patient population. Children referred to the hospital are more likely to exhibit more symptoms and be more ill. The prevalence of some symptoms is challenging to assess among young children since they are not objective or are difficult for a patient to describe and may be under- or overestimated by caregivers. All collaborating centers used the same questionnaire for data collection but clinical management, e.g., admission criteria, could vary. Especially during the second wave of the pandemic, access to primary medical care in Poland was limited and this might have affected decisions regarding hospitalization. The main advantages of our study include the prospective design and the inclusion of a substantial number of cases divided into age groups, which allowed us to demonstrate that the presentation of COVID-19 is age-related. In addition, to the best of our knowledge, this is the first description of differences in the clinical course of COVID-19 in children between the first and second waves of the pandemic. Since the vast majority of previous studies present data from the first months of the pandemic, our observations made for several months may extend experience with pediatric COVID-19.

In conclusion, based on our experience, the epidemiological characteristics of pediatric patients infected with SARS-CoV-2 and the clinical presentation of COVID-19 are age-related. Sources of infection seem to differ according to patient age. Younger children are more frequently infected by close relatives, and they more often suffer from pneumonia and gastrointestinal symptoms and require hospitalization, which is usually short. In addition, the clinical course of the disease differed significantly during the first two waves of the pandemic, suggesting the possible influence of new variants of SARS-CoV-2 on disease presentation.

Author Contributions: Conceptualization and methodology, M.P.-Ś., E.T., A.M. and M.M.; formal analysis, M.P.-Ś.; interpretation of the data, M.P.-Ś., E.T., A.M. and M.P.; Investigation, M.P.-Ś., E.T., A.M., M.P., J.P., K.Z., M.F., K.M.-M., K.F., P.C., J.Ł.-Z., J.R., B.H., M.S., P.F.-C., I.Z., L.S., K.T., A.S. (Artur Sulik), B.S., I.P.-B., I.K., A.S. (Adam Sybilski), M.S.-P., U.D., E.M.-S., S.N., E.K., B.K. and A.G.; writing—original draft preparation, review and editing, M.P.-Ś., E.T., A.M., M.P. and M.M.; visualization, M.P.-Ś. and E.T; supervision, M.P.-Ś. and M.M.; funding acquisition, M.P.-Ś. and E.T. All authors have collected the data. All authors have read and agreed to the published version of the manuscript.

Funding: Medical Research Agency, grant number 2020/ABM/COVID19/PTEILCHZ, and the Polish Association of Epidemiologists and Infectiologists.

Institutional Review Board Statement: The study was conducted according to the guidelines standards of the Declaration of Helsinki, and approved by the Ethics Committee of the Regional Medical Chamber in Warsaw (No KB/1270/20; date of approval: 3 April 2020).

Informed Consent Statement: Informed consent was obtained from all subjects involved in the study.

Data Availability Statement: The datasets used and analyzed during the current study are available from the corresponding author upon reasonable request.

Conflicts of Interest: The authors declare no conflict of interest.

References

1. World Health Organization. Coronavirus Disease 2019 (COVID-190 Situation Report-51. World Health Organization, 11 March 2020. Available online: https://www.who.int.docs/default-source/coronaviruse/situation-reports/20200311-sitrep-51--covid-19-pdf (accessed on 1 July 2021).
2. Jackowska, T.; Wrotek, A.; Jankowski, M.; Pinkas, J. Significant COVID-19 burden in Polish children. *Arch. Med Sci.* **2020**, *16*, 1–10. [CrossRef]
3. Lu, X.; Zhang, L.; Du, H.; Zhang, J.; Li, Y.Y.; Qu, J.; Zhang, W.; Wang, Y.; Bao, S.; Li, Y.; et al. SARS-CoV-2 Infection in Children. *N. Engl. J. Med.* **2020**, *382*, 1663–1665. [CrossRef]
4. Bialek, S.; Gierke, R.; Hughes, M.; McNamara, L.A.; Pilishvili, T.; Skoff, T. Coronavirus Disease 2019 in Children—United States, February 12—April 2, 2020. *Morb. Mortal. Wkly. Rep.* **2020**, *69*, 422–426.
5. Parri, N.; Lenge, M.; Buonsenso, D. Coronavirus Infection in Pediatric Emergency Departments (CONFIDENCE) Research Group. Children with Covid-19 in Pediatric Emergency Departments in Italy. *N. Engl. J. Med.* **2020**, *383*, 187–190. [CrossRef]
6. Pokorska-Śpiewak, M.; Talarek, E.; Popielska, J.; Nowicka, K.; Ołdakowska, A.; Zawadka, K.; Kowalik-Mikołajewska, B.; Tomasik, A.; Dobrzeniecka, A.; Lipińska, M.; et al. Comparison of clinical severity and epidemiological spectrum between coronavirus disease 2019 and influenza in children. *Sci. Rep.* **2021**, *11*, 5760. [CrossRef]
7. Graff, K.; Smith, C.; Silveira, L.; Jung, S.; Curran-Hays, S.; Jarjour, J.; Carpenter, L.; Pickard, K.; Mattiucci, M.; Fresia, J.; et al. Risk Factors for Severe COVID-19 in Children. *Pediatr. Infect. Dis. J* **2021**, *40*, e137–e145. [CrossRef] [PubMed]
8. Kim, L.; Whitaker, M.; O'Halloran, A.; Kambhampati, A.; Chai, S.J.; Reingold, A.; Armistead, I.; Kawasaki, B.; Meek, J.; Yousey-Hindes, K.; et al. Hospitalization Rates and Characteristics of Children Aged <18 Years Hospitalized with Laboratory-Confirmed COVID-19—COVID-NET, 14 States, March 1–July 25, 2020. *Morb. Mortal. Wkly. Rep.* **2020**, *69*, 1081–1088. [CrossRef] [PubMed]

9. Garazzino, S.; Montagnani, C.; Donà, D.; Meini, A.; Felici, E.; Vergine, G.; Bernardi, S.; Giacchero, R.; Vecchio, A.L.; Marchisio, P.; et al. Multicentre Italian study of SARS-CoV-2 infection in children and adolescents, preliminary data as at 10 April 2020. *Eurosurveillance* **2020**, *25*, 2000600. [CrossRef]
10. Zachariah, P.; Johnson, C.L.; Halabi, K.C.; Ahn, D.; Sen, A.I.; Fischer, A.; Banker, S.L.; Giordano, M.; Manice, C.S.; Diamond, R.; et al. Epidemiology, Clinical Features, and Disease Severity in Patients With Coronavirus Disease 2019 (COVID-19) in a Children's Hospital in New York City, New York. *JAMA Pediatr.* **2020**, *174*, e202430. [CrossRef] [PubMed]
11. Götzinger, F.; Santiago-García, B.; Noguera-Julián, A.; Lanaspa, M.; Lancella, L.; Carducci, F.I.C.; Gabrovska, N.; Velizarova, S.; Prunk, P.; Osterman, V.; et al. COVID-19 in children and adolescents in Europe: A multinational, multicentre cohort study. *Lancet Child Adolesc. Health* **2020**, *4*, 653–661. [CrossRef]
12. Dong, Y.; Mo, X.; Hu, Y.; Qi, X.; Jiang, F.; Jiang, Z.; Tong, S. Epidemiology of COVID-19 among Children in China. *Pediatrics* **2020**, *145*, e20200702. [CrossRef]
13. Castagnoli, R.; Votto, M.; Licari, A.; Brambilla, I.; Bruno, R.; Perlini, S.; Rovida, F.; Baldanti, F.; Marseglia, G.L. Severe Acute Respiratory Syndrome Coronavirus 2 (SARS-CoV-2) Infection in Children and Adolescents: A Systematic Review. *JAMA Pediatr.* **2020**, *174*, 882–889. [CrossRef] [PubMed]
14. Hoang, A.; Chorath, K.; Moreira, A.; Evans, M.; Burmeister-Morton, F.; Burmeister, F.; Naqvi, R.; Petershack, M.; Moreira, A. COVID-19 in 7780 pediatric patients: A systematic review. *EClinicalMedicine* **2020**, *24*, 100433. [CrossRef]
15. Mehta, N.S.; Mytton, O.T.; Mullins, E.W.; Fowler, T.A.; Falconer, C.L.; Murphy, O.B.; Langenberg, C.; Jayatunga, W.J.; Eddy, D.H.; Nguyen-Van-Tam, J.S.; et al. SARS-CoV-2 (COVID-19): What Do We Know About Children? A Systematic Review. *Clin. Infect. Dis.* **2020**, *71*, 2469–2479. [CrossRef] [PubMed]
16. Badal, S.; Bajgain, K.T.; Badal, S.; Thapa, R.; Bajgain, B.B.; Santana, M.J. Prevalence, clinical characteristics, and outcomes of pediatric COVID-19: A systematic review and meta-analysis. *J. Clin. Virol.* **2021**, *135*, 104715. [CrossRef] [PubMed]
17. Swann, O.V.; Holden, K.A.; Turtle, L.; Pollock, L.; Fairfield, C.J.; Drake, T.M.; Seth, S.; Egan, C.; Hardwick, H.E.; Halpin, S.; et al. Clinical characteristics of children and young people admitted to hospital with covid-19 in United Kingdom: Prospective multicentre observational cohort study. *BMJ* **2020**, *370*, m3249. [CrossRef] [PubMed]
18. Mania, A.; Mazur-Melewska, K.; Lubarski, K.; Kuczma-Napierała, J.; Mazurek, J.; Jończyk-Potoczna, K.; Służewski, W.; Figlerowicz, M. Wide spectrum of clinical picture of COVID-19 in children—From mild to severe disease. *J. Infect. Public Health* **2021**, *14*, 374–379. [CrossRef] [PubMed]
19. Antúnez-Montes, O.Y.; Escamilla, M.I.; Figueroa-Uribe, A.F.; Arteaga-Menchaca, E.; Lavariega-Saráchaga, M.; Salcedo-Lozada, P.; Melchior, P.; De Oliveira, R.B.; Tirado Caballero, J.C.; Redondo, H.P.; et al. COVID-19 and Multisystem Inflammatory Syndrome in Latin American Children: A Multinational Study. *Pediatr. Infect. Dis. J.* **2021**, *40*, e1–e6. [CrossRef]
20. Group ICC. COVID-19 symptoms at hospital admission vary with age and sex: Results from the ISARIC prospective multinational observational study. *Infection* **2021**, *49*, 889–905. [CrossRef]
21. Siebach, M.K.; Piedimonte, G.; Ley, S.H. COVID-19 in childhood: Transmission, clinical presentation, complications and risk factors. *Pediatr. Pulmonol.* **2021**, *56*, 1342–1356. [CrossRef] [PubMed]
22. Foust, A.M.; Phillips, G.S.; Chu, W.C.; Daltro, P.; Das, K.M.; Garcia-Peña, P.; Kilborn, T.; Winant, A.J.; Lee, E.Y. International Expert Consensus Statement on Chest Imaging in Pediatric COVID-19 Patient Management: Imaging Findings, Imaging Study Reporting, and Imaging Study Recommendations. *Radiol. Cardiothorac. Imaging* **2020**, *2*, e200214. [CrossRef] [PubMed]
23. Vargas-Gandica, J.; Winter, D.; Schnippe, R.; Rodriguez-Morales, A.G.; Mondragon, J.; Antezana, J.P.E.; Trelles-Thorne, M.D.P.; Bonilla-Aldana, D.K.; Rodriguez-Morales, A.J.; Paniz-Mondolfi, A. Ageusia and anosmia, a common sign of COVID-19? A case series from four countries. *J. Neurovirol.* **2020**, *26*, 785–789. [CrossRef]
24. Lechien, J.R.; Chiesa-Estomba, C.M.; De Siati, D.R.; Horoi, M.; Le Bon, S.D.; Rodriguez, A.; Dequanter, D.; Blecic, S.; El Afia, F.; Distinguin, L.; et al. Olfactory and gustatory dysfunctions as a clinical presentation of mild-to-moderate forms of the coronavirus disease (COVID-19): A multicenter European study. *Eur. Arch. Otorhinolaryngol.* **2020**, *277*, 2251–2261. [CrossRef] [PubMed]
25. Mak, P.Q.; Chung, K.-S.; Wong, J.S.-C.; Shek, C.-C.; Kwan, M.Y.-W. Anosmia and Ageusia: Not an Uncommon Presentation of COVID-19 Infection in Children and Adolescents. *Pediatr. Infect. Dis. J.* **2020**, *39*, e199–e200. [CrossRef] [PubMed]

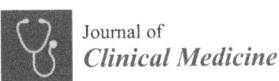

Article

Prevalence and Prognostic Impact of Deranged Liver Blood Tests in COVID-19: Experience from the Regional COVID-19 Center over the Cohort of 3812 Hospitalized Patients

Frane Paštrovic [1], Marko Lucijanic [2,3], Armin Atic [4], Josip Stojic [4], Mislav Barisic Jaman [1], Ida Tjesic Drinkovic [1], Marko Zelenika [1], Marko Milosevic [1], Barbara Medic [1], Jelena Loncar [1], Maja Mijic [5], Tajana Filipec Kanizaj [3,5], Dominik Kralj [6], Ivan Lerotic [6], Lucija Virovic Jukic [3,6], Neven Ljubicic [3,6], Kresimir Luetic [7], Dora Grgic [8], Matea Majerovic [8], Rajko Ostojic [3,8], Zeljko Krznaric [3,8], Ivica Luksic [3,9], Nevenka Piskac Zivkovic [10], Tatjana Keres [11], Vlatko Grabovac [4,11], Jasminka Persec [12,13], Bruno Barsic [3,11] and Ivica Grgurevic [1,3,14,*]

1. Department of Gastroenterology, Hepatology and Clinical Nutrition, University Hospital Dubrava, 10000 Zagreb, Croatia; fpastrovic@gmail.com (F.P.); mislav.barisic.jaman@gmail.com (M.B.J.); ida.tjesicdrinkovic@gmail.com (I.T.D.); markozelenika@gmail.com (M.Z.); markom342@gmail.com (M.M.); barby.medic@gmail.com (B.M.); jloncarzg@gmail.com (J.L.)
2. Department of Hematology, University Hospital Dubrava, 10000 Zagreb, Croatia; markolucijanic@yahoo.com
3. Department of Gastroenterology, Hepatology and Clinical Nutrition, School of Medicine, University of Zagreb, 10000 Zagreb, Croatia; tajana.filipec@gmail.com (T.F.K.); lucija.jukic@gmail.com (L.V.J.); neven.ljubicic@kbcsm.hr (N.L.); rajko.ostojic@gmail.com (R.O.); zeljko.krznaric1@zg.ht.hr (Z.K.); luksic.ivica@gmail.com (I.L.); barsicbruno@gmail.com (B.B.)
4. Department of Emergency Medicine, University Hospital Dubrava, 10000 Zagreb, Croatia; aticarmin@gmail.com (A.A.); josip.stojic95@gmail.com (J.S.); gr.vlatko@gmail.com (V.G.)
5. Department of Gastroenterology and Hepatology, University Hospital Merkur, 10000 Zagreb, Croatia; mijic.maja@gmail.com
6. Department of Gastroenterology and Hepatology, University Hospital Sestre Milosrdnice, 10000 Zagreb, Croatia; dominik.rex@gmail.com (D.K.); ivanlerotic@yahoo.com (I.L.)
7. Department of Gastroenterology and Hepatology, University Hospital Sveti Duh, 10000 Zagreb, Croatia; kresimir.luetic@hlk.hr
8. Department of Gastroenterology and Hepatology, University Hospital Center Zagreb, 10000 Zagreb, Croatia; dora.grgic1@gmail.com (D.G.); matea.majerovic@gmail.com (M.M.)
9. Department of Maxillofacial Surgery, University Hospital Dubrava, 10000 Zagreb, Croatia
10. Department of Pulmology, University Hospital Dubrava, 10000 Zagreb, Croatia; npiskac@gmail.com
11. Intensive Care Unit, Department of Internal Medicine, University Hospital Dubrava, 10000 Zagreb, Croatia; tatjana.keres@gmail.com
12. Intensive Care Unit, Department of Anesthesiology, Renimatology and Intensive Care, University Hospital Dubrava, 10000 Zagreb, Croatia; anestezija.predstojnica@kbd.hr
13. Department of Anesthesiology, Renimatology and Intensive Care, School of Dental Medicine, University of Zagreb, 10000 Zagreb, Croatia
14. Faculty of Pharmacy and Biochemistry, University of Zagreb, 10000 Zagreb, Croatia
* Correspondence: ivica.grgurevic@zg.htnet.hr; Tel.: +385-12903434; Fax: +385-12902550

Citation: Paštrovic, F.; Lucijanic, M.; Atic, A.; Stojic, J.; Barisic Jaman, M.; Tjesic Drinkovic, I.; Zelenika, M.; Milosevic, M.; Medic, B.; Loncar, J.; et al. Prevalence and Prognostic Impact of Deranged Liver Blood Tests in COVID-19: Experience from the Regional COVID-19 Center over the Cohort of 3812 Hospitalized Patients. *J. Clin. Med.* 2021, 10, 4222. https://doi.org/10.3390/jcm10184222

Academic Editor: Robert Flisiak

Received: 4 August 2021
Accepted: 14 September 2021
Published: 17 September 2021

Publisher's Note: MDPI stays neutral with regard to jurisdictional claims in published maps and institutional affiliations.

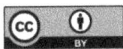

Copyright: © 2021 by the authors. Licensee MDPI, Basel, Switzerland. This article is an open access article distributed under the terms and conditions of the Creative Commons Attribution (CC BY) license (https://creativecommons.org/licenses/by/4.0/).

Abstract: Background: Derangement of liver blood tests (LBT) is frequent in patients with Coronavirus disease 2019 (COVID-19). We aimed to evaluate (a) the prevalence of deranged LBT as well as their association with (b) clinical severity at admission and (c) 30-day outcomes among the hospitalized patients with COVID-19. Methods: Consecutive patients with COVID-19 hospitalized in the regional referral center over the 12-month period were included. Clinical severity of COVID-19 at hospital admission and 30-day outcomes (need for intensive care, mechanical ventilation, or death) were analyzed. Results: Derangement of LBT occurred in 2854/3812 (74.9%) of patients, most frequently due to elevation of AST (61.6%), GGT (46.1%) and ALT (33.4%). Elevated AST, ALT, GGT and low albumin were associated with more severe disease at admission. However, in multivariate Cox regression analysis, when adjusted for age, sex, obesity and presence of chronic liver disease, only AST remained associated with the risk of dying (HR 1.5081 and 2.1315, for elevations 1–3 × ULN and >3 × ULN, respectively) independently of comorbidity burden and COVID-19 severity at admission. Patients with more severe liver injury more frequently experienced defined adverse outcomes.

Conclusions: Deranged LBTs are common among patients hospitalized with COVID-19 and might be used as predictors of adverse clinical outcomes.

Keywords: COVID-19; liver functional tests; mortality

1. Introduction

Coronavirus disease 2019 (COVID-19) is a multisystemic disease, with pandemic features [1]. The clinical picture is characterized by respiratory symptoms of various severity, including the development of pneumonia and respiratory failure with the need for oxygen supplementation, and these patients require hospital admission. Further deterioration in the form of acute respiratory distress syndrome (ARDS) and need for mechanical ventilation (MV) occurs in around 15–20% of hospitalized patients [1–3]. Along with respiratory illness other organs and systems are affected, including coagulation with the development of thromboembolic incidents, bleeding, myocarditis, central and peripheral nervous system affection, musculoskeletal symptoms, gastrointestinal and hepatobiliary problems [3].

Whereas elevation of aminotransferases has been commonly seen in hospitalized patients with COVID-19, liver failure represents a rare development usually encountered among patients with already known liver cirrhosis, or as the part of multiorgan failure caused by severe inflammatory response syndrome and septic shock [4–9]. In some previous reports deranged liver blood tests (LBT) were associated with more severe forms of COVID-19 and adverse clinical outcomes, although not all the authors came to the same conclusion [10–14]. As elevated aminotransferases are not organ specific, they might originate not only from the liver but also from muscles and other sources, and in line with rare occurrence of liver failure, some authors argue about the clinical importance of elevated aminotransferases and about the potential liver involvement in COVID-19 [15,16]. This view is supported by the lack of larger series of liver biopsies, and the microinjury of muscles in COVID-19 leading to the elevation of aminotransferases [17]. Additionally, studies that were using liver dedicated non-invasive diagnostic devices such of Fibroscan came to conflicting conclusions in terms of liver involvement and prognostic impact of the indicators of liver health among patients with COVID-19 [18,19].

Therefore, we aimed to evaluate (a) prevalence of deranged LBT at admission to hospital, as well as their association with (b) clinical severity, and (c) 30-day outcomes among the hospitalized patients with COVID-19, reflecting the real-life experience from the largest regional COVID-19 hospital in Croatia.

2. Patients and Methods

2.1. Patients

This study included 3.812 consecutive patients with COVID-19 who were hospitalized in Dubrava University Hospital over the period from 19 March 2020 to 19 March 2021. Dubrava University Hospital was completely re-purposed to serve exclusively as the regional tertiary COVID-19 center during COVID-19 pandemic.

All patients had a positive nasopharyngeal swab on severe acute respiratory syndrome coronavirus 2 (SARS-CoV-2) by polymerase chain reaction (PCR) or antigen test and were admitted through the hospital's emergency department. Standardized clinical work-up was performed for each patient, including medical history taking, clinical examination, obtaining blood biochemistry, peripheral oxygen saturation, chest X-ray, and electrocardiogram. Other examinations were performed as indicated based on the clinical picture and decision of the attending physician. Included were the patients with available laboratory and clinical parameters collected within the 24 h from admission, sufficient to assess the severity of COVID-19, presence of comorbidity, along with LBTs (aspartate aminotransferase (AST), alanine aminotransferase (ALT), gamma-glutamyl transferase (GGT), alkaline phosphatase (ALP), total bilirubin (Bil), serum albumin (alb), prothrombin time (PT)), complete blood count (CBC), who were followed for 30-day from the admission to hospital.

Patients were admitted to the intensive care unit (ICU), or to the regular ward based on the severity of clinical picture at presentation, as assessed in emergency department according to the national guidelines that incorporated severity of pneumonia and modified early warning score (MEWS) [20,21]. Upon admission to the ward, patients were treated with corticosteroids, antivirals (hydroxychloroquine, ritonavir/lopinavir or remdesivir), low molecular weight heparin (LMWH) and oxygen supplementation as needed according to the national guidelines. LMWH was prescribed in prophylactic doses to all patients without contraindication, whereas therapeutic doses were used in patients with documented thromboembolic events, as well as in those with elevated D-dimers upon judgement of the attending physician, especially in more severe forms of COVID-19. Other medications (for chronic medical conditions and acute complications, including antimicrobials) were administered upon the decision of the attending physician on the ward. Antibiotics were not a part of the standardized initial treatment of COVID-19. Oxygen was delivered by bi-nasal catheters, masks (up to 15 L/min) or high-flow nasal cannula (HFNC, if >15 L/min was needed). All presented patients completed their hospitalization for acute COVID-19. This paper is a part of the project "Registar hospitalno liječenih bolesnika u Respiracijskom centru KB Dubrava"/"Registry of patients hospitalized in University Hospital Dubrava Respiratory center".

2.2. Methods

Severity of COVID-19 at admission was graded using the classification from the national guidelines for treatment of COVID-19, version 2, issued on 19 November 2020 by the Ministry of Health [20]. Severe COVID-19 was considered in patients presenting with (a) bilateral pneumonia accompanied by either of the following features: (i) respiration rate (RR) $\geq$ 30/min; (ii) respiratory failure, (iii) peripheral oxygen saturation $\leq$ 93% (in resting state, room air); or (b) MEWS 3–4. Critical form of disease was considered in patients with (a) ARDS (partial pressure of arterial oxygen/fraction of inspired oxygen (PaO_2)/FiO_2) $\leq$ 300 mmHg), (b) presence of sepsis or septic shock, with/without organs' failure, or (c) MEWS $\geq$ 5, and these patients required ICU admission. Comorbidities were assessed as individual entities and were summarized using the Charlson comorbidity index [22]. Eastern Cooperative Oncology Group (ECOG) score was used to assess the overall physical performance [23]. Obesity was defined as body mass index (BMI) > 30 kg/m^2. All LBTs were recorded at hospital admission. The following were considered as normal ranges: Bilirubin $\leq$ 20 µmol/L, AST $\leq$ 30 IU/L in females and $\leq$ 38 IU/L for males, ALT $\leq$ 36 for females and $\leq$48 for males, GGT $\leq$ 35 IU/L for females and $\leq$ 55 IU/L for males, ALP $\leq$ 153 IU/L for females and $\leq$ 142 IU/L for males, albumin $\geq$ 35 g/L, and PT (quick) $\geq$ 70%. In accordance to the proposed nomenclature, the term LBT referred to all these tests, whereas the term "liver enzymes" referred to AST, ALT, GGT and AP [24]. "Liver injury" was considered in patients having deranged any of the liver enzymes accompanied by the elevated bilirubin. We did not use albumin or PT to define the presence of liver injury, as the duration of the disease at presentation was too short to result in decreased level of albumin, and many of patients had low albumin level and PT due to co-morbidity or nutritional issues. In addition, many patients used oral anticoagulants. Venous (pulmonary embolism, deep vein thrombosis) and arterial (myocardial infarction, cerebrovascular insult, peripheral embolization, mesenterial thrombosis) thrombotic events were considered only if documented by objective imaging and laboratory methods. Bleeding (gastrointestinal, epistaxis/hemoptysis, intramuscular, hematuria, retroperitoneal, intracranial) was considered as clinically relevant if documented in medical documentation. Thirty-day mortality was assessed from the date of hospital admission.

2.3. Statistical Methods

The presented analyses are retrospective in nature. Normality of distribution of numerical variables was tested using the Kolmogorov–Smirnov test. All numerical variables were non-normally distributed and were presented as median and interquartile range (IQR) and were compared between groups using the Mann–Whitney U or the Kruskal–Wallis ANOVA test where appropriate. The Jonckheere–Terpstra test for trend was used to assess rising or degrading trends of specific parameters over disease severity categories. Correlation between numerical variables was assessed using the Spearman rank correlation, relationships with Rho ≥ 0.2 considered as meaningful. Categorical variables are presented as frequency and percentage and were compared between groups using the X^2 test and the X^2 test for trend. Survival analyses were based on the Kaplan–Meier method. Survival curves were compared using the Cox–Mantel version of the log-rank test for univariate and the Cox regression analysis for multivariate analyses. The log-rank test for trend was used for assessing the trend of gradual increase in mortality with higher degree of derangement of liver specific parameters. p-values < 0.05 were considered statistically significant. All analyses were performed using the MedCalc statistical software version 20 (MedCalc Software Ltd., Ostend, Belgium).

2.4. Ethical Issues

This study was conducted in accordance with the World Medical Association Declaration of Helsinki and the study protocol was approved by the Institutional Ethics Committee, No 2020/1012-10. Due to retrospective design signed informed consent was waived by the Ethics Committee.

3. Results

3.1. Patients' Characteristics

A total of 3812 COVID-19 patients were analyzed. Median age was 74 years, IQR (64–82). There were 2148/3812 (56.3%) males and 1664/3812 (43.7%) females, and 1023 (28.6%) of patients were obese. There was a significant burden of co-morbidities as 2658 (69.7%), 1154 (30.3%), 617 (16.2%) and 474 (12.4%) patients had arterial hypertension, diabetes, congestive heart failure and chronic kidney disease, respectively. One hundred and six (2.8%) of the patients had history of chronic liver disease, and of them 49 (1.3%) had cirrhosis. Four hundred and thirty-four (11.4%) patients were current smokers. A total of 3390 (88.9%) patients had pneumonia at admission, and of them 3136 (82.3%) required oxygen supplementation. Median length of hospitalization was 10 days IQR (6–16). Rates of ICU admission, need for HFNC oxygenation and MV were 23.1%, 19.9% and 17.3%, respectively. A total of 1315 (34.5%) patients died during the 30-day period. Patients' characteristics at admission to hospital and their outcomes are shown in Table 1. The relationship between the patients' characteristics with LBT profile is shown in Supplementary Table S1.

Table 1. Characteristics of the analyzed cohort of patients with COVID-19 at admission to hospital.

	N (%), Median (IQR)
Total number of patients	3812
Age (years)	74 (64–82)
Sex	
Female	1664 (43.7%)
Male	2148 (56.3%)
Arterial hypertension	
Yes	2658 (69.7%)
No	1154 (30.3%)

Table 1. *Cont.*

	N (%), Median (IQR)
Diabetes mellitus	
Yes	1154 (30.3%)
No	2658 (69.7%)
Obesity (Body mass index ≥ 30 kg/m^2)	
Yes	1023 (28.6%)
No	2554 (71.4%)
Congestive heart failure	
Yes	617 (16.2%)
No	3195 (82.8%)
Chronic kidney disease	
Yes	474 (12.4%)
No	3338 (87.6%)
Chronic liver disease	
Yes	106 (2.8%)
No	3706 (97.2%)
Liver cirrhosis	
Yes	49 (1.3%)
No	3763 (98.7%)
Charlson comorbidity index	4 IQR (3–6)
Alcohol use	
Yes	207 (5.4%)
No	3605 (94.6%)
Smoking	
Yes	434 (11.4%)
No	3378 (88.6%)
Number of drugs in chronic therapy	5 (3–8)
Statin use	
Yes	911 (23.9%)
No	2901 (76.1%)
Antibiotic therapy before admission	
Yes	1285 (33.7%)
No	2527 (66.3%)
Oral anticoagulant therapy	
Yes	1049 (27.5%)
No	2763 (72.5%)
AST (U/L)	41 (28–64)
ALT (U/L)	31 (19–52)
GGT (U/L)	42 (24–81)
ALP (U/L)	72 (56–97)
Total bilirubin (umol/L)	11.4 (8.6–15.9)
Albumin (g/L)	32 (28–35)
Prothrombin time (%, Quick) *	100% (89–109%)
Liver blood tests (any)	
Normal level	958 (25.1%)
Deranged	2854 (74.9%)
White blood cell count ($\times 10^9$/L)	8 (5.8–11.2)
Hemoglobin (g/L)	128 (113–141)
Platelets ($\times 10^9$/L)	221 (163–297)

Table 1. Cont.

	N (%), Median (IQR)
C-reactive protein (mg/L)	88.7 (39.5–151)
Ferritin (ug/L)	711 (386–1289)
D-dimers (mg/L)	1.42 (0.73–3.6)
Day of disease on admission	5 (1–9)
ECOG status	3 (1–4)
Pneumonia	
Yes	3390 (88.9%)
No	422 (11.1%)
Oxygen therapy	
Yes	3136 (82.3%)
No	676 (17.7%)
MEWS severity	
Mild	392 (10.3%)
Moderate	196 (5.1%)
Severe	2652 (69.6%)
Critical	572 (15%)
ICU admission	
Yes	881 (23.1%)
No	2931 (76.9%)
Mechanical ventilation	
Yes	659 (17.3%)
No	3153 (82.7%)
30-day mortality	
Yes	1315 (34.5%)
No	2497 (65.5%)

Table legend: AST—aspartate aminotransferase, ALT—alanine aminotransferase, GGT—gamma-glutamyl transferase, ALP—alkaline phosphatase, IQR—interquartile range, ICU—intensive care unit, MEWS—modified early warning score, ECOG—Eastern Cooperative Oncology Group. * Prothrombin time values calculated for the patients not receiving oral anticoagulants.

3.2. Relationship between Patients' Characteristics and the Profile of LBTs at Admission

Median AST levels were 41 IQR (28–64). A total of 1432 (38.4%), 1922 (51.5%) and 377 (10.1%) patients presented with normal, 1–3 × elevated and >3 × elevated AST levels on admission, respectively. Higher AST was significantly associated with male sex, obesity, presence of chronic liver disease and liver cirrhosis, higher CRP, and higher ferritin ($p < 0.05$ for all analyses).

Median ALT levels were 31 IQR (19–52). A total of 2521 (67.4%), 1049 (28%) and 172 (4.6%) patients presented with normal, 1–3 × elevated and >3 × elevated ALT levels on admission, respectively. Higher ALT was significantly associated with male sex, younger age, obesity, with active or previous smoking, higher hemoglobin, and higher ferritin ($p < 0.05$ for all analyses).

Median GGT levels were 42 IQR (24–81). A total of 1934 (53.9%), 1212 (33.8%) and 441 (12.3%) patients presented with normal, 1–3 × elevated and >3 × elevated GGT levels on admission, respectively. Higher GGT was significantly associated with younger age, male sex, obesity, presence of chronic liver disease and liver cirrhosis, alcohol use, active or previous smoking, use of pre-admission antibiotic therapy, and with higher ferritin ($p < 0.05$ for all analyses).

Median ALP levels were 72 IQR (56–97). A total of 2862 (90.3%), 270 (8.5%) and 39 (1.2%) patients presented with normal, 1–3 × elevated and >3 × elevated ALP levels on admission, respectively. Higher ALP was significantly associated with non-obesity, presence of chronic kidney disease, presence of chronic liver disease and liver cirrhosis, use of oral anticoagulant therapy, use of pre-admission antibiotic therapy, and with higher D-dimers ($p < 0.05$ for all analyses).

Median total bilirubin levels were 11.4 IQR (8.6–15.9). A total of 2586 (85.3%), 375 (12.4%) and 69 (2.3%) patients presented with normal, 1–3 × elevated and >3 × elevated total bilirubin levels on admission, respectively. Higher total bilirubin was significantly associated with male sex, presence of congestive heart failure, presence of chronic liver disease and liver cirrhosis, alcohol use, oral anticoagulant therapy use ($p < 0.05$ for all analyses).

Median albumin levels were 32 g/L IQR (28–35). A total of 114 (4.9%), 515 (22.1%) and 1698 (73%) patients presented with albumin levels of ≥ 40 g/L, 35–39 g/L and <35 g/L, respectively. Lower albumin was significantly associated with older age, female sex, arterial hypertension, congestive heart failure, chronic kidney disease, chronic liver disease and liver cirrhosis, higher Charlson comorbidity index, active or previous smoking, use of oral anticoagulant therapy, use of pre-admission antibiotic therapy, higher WBC, lower hemoglobin, higher CRP, higher ferritin, and higher D-dimers ($p < 0.05$ for all analyses).

Median PT values were 100% IQR (89–109%). Considering that 27.5% of patients were receiving oral anticoagulant therapy, further analysis was narrowed to the subgroup without exposure to these drugs. Accordingly, lower PT values were significantly associated with male sex, presence of congestive heart failure, presence of chronic liver disease and liver cirrhosis, use of pre-admission antibiotic therapy, lower hemoglobin, and higher D-dimers ($p < 0.05$ for all analyses).

Associations of each of the analyzed LBTs with other parameters were either non-significant or associated with very low coefficient of correlation (<0.2) to be considered meaningful.

3.3. Relationship of LBTs with COVID-19 Severity at Admission

Median time from the first symptoms of COVID-19 to admission was 5 days IQR (1–9). Only higher ALT was associated with longer disease duration prior to admission, whereas lower albumin was associated with worse ECOG functional status. Higher AST, ALT, GGT and lower ALP, albumin and PT were associated with severe clinical presentation of COVID-19 ($p < 0.05$ for all analyses). However, total bilirubin showed no association with the COVID-19 severity at admission.

3.4. Associations between Deranged LBTs at Admission and Clinical Outcomes

Associations of clinical outcomes with LBTs are shown in Table 2. Higher AST, ALT, GGT and lower albumin were significantly associated with ICU admission, need for HFNC oxygenation and MV, higher total bilirubin was associated with the ICU admission only ($p < 0.05$ for all analyses), whereas ALP and PT show no associations with these outcomes ($p > 0.05$). When analyzed as continuous variables, higher AST, ALP, bilirubin and lower albumin and PT were associated with inferior 30-day survival, while ALT and GGT were not associated with inferior 30-day survival ($p < 0.05$ for all analyses).

We further investigated associations of LBTs with 30-day mortality using the time to event survival analyses stratified by the degree of derangement from normal values (normal, 1–3 × elevated and >3 × elevated for AST, ALT, GGT, ALP and bilirubin; ≥ 40 g/L, 35–39 g/L and <35 g/L for albumin, and ≥ 100%, 80–99% and <80% for PT). As depicted in Figure 1A–F, significant gradual increase in mortality was observed with higher degree of derangement of all investigated parameters except for ALT (p for trend <0.05 for all analyses except for ALT). Hazard ratios and confidence intervals for the associations of each LBT with 30-day mortality stratified categorically by the degree of derangement are presented in Table 3.

Table 2. Relationship of liver blood tests with the clinical outcomes of hospitalized patients with COVID-19.

	Overall/Any Enzyme	AST (U/L)	ALT (U/L)	GGT (U/L)	ALP (U/L)	Bilirubin (umol/L)	Albumin (g/L)	PT (%, Quick)
Length of hospitalization	10 IQR (6–16)	Rho = 0; p = 0.852	Rho = −0.01; p = 0.516	Rho = 0.03; p = 0.111	Rho = 0; p = 0.965	Rho = −0.02; p = 0.141	Rho = −0.06; p = 0.008 *	Rho = 0.01; p = 0.534
Intensive care unit		Median	Median	Median	Median	Median	Median	Median
Yes	879 (23.1%)	47.5	34	47	72	11.7	30	100%
No	2933 (76.9%)	39	29	40	72	11.3	32	101%
		p < 0.001 *	p < 0.001 *	p < 0.001 *	p = 0.486	p = 0.022 *	p < 0.001 *	p = 0.283
High-flow oxygenation		Median	Median	Median	Median	Median	Median	Median
Yes	758 (19.9%)	49	35	51	72	11.5	31	102%
No	3054 (80.1%)	39	29	40	72	11.3	32	101%
		p < 0.001 *	p < 0.001 *	p < 0.001 *	p = 0.829	p = 0.481	p < 0.001 *	p = 0.528
Mechanical ventilation		Median	Median	Median	Median	Median	Median	Median
Yes	660 (17.3%)	48	34	49	73	11.8	30	101%
No	3152 (82.7%)	40	30	40	72	11.3	32	101%
		p < 0.001 *	p < 0.001 *	p < 0.001 *	p = 0.606	p = 0.109	p < 0.001 *	p = 0.698
Venous thrombosis		Median	Median	Median	Median	Median	Median	Median
Yes	207 (5.4%)	38	30	46	75	11.9	30.5	94%
No	3605 (94.6%)	41	31	42	72	11.3	32	101%
		p = 0.011 *	p = 0.608	p = 0.665	p = 0.035 *	p = 0.214	p = 0.009 *	p < 0.001 *
Arterial thrombosis		Median	Median	Median	Median	Median	Median	Median
Yes	213 (5.6%)	42.5	29	36	74	11.8	32	100%
No	3599 (94.4%)	41	31	42	72	11.4	32	101%
		p = 0.688	p = 0.204	p = 0.061	p = 0.461	p = 0.664	p = 0.225	p = 0.848
Bleeding		Median	Median	Median	Median	Median	Median	Median
Yes	304 (8%)	39	29	41	75	11.3	30	98%
No	3508 (92%)	41	31	42	72	11.4	32	101%
		p = 0.310	p = 0.085	p = 0.210	p = 0.042 *	p = 0.835	p < 0.001 *	p = 0.018 *
30-day death		Median	Median	Median	Median	Median	Median	Median
Yes	1315 (34.5%)	48	30	43	77.5	12.3	30	97.5%
No	2497 (65.5%)	38	31	41	69	11	33	102%
		p < 0.001 *	p = 0.812	p = 0.199	p < 0.001 *	p < 0.001 *	p < 0.001 *	p < 0.001 *

* Statistically significant at level p < 0.05; albumin was graded as normal ≥40 g/L, 35–39 g/L and <35 g/L; PT values were considered only in patients not receiving oral anticoagulant therapy.

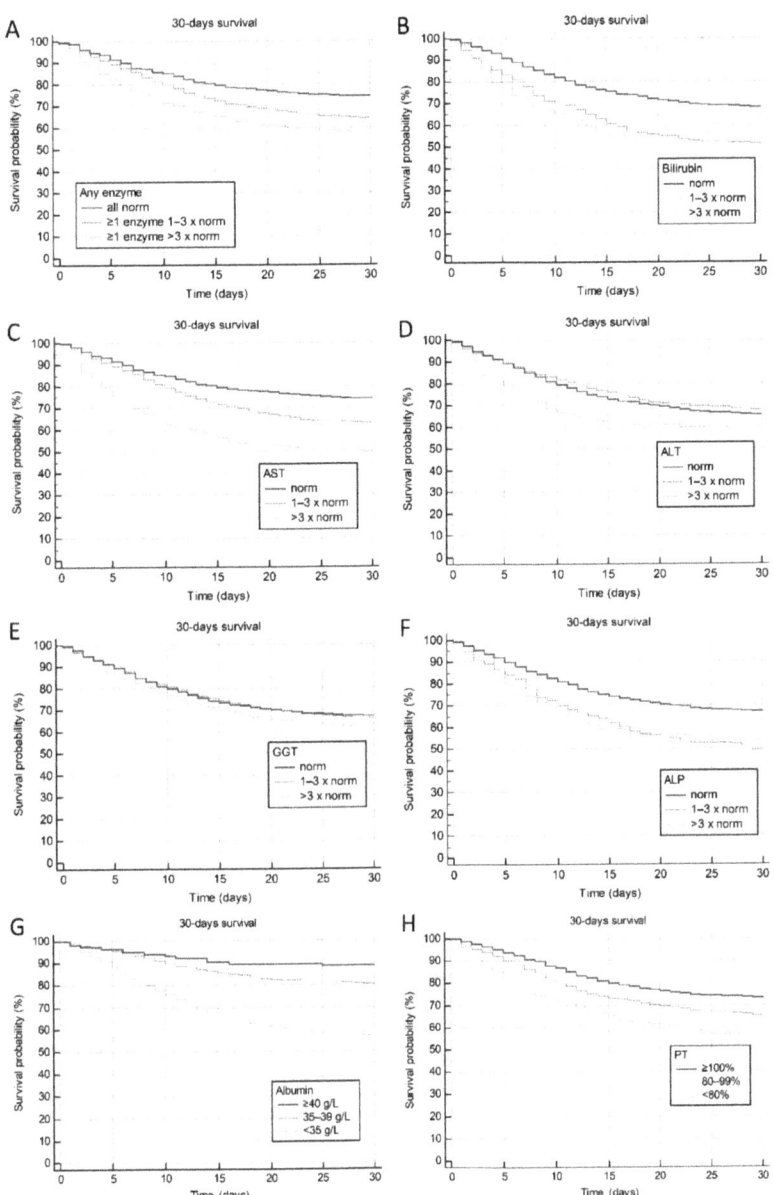

Figure 1. Association of the degree of liver blood tests derangement and 30-day mortality. (**A**) elevation in any of AST, ALT, GGT, ALP, total bilirubin. Elevation in (**B**) total bilirubin, (**C**) AST, (**D**) ALT, (**E**) GGT, (**F**) ALP, (**G**) reduction in albumin and (**H**) PT. Legend: AST—aspartate aminotransferase, ALT—alanine aminotransferase, GGT—gamma-glutamyl transferase, ALP—alkaline phosphatase, PT—prothrombin time (quick, %).

Table 3. Associations of liver blood tests with 30-day survival.

LBT	× ULN	30-Day Survival (%)	Hazard Ratio vs. Normal (95% CI)	p for Trend	p for Difference
AST (U/L)	N	74	Reference	<0.001	<0.001
	1–3	63	1.5 (1.33–1.68)		
	>3	50	2.42 (1.97–2.98)		
ALT (U/L)	N	66	Reference	0.631	0.021
	1–3	68	0.92 (0.82–1.04)		
	>3	59	1.32 (0.99–1.74)		
GGT (U/L)	N	67	Reference	0.034	0.056
	1–3	66	1.03 (0.92–1.17)		
	>3	61	1.23 (1.03–1.47)		
ALP (U/L)	N	67	Reference	<0.001	<0.001
	1–3	50	1.72 (1.37–2.14)		
	>3	54	1.61 (0.91–2.85)		
Bilirubin (umol/L)	N	68	Reference	<0.001	<0.001
	1–3	52	1.73 (1.42–2.09)		
	>3	52	1.79 (1.15–2.78)		
Albumin (g/L)	>40	89	Reference	<0.001	<0.001
	35–40	80	1.77 (1.29–2.43)		
	<35	57	4.55 (3.39–6.12)		
PT (%, Quick)	≥100	73	Reference	<0.001	<0.001
	80–99	66	1.36 (1.19–1.57)		
	<80	56	1.92 (1.52–2.43)		

AST—aspartate aminotransferase, ALT—alanine aminotransferase, GGT—gamma-glutamyl transferase, ALP—alkaline phosphatase, CI—confidence interval, LBT—liver blood tests, PT—prothrombin time (Quick, %), ULN—upper limit of normal.

Considering the relationship of LBTs with 30-day mortality, a Cox regression analysis model controlling for age, sex, obesity, Charlson comorbidity index, MEWS severity, chronic liver disease, liver cirrhosis, AST, ALT, GGT, ALP, total bilirubin, albumin and PT was created to assess independent associations. Model is shown in Table 4. As presented, AST elevation 1–3 × ULN and >3 × ULN was negatively and ALT elevation 1–3 × ULN was positively associated with 30-day survival independently of each other and age, comorbidity burden and disease severity at presentation.

3.5. Associations between the Presence of Liver Injury at Admission and Clinical Outcomes

A total of 2650 patients had available synchronous data on all liver enzymes (AST, ALT, GGT, ALP) and bilirubin among whom a total of 314 (11.8%) had combined elevation of both bilirubin and any of the enzymes corresponding to the liver injury, 1732 (65.4%) had enzyme elevation without elevated bilirubin, and in 604 (22.8%) neither enzymes nor bilirubin were elevated. There was a significant trend of increased frequency of adverse outcomes (MV, ICU admission, 30-day mortality) over higher degree of liver lesion ($p < 0.001$ for overall difference and $p < 0.001$ for trend for all outcomes, Figure 2). Patients with normal levels of liver enzymes and bilirubin, those with elevated enzymes but not bilirubin, and patients with liver injury needed MV in 10.6%, 18.9% and 22.9% cases, respectively, were transferred to ICU in 14.4%, 24.5% and 29.6% cases, respectively and experienced death during 30-days of hospitalization in 23.7%, 34.2% and 51.6% cases, respectively.

Table 4. Cox regression model investigating independent contribution of investigated parameters to 30-day mortality.

Covariate	p	HR	95% CI for HR
Age (years)	<0.001 *	1.0311	1.0207 to 1.0416
Male sex	0.137	1.1593	0.9542 to 1.4086
Obesity	0.796	1.0272	0.8385 to 1.2582
Charlson comorbidity index	<0.001 *	1.1270	1.0831 to 1.1727
COVID severity severe vs. mild	<0.001 *	13.1424	4.1771 to 41.3497
COVID severity critical vs. mild	<0.001 *	28.2629	8.8608 to 90.1489
AST 1–3 × elevated vs. normal	<0.001 *	1.5081	1.2089 to 1.8814
AST >3 × elevated vs. normal	<0.001 *	2.1315	1.3957 to 3.2552
ALT 1–3 × elevated vs. normal	<0.001 *	0.6432	0.5042 to 0.8206
ALT >3 × elevated vs. normal	0.053	0.5762	0.3296 to 1.0072
GGT 1–3 × elevated vs. normal	0.236	1.1393	0.9185 to 1.4131
GGT >3 × elevated vs. normal	0.727	1.0735	0.7207 to 1.5990
ALP 1–3 × elevated vs. normal	0.142	1.3301	0.9088 to 1.9467
ALP >3 × elevated vs. normal	0.129	2.0607	0.8090 to 5.2489
Total bilirubin 1–3 × elevated vs. normal	0.066	1.3087	0.9819 to 1.7443
Total bilirubin >3 × elevated vs. normal	0.881	1.0668	0.4577 to 2.4863
Albumin 35–39 g/L vs. ≥40 g/L	0.759	1.1403	0.4915 to 2.6459
Albumin <35 g/L g/L vs. ≥40 g/L	0.351	1.4787	0.6503 to 3.3624
PT 80–89% vs. ≥100%	0.388	1.0933	0.8929 to 1.3387
PT < 80% vs. ≥100%	0.056	1.3417	0.9920 to 1.8148
Chronic liver disease	0.246	0.5553	0.2057 to 1.4990
Liver cirrhosis	0.610	1.4051	0.3798 to 5.1976

* Statistically significant at level $p < 0.05$. AST—aspartate aminotransferase, ALT—alanine aminotransferase, GGT—gamma-glutamyl transferase, ALP—alkaline phosphatase, CI—confidence interval, PT—prothrombin time (quick, %).

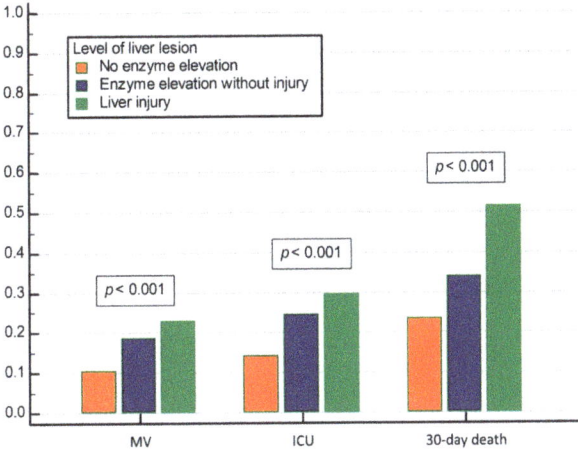

Figure 2. Relationship between the level of liver lesion and clinical outcomes (mechanical ventilation (MV), Intensive care unit (ICU) admission, and 30-day mortality). Liver injury was defined as the elevation of any liver enzyme plus elevated bilirubin. Liver enzymes: aspartate aminotransferase, alanine aminotransferase, gamma-glutamyl transferase, alkaline phosphatase.

4. Discussion

This study analyzed derangements of LBTs in one of the largest cohort of patients hospitalized with COVID-19 reported so far, as well as their association with the clinical severity at admission and 30-day outcomes. Derangement of LBTs occurred in 3/4 of patients at admission to hospital, most frequently due to the elevation of AST, followed by GGT and ALT. Elevated AST, ALT, GGT and low ALP, albumin and PT were associated with more severe disease at admission, whereas only elevated AST was independent predictor of death. There is incremental trend for higher rates of ICU admission, MV and 30-day mortality among the patients with liver injury when compared to those with only deranged liver enzymes and those with normal liver biochemistry.

According to the presented results elevated LBTs are frequently observed among patients with COVID-19 at admission to hospital. Elevation of at least one LBT was observed in almost 75% of patients in our cohort at admission. In line with other reports AST was the most frequently elevated (in 61.6%), followed by GGT in 46.1% and ALT in 33.4% of patients. This is much higher prevalence of deranged LBTs than initially reported in studies coming from China (14.9%), but comparable to data from United States ranging from 40–67% [1–3,25,26]. The observed differences in the rates of elevated LBTs might be due to some racial specificities, different threshold for hospital admission and the prevalence of severe cases, but also due to demographic features including age, prevalence of obesity, drinking habits, chronic medication use, just to mention the most obvious reasons. Indeed, three most frequently elevated LBTs in our population (AST, GGT, ALT) share the common denominators as they were all associated with male sex, presence of obesity and elevated ferritin level. In addition, elevated GGT was associated with alcohol use, and both ALT and GGT with smoking. These associations might point to the underreported alcohol consumption and unrecognized prevalence of non-alcoholic fatty liver disease in the analyzed cohort, reflecting their prevalence in general population. On the other hand, association with the inflammatory mediators (ferritin, and in case of AST with CRP as well), may link these enzymes with the liver involvement in the inflammatory response to COVID-19. The source of elevated LBTs in COVID-19 has been repeatedly discussed, as they are not completely liver-specific and may originate from other tissues, such as muscles [15,16]. However, other authors did not find consistent correlation between elevated AST and markers of muscle injury, leading to conclusion that the liver was the most likely source of elevated LBTs [4]. This liver lesion seems not to be clinically significant in majority of cases, as liver failure develops only exceptionally, usually among the patients with already compromised liver function due to existing cirrhosis, or as the part of multiorgan failure in most severe cases of COVID-19 [6,7,17].

Deranged LBTs are associated with more severe clinical presentation of COVID-19, which is in keeping with the reports from other authors [5,10,25]. In our cohort, more severe clinical presentation of COVID-19 at admission was observed among patients with elevated AST, ALT, GGT and low ALP, albumin and PT. Whereas elevated liver enzymes suggest the presence of strong inflammatory response with liver involvement, decreased PT and albumin most probably reflect the presence of comorbidity, worse nutritional and overall performance status, and therefore these associations appear logical. However, a word of caution is needed, as the design of this study does not allow for definitive conclusion about the association between deranged LBTs and severity of COVID-19. Namely, LBTs were analyzed only at the admission to hospital and not at the peak hospitalization/peak of illness. In some previous studies, further increase in frequency and the level of LBTs was reported in patients who developed more severe clinical picture, even if they had mild disease at admission. Additionally, patients presented with variable durations of symptoms before admission (IQR 1–9 days), which represents additional bias.

The most important result of our study is clear association between the serum levels of LBTs and clinical outcomes, indicating strongly for their prognostic significance. Indeed, significant gradual increase in mortality was observed with higher degree of derangement of all investigated LBTs, except for ALT (Figure 1). However, the risk of dying from

COVID-19 was independently increased only among the patients with elevated AST at admission (depending on the magnitude of AST elevation), and this association persisted after adjustment for age, sex, obesity, comorbidity, disease severity at admission, and other investigated LBTs. Interestingly, mild (<3 × ULN) elevation of ALT was found protective in terms of mortality, whereas ALT > 3 × ULN re-gained detrimental effect on survival. We do not see a mechanistic explanation for this protective effect of mildly elevated ALT, and the same phenomenon was reported in a recently published study from China [27].

Conflicting data have been published regarding the prognostic impact of elevated LBTs. Whereas in some studies, elevated LBTs were associated with more severe clinical presentation but they were lacking follow-up data to analyze mortality, and others reported various associations to ICU admission, need for mechanical ventilation and death [5,7,10–14,25]. In the study conducted over the 1827 hospitalized patients in United States, higher risk of dying was observed only among patients with elevated baseline bilirubin, whereas both elevated bilirubin and AST as recorded at the peak hospitalization were associated with death, and other LBTs were not [25]. However, abnormal AST, Bil and albumin at admission were all associated with the higher risk of ICU admission and mechanical ventilation.

The pathophysiological role of the liver in COVID-19 remains still not fully elucidated, as histological data are scarce, due to very infrequent liver biopsy taking. Whereas ACE2 receptors, as the gate for SARS-CoV-2 entry in the cell, are most abundantly expressed on the cholangiocytes, hepatocellular profile of elevated LBTs has been commonly reported, and histological changes (in the limited series of patients) were more in favor of deranged liver circulation (microthrombosis), mitochondrial dysfunction and mild hepatitis, rather than biliary injury [4,6,28,29]. In keeping with these findings, it is not unexpected that AST is most frequently elevated in patients with COVID-19, as it has been considered specific for liver ischemia, mitochondrial dysfunction and alcohol related liver disease [4,6]. Yet, reliable evidence of viral replication within hepatocytes has not been confirmed, so there is still doubt if liver lesion is caused by virus itself or is it immune-mediated [6,30,31]. As for the biliary injury, cases of severe post-COVID cholangiopathy with some distinct pathological features have recently been reported among patients who suffered from critical disease and were mechanically ventilated [32].

Liver involvement in pathogenesis of COVID-19 and prognostic importance of LBTs is furtherly supported by our results showing incremental increase in frequency of adverse outcomes (ICU admission, MV or death) when patients were assessed according to the severity of liver lesion. Indeed, patients with liver injury (defined here by elevated bilirubin in addition to elevated liver enzymes) had worse prognosis when compared to patients with the isolated elevation of liver enzymes (not accompanied by the elevated bilirubin), and to patients with normal both liver enzymes and bilirubin. Based on our results and available data from other studies we believe it is still not possible to claim if liver contributes to the severity of inflammatory response to SARS CoV-2 infection, and hence to the severity of COVID-19, or is it only indicator and the part of generalized severe inflammatory response to the virus. In any case, patients with biochemical indicators of more severe liver injury appear to be under increased risk of severe clinical course including the need for ICU treatment, MV and death.

In contrast to the high prevalence of biochemical abnormalities suggestive of liver involvement in COVID-19, the prevalence of chronic liver disease (2.8%) and cirrhosis (1.3%) observed in our cohort was low [3,19]. We assume this might be due to the awareness of the risks of acquiring COVID-19 among liver patients and preventive measures taken to avoid exposure to infection.

Interestingly, the association between the presence of cirrhosis and mortality risk was not independent when adjusted to other covariables in multivariate regression analysis as shown in Table 4. We assume that cirrhosis could not achieved statistical significance in the context of deranged LBT, probably due to overlapping prognostic properties and insufficient statistical power as the result of low number of patients with cirrhosis ($n = 49$), as compared to the entire cohort of 3812 patients analyzed here.

High mortality in our cohort might result from the selection criteria for the admission, as our hospital was the major tertiary referral center taking care of patients with most severe forms of COVID-19, as well as for those with other urgent conditions complicated with COVID-19. Indeed, almost 90% of patients had pneumonia, 82% required oxygen supplementation, and at peak pandemic almost 25% needed ICU admission or were receiving HFNC oxygenation outside ICU. In addition, the analyzed population was old, with median age of 74 and burdened by multiple co-morbidities.

The limitations of our study are single center experience, selection of most severe/critical COVID-19 cases, or COVID-19 cases with comorbidities that required hospital level of care, which are representative of the tertiary COVID-19 hospital, and inability to longitudinally assess dynamics of particular measurements over time. In addition to this, we did not regularly perform liver imaging in patients with deranged LBT to furtherly explore liver status, given almost universal prevalence and self-limited course of deranged liver biochemistry in typical cases. Nevertheless, this study was performed in the one of the largest cohort of patients reported so far, representative for the Caucasian population with almost universal prevalence of pneumonia, all of whom underwent standardized diagnostic procedures and therapy. Therefore, the obtained results might be considered robust, with high statistical power.

In conclusion, patients who are hospitalized due to COVID-19 usually have elevated LBTs at admission. Only elevated AST is the independent predictor of death. There is an incremental trend for higher rates of ICU admission, MV and 30-day mortality among the patients with more severe liver injury when compared to those with normal liver biochemistry.

Supplementary Materials: The following are available online at https://www.mdpi.com/article/10.3390/jcm10184222/s1, Table S1. Patients' characteristics at admission and their relationship with liver blood tests.

Author Contributions: Conceptualization, M.L., I.G.; methodology, M.L., I.G.; software, F.P., M.L., A.A., J.S.; validation, F.P., M.L., T.F.K., L.V.J., N.L., K.L., R.O., Z.K., I.L. (Ivica Luksic), N.P.Z., B.B., I.G.; formal analysis, M.L., I.G.; investigation, F.P., M.L., A.A., J.S., M.B.J., I.T.D., M.Z., M.M. (Marko Milosevic), B.M., J.L., M.M. (Maja Mijic), T.F.K., D.K., I.L. (Ivan Lerotic), L.V.J., N.L., K.L., D.G., M.M. (Matea Majerovic), R.O., Z.K., I.L. (Ivica Luksic), N.P.Z., T.K., V.G., J.P., B.B., I.G.; data curation, F.P., A.A., J.S., M.B.J., I.T.D., M.Z., M.M. (Marko Milosevic), B.M.; writing—original draft preparation, F.P., M.L., I.G.; writing—review and editing, F.P., M.L., A.A., J.S., M.B.J., I.T.D., M.Z., M.M. (Marko Milosevic), B.M., J.L., M.M. (Maja Mijic), T.F.K., D.K., I.L. (Ivan Lerotic), L.V.J., N.L., K.L., D.G., M.M. (Matea Majerovic), R.O., Z.K., I.L. (Ivica Luksic), N.P.Z., T.K., V.G., J.P., B.B., I.G.; visualization, F.P., M.L., I.G.; supervision, I.G., B.B., I.L. (Ivan Lerotic); project administration, F.P. All authors have read and agreed to the published version of the manuscript.

Funding: The authors disclose no funding sources for this research.

Institutional Review Board Statement: This study was conducted in accordance with the World Medical Association Declaration of Helsinki and the study protocol was approved by the Institutional Ethics Committee, No. 2020/1012-10. Due to retrospective design signed informed consent was waived by the Ethics Committee.

Informed Consent Statement: Due to retrospective design signed informed consent was waived by the Institutional Ethics Committee.

Data Availability Statement: Data from this investigation are available from the corresponding author upon the reasonable request, after the approval of the University hospital Dubrava who is the founder and the owner of the Registry.

Conflicts of Interest: The authors declare no conflict of interest.

References

1. Guan, W.J.; Ni, Z.Y.; Hu, Y.; Liang, W.H.; Ou, C.Q.; He, J.X.; Liu, L.; Shan, H.; Lei, C.L.; Hui, D.S.C.; et al. China Medical Treatment Expert Group for Covid-19. Clinical Characteristics of Coronavirus Disease 2019 in China. *N. Engl. J. Med.* **2020**, *382*, 1708–1720. [CrossRef]
2. Wiersinga, W.J.; Rhodes, A.; Cheng, A.C.; Peacock, S.J.; Prescott, H.C. Pathophysiology, Transmission, Diagnosis, and Treatment of Coronavirus Disease 2019 (COVID-19): A Review. *JAMA* **2020**, *324*, 782–793. [CrossRef]
3. Richardson, S.; Hirsch, J.S.; Narasimhan, M. Presenting Characteristics, Comorbidities, and Outcomes among 5700 Patients Hospitalized with COVID-19 in the New York City Area. *JAMA* **2020**, *323*, 2052–2059. [CrossRef]
4. Bloom, P.P.; Meyerowitz, E.A.; Reinus, Z.; Daidone, M.; Gustafson, J.; Kim, A.Y.; Schaefer, E.; Chung, R.T. Liver Biochemistries in Hospitalized Patients with COVID-19. *Hepatology* **2021**, *73*, 890–900. [CrossRef]
5. Cai, Q.; Huang, D.; Yu, H.; Zhu, Z.; Xia, Z.; Su, Y.; Li, Z.; Zhou, G.; Gou, J.; Qu, J.; et al. COVID-19: Abnormal liver function tests. *J. Hepatol.* **2020**, *73*, 566–574. [CrossRef]
6. Marjot, T.; Webb, G.J.; Barritt, A.S., 4th; Moon, A.M.; Stamataki, Z.; Wong, V.W.; Barnes, E. COVID-19 and liver disease: Mechanistic and clinical perspectives. *Nat. Rev. Gastroenterol. Hepatol.* **2021**, *18*, 348–364. [CrossRef] [PubMed]
7. Chew, M.; Tang, Z.; Radcliffe, C.; Caruana, D.; Doilicho, N.; Ciarleglio, M.M.; Deng, Y.; Garcia-Tsao, G. Significant Liver Injury during Hospitalization for COVID-19 Is Not Associated with Liver Insufficiency or Death. *Clin. Gastroenterol. Hepatol.* **2021**, *19*, 2182–2191.e7. [CrossRef] [PubMed]
8. Marjot, T.; Moon, A.M.; Cook, J.A.; Abd-Elsalam, S.; Aloman, C.; Armstrong, M.J.; Pose, E.; Brenner, E.J.; Cargill, T.; Catana, M.A.; et al. Outcomes following SARS-CoV-2 infection in patients with chronic liver disease: An international registry study. *J. Hepatol.* **2021**, *74*, 567–577. [CrossRef] [PubMed]
9. Sarin, S.K.; Choudhury, A.; Lau, G.K.; Zheng, M.H.; Ji, D.; Abd-Elsalam, S.; Hwang, J.; Qi, X.; Cua, I.H.; Suh, J.I.; et al. APASL COVID Task Force, APASL COVID Liver Injury Spectrum Study (APCOLIS Study-NCT 04345640). Pre-existing liver disease is associated with poor outcome in patients with SARS CoV2 infection; The APCOLIS Study (APASL COVID-19 Liver Injury Spectrum Study). *Hepatol. Int.* **2020**, *14*, 690–700. [CrossRef] [PubMed]
10. Ding, Z.Y.; Li, G.X.; Chen, L.; Shu, C.; Song, J.; Wang, W.; Wang, Y.W.; Chen, Q.; Jin, G.N.; Liu, T.T.; et al. Tongji Multidisciplinary Team for Treating COVID-19 (TTTC) Association of liver abnormalities with in-hospital mortality in patients with COVID-19. *J. Hepatol.* **2021**, *74*, 1295–1302. [CrossRef] [PubMed]
11. Mao, R.; Qiu, Y.; He, J.S.; Tan, J.Y.; Li, X.H.; Liang, J.; Shen, J.; Zhu, L.R.; Chen, Y.; Iacucci, M.; et al. Manifestations and prognosis of gastrointestinal and liver involvement in patients with COVID-19: A systematic review and meta-analysis. *Lancet Gastroenterol. Hepatol.* **2020**, *5*, 667–678. [CrossRef]
12. Ponziani, F.R.; Del Zompo, F.; Nesci, A.; Santopaolo, F.; Ianiro, G.; Pompili, M.; Gasbarrini, A.; "Gemelli against COVID-19" Group. Liver involvement is not associated with mortality: Results from a large cohort of SARS-CoV-2-positive patients. *Aliment. Pharmacol. Ther.* **2020**, *52*, 1060–1068. [CrossRef] [PubMed]
13. Zhang, Y.; Zheng, L.; Liu, L.; Zhao, M.; Xiao, J.; Zhao, Q. Liver impairment in COVID-19 patients: A retrospective analysis of 115 cases from a single centre in Wuhan city, China. *Liver Int.* **2020**, *40*, 2095–2103. [CrossRef] [PubMed]
14. Piano, S.; Dalbeni, A.; Vettore, E.; Benfaremo, D.; Mattioli, M.; Gambino, C.G.; Framba, V.; Cerruti, L.; Mantovani, A.; Martini, A.; et al. COVID-LIVER study group. Abnormal liver function tests predict transfer to intensive care unit and death in COVID-19. *Liver Int.* **2020**, *40*, 2394–2406. [CrossRef] [PubMed]
15. Bangash, M.N.; Patel, J.M.; Parekh, D.; Murphy, N.; Brown, R.M.; Elsharkawy, A.M.; Mehta, G.; Armstrong, M.J.; Neil, D. SARS-CoV-2: Is the liver merely a bystander to severe disease? *J. Hepatol.* **2020**, *73*, 995–996. [CrossRef]
16. Bangash, M.N.; Patel, J.; Parekh, D. COVID-19 and the liver: Little cause for concern. *Lancet Gastroenterol. Hepatol.* **2020**, *5*, 529–530. [CrossRef]
17. Jothimani, D.; Venugopal, R.; Abedin, M.F.; Kaliamoorthy, I.; Rela, M. COVID-19 and the liver. *J. Hepatol.* **2020**, *73*, 1231–1240. [CrossRef] [PubMed]
18. Demirtas, C.O.; Keklikkiran, C.; Ergenc, I.; Sengel, B.E.; Eskidemir, G.; Cinel, I.; Odabasi, Z.; Korten, V.; Yilmaz, Y. Liver stiffness is associated with disease severity and worse clinical scenarios in coronavirus disease 2019: A prospective transient elastography study. *Int. J. Clin. Pract.* **2021**, *75*, e14363. [CrossRef]
19. Campos-Varela, I.; Villagrasa, A.; Simon-Talero, M.; Riveiro-Barciela, M.; Ventura-Cots, M.; Aguilera-Castro, L.; Alvarez-Lopez, P.; Nordahl, E.A.; Anton, A.; Bañares, J.; et al. The role of liver steatosis as measured with transient elastography and transaminases on hard clinical outcomes in patients with COVID-19. *Therap. Adv. Gastroenterol.* **2021**, *14*, 17562848211016567. [CrossRef]
20. The Ministry of Health of the Republic of Croatia. Guidelines for Treatment of Patients with COVID-19, Version 2. 2020. Available online: https://zdravlje.gov.hr/UserDocsImages//2020%20CORONAVIRUS//Smjernice%20za%20lije%C4%8Denje%20oboljelih%20od%20koronavirusne%20bolesti%202019%20(COVID-19),%20verzija%202%20od%2019.%20studenoga%202020.pdf (accessed on 15 June 2021).
21. Subbe, C.P.; Kruger, M.; Rutherford, P.; Gemmel, L. Validation of a modified Early Warning Score in medical admissions. *QJM* **2001**, *94*, 521–526. [CrossRef]
22. Charlson, M.E.; Pompei, P.; Ales, K.L.; MacKenzie, C.R. A new method of classifying prognostic comorbidity in longitudinal studies: Development and validation. *J. Chronic Dis.* **1987**, *40*, 373–383. [CrossRef]

23. Oken, M.M.; Creech, R.H.; Tormey, D.C.; Horton, J.; Davis, T.E.; McFadden, E.T.; Carbone, P.P. Toxicity and response criteria of the Eastern Cooperative Oncology Group. *Am. J. Clin. Oncol.* **1982**, *5*, 649–655. [CrossRef] [PubMed]
24. Newsome, P.N.; Cramb, R.; Davison, S.M.; Dillon, J.F.; Foulerton, M.; Godfrey, E.M.; Hall, R.; Harrower, U.; Hudson, M.; Langford, A.; et al. Guidelines on the management of abnormal liver blood tests. *Gut* **2018**, *67*, 6–19. [CrossRef] [PubMed]
25. Hundt, M.A.; Deng, Y.; Ciarleglio, M.M.; Nathanson, M.H.; Lim, J.K. Abnormal Liver Tests in COVID-19: A Retrospective Observational Cohort Study of 1,827 Patients in a Major U.S. Hospital Network. *Hepatology* **2020**, *72*, 1169–1176. [CrossRef] [PubMed]
26. Sultan, S.; Altayar, O.; Siddique, S.M.; Davitkov, P.; Feuerstein, J.D.; Lim, J.K.; Falck-Ytter, Y.; El-Serag, H.B.; AGA Institute. AGA Institute Rapid Review of the Gastrointestinal and Liver Manifestations of COVID-19, Meta-Analysis of International Data, and Recommendations for the Consultative Management of Patients with COVID-19. *Gastroenterology* **2020**, *159*, 320–334.e27. [CrossRef] [PubMed]
27. Lv, Y.; Zhao, X.; Wang, Y.; Zhu, J.; Ma, C.; Feng, X.; Ma, Y.; Zheng, Y.; Yang, L.; Han, G.; et al. Abnormal Liver Function Tests Were Associated with Adverse Clinical Outcomes: An Observational Cohort Study of 2912 Patients with COVID-19. *Front. Med.* **2021**, *8*, 639855. [CrossRef] [PubMed]
28. Pirola, C.J.; Sookoian, S. SARS-CoV-2 virus and liver expression of host receptors: Putative mechanisms of liver involvement in COVID-19. *Liver Int.* **2020**, *40*, 2038–2040. [CrossRef]
29. Sonzogni, A.; Previtali, G.; Seghezzi, M.; Grazia Alessio, M.; Gianatti, A.; Licini, L.; Morotti, D.; Zerbi, P.; Carsana, L.; Rossi, R.; et al. Liver histopathology in severe COVID 19 respiratory failure is suggestive of vascular alterations. *Liver Int.* **2020**, *40*, 2110–2116. [CrossRef] [PubMed]
30. Nie, X.; Qian, L.; Sun, R.; Huang, B.; Dong, X.; Xiao, Q.; Zhang, Q.; Lu, T.; Yue, L.; Chen, S.; et al. Multi-organ proteomic landscape of COVID-19 autopsies. *Cell* **2021**, *184*, 775–791.e14. [CrossRef]
31. Wang, Y.; Liu, S.; Liu, H.; Li, W.; Lin, F.; Jiang, L.; Li, X.; Xu, P.; Zhang, L.; Zhao, L.; et al. SARS-CoV-2 infection of the liver directly contributes to hepatic impairment in patients with COVID-19. *J. Hepatol.* **2020**, *73*, 807–816. [CrossRef]
32. Roth, N.C.; Kim, A.; Vitkovski, T.; Xia, J.; Ramirez, G.; Bernstein, D.; Crawford, J.M. Post-COVID-19 Cholangiopathy: A Novel Entity. *Am. J. Gastroenterol.* **2021**, *116*, 1077–1082. [CrossRef] [PubMed]

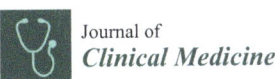

Article

Proinflammatory and Hepatic Features Related to Morbidity and Fatal Outcomes in COVID-19 Patients

Omar Ramos-Lopez [1,†], Rodrigo San-Cristobal [2,†], Diego Martinez-Urbistondo [3], Víctor Micó [4], Gonzalo Colmenarejo [5], Paula Villares-Fernandez [3], Lidia Daimiel [4] and J. Alfredo Martinez [2,6,7,8,*]

1. Medicine and Psychology School, Autonomous University of Baja California, Tijuana 22390, Mexico; oscar.omar.ramos.lopez@uabc.edu.mx
2. Precision Nutrition and Cardiometabolic Health, IMDEA Food Institute, CEI UAM+CSIC, 28049 Madrid, Spain; rodrigo.sancristobal@imdea.org
3. Hospital Universitario HM Sanchinarro, 28050 Madrid, Spain; dmurbistondo@gmail.com (D.M.-U.); pvillares@hmhospitales.com (P.V.-F.)
4. Nutritional Control of the Epigenome Group, IMDEA Food Institute, CEI UAM+CSIC, 28049 Madrid, Spain; victor.mico@imdea.org (V.M.); lidia.daimiel@imdea.org (L.D.)
5. Biostatistics and Bioinformatics Unit, IMDEA Food Institute, CEI UAM+CSIC, 28049 Madrid, Spain; gonzalo.colmenarejo@imdea.org
6. Department of Nutrition, Food Science, Physiology and Toxicology, Centre for Nutrition Research, University of Navarra, 31009 Pamplona, Spain
7. Navarra Institute for Health Research (IdiSNA), 31009 Pamplona, Spain
8. Spanish Biomedical Research Centre in Physiopathology of Obesity and Nutrition (CIBERobn), 28029 Madrid, Spain
* Correspondence: jalfredo.martinez@imdea.org; Tel.: +34-948-425600
† Both authors contributed equally to this work.

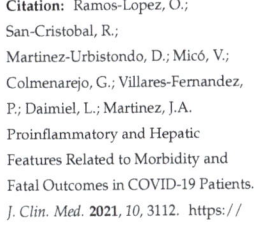

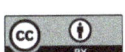

Copyright: © 2021 by the authors. Licensee MDPI, Basel, Switzerland. This article is an open access article distributed under the terms and conditions of the Creative Commons Attribution (CC BY) license (https://creativecommons.org/licenses/by/4.0/).

Abstract: Objective: to screen putative associations between liver markers and proinflammatory-related features concerning infectious morbidity and fatal outcomes in COVID-19 patients. Methods: a total of 2094 COVID-19 positive patients from the COVID-DATA-SAFE-LIFES cohort (HM hospitals consortium) were classified according to median values of hepatic, inflammatory, and clinical indicators. Logistic regression models were fitted and ROC cures were generated to explain disease severity and mortality. Results: intensive care unit (ICU) assistance plus death outcomes were associated with liver dysfunction, hyperinflammation, respiratory insufficiency, and higher associated comorbidities. Four models including age, sex, neutrophils, D-dimer, oxygen saturation lower than 92%, C-reactive protein (CRP), Charlson Comorbidity Index (CCI), FIB-4 and interactions with CRP, neutrophils, and CCI explained ICU plus death variance in more than 28%. The predictive values of ROC curves were: FIB-4 (0.7339), AST/ALT ratio (0.7107), CRP (0.7003), CCI index (0.6778), neutrophils (0.6772), and platelets (0.5618) concerning ICU plus death outcomes. Conclusions: the results of this research revealed that liver and proinflammatory features are important determinants of COVID-19 morbidity and fatal outcomes, which could improve the current understanding of the COVID-19 physiopathology as well as to facilitate the clinical management and therapy decision-making of this disease under a personalized medicine scope.

Keywords: liver markers; inflammation; morbidity; mortality; personalized medicine

1. Introduction

Coronavirus disease 2019 (COVID-19), caused by the Severe Acute Respiratory Syndrome Coronavirus 2 (SARS-COV-2), has being declared as a pandemic by the World Health Organization (WHO) in March 2020 based on the rises in the daily number of new cases, fast and ample spread, lethality, and the lack of effective antiviral treatments [1]. Since COVID-19 emergence in Wuhan, China, in December 2019, millions of COVID-19 cases have been reported worldwide, with a wide spectrum of respiratory presentations and multisystemic complications [2].

The excessive immunological reaction to the virus (known as "cytokine storm") by the host is largely responsible for the respiratory manifestations of COVID-19, encompassing pneumonia and acute respiratory distress syndrome (ARDS); however, in some patients this response may also involve hepatic, gastrointestinal, cardiac, renal, neurological, and hematological affectations [3]. Concerning liver injuries, large-scale case studies indicate that up to 11% of patients developed liver comorbidities, and more than 50% of cases reported abnormal levels of transaminases during disease progression, whereas liver dysfunction was more prevalent in severe COVID-19 patients [4]. In such patients, liver damage seems to be directly caused by the viral infection of liver cells, drug toxicity, and immune-mediated inflammation [5]. However, further studies are needed to understand and elucidate the precise causes of liver disease in COVID-19.

Until now, certain clinical, demographic, and phenotypical factors have been reported to be associated with the evolution and severity of COVID-19, encompassing age, sex, ethnicity, underlying medical conditions such as obesity, diabetes, and hypertension, poverty and crowding, pregnancy, and the use of certain medications and genetics [6,7]. Others include elevated levels of proinflammatory cytokines, liver enzymes, coagulation factors, body temperature, and unhealthy lifestyle such as smoking and alcoholic drinks consumption [8]. Nonetheless, there is a constant need for the search for easily accessible, rapid and accurate markers related to the course of COVID-19, which could contribute to improving the individualized clinical management and monitoring of the progression of this infection through an integrative precision medicine approach [9]. The aim of this research was to screen putative associations between available liver markers and proinflammatory-related features concerning infectious morbidity and fatal outcomes in COVID-19 patients.

2. Methods

2.1. Database and Study Variables

In this retrospective study, data from emergency admission of 2094 COVID-19 positive patients from the COVID-DATA-SAFE-LIFES cohort were analyzed. This cohort contains data on 2226 patients treated for COVID-19 in the HM group hospitals in the first wave of infections (March–May 2020), which has been made available to the international scientific community for study upon appropriate request and approval by a Committee expressly appointed by the hospital consortium (CEIm HM Hospitales Ref No. 20.05.1627-GHM) and under appropriate ethical protocols (Helsinki Declaration).

All data were recorded according to in-hospital protocols, which were harmonized and curated for further analysis in the R software (version 4.0.3). The study variables analyzed in this investigation at baseline comprised age, sex, oxygen saturation, leukocytes, lymphocytes, neutrophils, platelets, basophils, eosinophils, monocytes, C-reactive protein (CRP), D-dimer, fibrinogen, ferritin, procalcitonin, glucose, cholesterol, lactate dehydrogenase (LDH), gamma glutamyl transferase (GGT), aspartate aminotransferase or glutamic oxaloacetic transaminase (AST/GOT), and alanine transaminase or glutamate pyruvate transaminase (ALT/GPT). The following inflammatory-related ratios were calculated: international normalized ratio (INR), AST/ALT ratio (AAR), basophil-to-lymphocyte ratio (BLR), neutrophil-to-lymphocyte ratio (NLR), platelet-to-lymphocyte ratio (PLR), eosinophil-to-basophil ratio (EBR), eosinophil-to-lymphocyte ratio (ELR), and lymphocyte-to-monocyte ratio (LMR). Moreover, the Charlson Comorbidity Index (CCI) was computed to express the sum of co-morbidities. As non-invasive methods for predicting liver fibrosis [10], the following scores were calculated:

AST to Platelet Ratio Index (APRI): APRI = [(AST/upper limit of the normal AST range) × 100]/Platelet Count.

Fibrosis-4 index (FIB-4): FIB-4 = Age (years) × AST (U/L)/[platelet count(10^9/L) × ALT$^{1/2}$ (U/L)].

2.2. Statistical Analyses

Quantitative and qualitative variables were expressed as means ± standard deviations (SD) and as number and percentage, respectively. Chi-square and Student's t-test were applied to analyze differences between qualitative and quantitative variables, as appropriate. Death and ICU were combined and used as main outcomes since these are objective criteria of poor prognosis, as reported elsewhere [11]. Phenotypical and metabolic characteristics of the COVID-19 patients were compared by the median values of hepatic (FIB-4), inflammatory (CRP, neutrophils), and clinical markers (CCI index and oxygen saturation) by Student's *t*-test. Multivariable logistic regression models were fitted to explain disease severity and mortality, with age and sex as covariates. Age was excluded from the CCI index in the models to avoid colinearity. Statistical associations were calculated by univariate logistic regression tests. In addition, area under the receiver operating characteristic (ROC) curves were built to evaluate the predictive values of clinically relevant variables. Statistical analyses were performed in the statistical program Stata 12 (StataCorp LLC, College Station, TX, USA; www.stata.com (accessed on 2 May 2021)) and IBM SPSS 20 (IBM Inc., Armonk, NY, USA). Statistical significance was set at p value lower than 0.05, with bilateral test.

3. Results

The clinical and phenotypical characteristics of COVID-19 patients based on respiratory insufficiency, comorbidity, or need of intensive care plus mortality risk are reported (Table 1). On average, individuals with oxygen saturation lower than 92%, CCI index equal or higher than 3, and those who underwent ICU or who died were male, older and presented higher levels of leukocytes, neutrophils, CRP, D-dimer, LDH, FIB-4 as well as elevated ratios of AAR, basophil-to-lymphocyte, neutrophil-to-lymphocyte, platelet-to-lymphocyte, and lymphocyte-to-monocyte than their counterparts. Conversely, no differences between groups were observed for basophils, procalcitonin, glucose, cholesterol, and GPT measurements.

Similar features were found when compared the median values of inflammatory (CRP and neutrophils) and liver (FIB-4) markers in COVID-19 patients (Table 2).

Logistic regression models using relevant biochemical and clinical variables to predict ICU plus death outcome were constructed, with age and sex as covariates. Interestingly, four models were statistically significant ($p < 0.001$) and explained ICU plus death variance in more than 28% (Table 3a–d). The models included age, sex, neutrophils, D-dimer, oxygen saturation < 92%, CRP, CCI index, FIB-4, and the following interactions: CCI index × CRP (Table 3a); FIB-4 * CCI index (Table 3b); FIB-4 * CRP (Table 3c); and FIB-4 * neutrophils (Table 3d), respectively. The four interactions were statistically significant in the corresponding models.

Table 1. Clinical and phenotypical characteristics of COVID-19 patients based on respiratory insufficiency (oxygen saturation), comorbidities (CCI), and ICU plus death outcomes.

Variable	Oxygen Saturation (SO$_2$%)			CCI			ICU and Death		
	≥92% (n = 494)	<92% (n = 1314)	p	<3 (n = 781)	≥3 (n = 994)	p	No ICU + No Death (n = 1645)	ICU + Death (n = 449)	p
Age	66.7 ± 16.7	72.8 ± 13.4	<0.001	52.2 ± 13.4	76.3 ± 10.7	<0.001	64.4 ± 16.0	76.2 ± 14.1	<0.001
Sex (F/M)	548/766	176/318	0.019	281/500	428/566	0.003	677/968	148/301	0.002
CCI	2.90 ± 2.38	4.01 ± 2.41	<0.001	1.00 ± 0.83	4.87 ± 1.93	<0.001	2.70 ± 2.21	5.15 ± 2.55	<0.001
Oxygen saturation (SO$_2$%)	95.4 ± 2.0	84.4 ± 9.1	<0.001	94.0 ± 4.3	91.0 ± 8.3	<0.001	93.6 ± 5.1	87.2 ± 10.8	<0.001
Leukocytes (×10^9/L)	7.13 ± 3.77	9.09 ± 6.04	<0.001	6.89 ± 3.15	8.00 ± 5.32	<0.001	7.14 ± 3.63	9.62 ± 6.65	<0.001
Lymphocytes (×10^9/L)	1.27 ± 1.51	1.01 ± 0.79	<0.001	1.23 ± 0.60	1.15 ± 1.61	0.172	1.24 ± 1.30	1.04 ± 1.27	0.007
Neutrophils (×10^9/L)	5.22 ± 3.13	7.37 ± 4.55	<0.001	5.08 ± 2.98	6.16 ± 4.10	<0.001	5.30 ± 3.20	7.79 ± 4.90	<0.001
Platelets (×10^9/L)	219.4 ± 93.5	231.2 ± 98.4	0.023	225.6 ± 91.4	218.1 ± 94.9	0.107	227.4 ± 95.7	210.6 ± 100.1	0.004
Basophils (×10^9/L)	0.022 ± 0.021	0.022 ± 0.021	0.526	0.021 ± 0.022	0.022 ± 0.020	0.475	0.021 ± 0.020	0.022 ± 0.021	0.400
Eosinophils (×10^9/L)	0.05 ± 0.26	0.02 ± 0.06	0.032	0.04 ± 0.08	0.04 ± 0.29	0.527	0.05 ± 0.23	0.02 ± 0.05	0.036
Monocytes (×10^9/L)	0.56 ± 0.37	0.68 ± 3.30	0.254	0.52 ± 0.29	0.63 ± 2.44	0.241	0.54 ± 0.30	0.75 ± 3.67	0.044
CRP (mg/L)	79.3 ± 83.2	158.4 ± 113.8	<0.001	83.4 ± 85.0	114.7 ± 107.5	<0.001	87.3 ± 87.1	161.3 ± 124.8	<0.001
D-dimer (μg/mL)	1.97 ± 6.72	3.33 ± 8.80	0.003	1.08 ± 2.56	3.19 ± 10.04	<0.001	1.75 ± 5.5	4.92 ± 13.21	<0.001
Fibrinogen (mg/dL)	638.5 ± 175.3	772.9 ± 348.4	0.035	696.1 ± 209.6	683.4 ± 193.8	0.763	646.8 ± 176.3	776.4 ± 307.0	0.002
Ferritin (ng/mL)	867 ± 701	2870 ± 2931	<0.001	2030 ± 3427	1313 ± 1345	0.226	1363 ± 2213	1812 ± 1484	0.392
Procalcitonin (ng/mL)	0.08 ± 0.03	1.02 ± 2.01	0.157	0.33 ± 0.89	1.00 ± 1.76	0.142	0.41 ± 0.89	0.89 ± 1.64	0.209
Glucose (mg/dL)	208.0 ± 97.6	177.0 ± 30.7	0.545	128.5 ± 34.1	216.8 ± 102.5	0.117	200.2 ± 105.7	169.0 ± 60.0	0.545
Cholesterol (mg/dL)	142.7 ± 31.5	144.5 ± 2.1	0.943	142.0 ± 4.2	142.8 ± 25.7	0.971	145.0 ± 39.6	133.1 ± 31.1	0.734
LDH (U/L)	546.1 ± 257.7	786.6 ± 411.2	<0.001	562.3 ± 256.0	646.9 ± 406.9	<0.001	563.5 ± 249.3	816.1 ± 570.5	<0.001
GGT (U/L)	74.2 ± 91.4	157.0 ± 345.4	0.025	74.5 ± 93.3	74.0 ± 170.0	0.978	74.4 ± 90.1	89.2 ± 211.7	0.420
GOT (U/L)	43.1 ± 110.9	58.7 ± 90.9	0.012	44.3 ± 32.9	50.9 ± 141.6	0.265	42.4 ± 32.8	66.6 ± 208.2	<0.001
GPT (U/L)	37.5 ± 82.5	46.3 ± 66.0	0.054	45.7 ± 46.1	38.5 ± 100.2	0.108	39.5 ± 40.6	45.9 ± 144.1	0.178
INR ratio	1.43 ± 1.25	1.43 ± 1.18	0.995	1.25 ± 0.49	1.55 ± 1.75	<0.001	1.34 ± 0.99	1.69 ± 2.10	<0.001
AAR ratio	1.39 ± 0.72	1.56 ± 0.74	<0.001	1.17 ± 0.51	1.58 ± 0.76	<0.001	1.32 ± 0.66	1.74 ± 0.76	<0.001
APRI score	0.59 ± 1.34	0.72 ± 0.77	0.073	0.57 ± 0.54	0.68 ± 1.55	0.105	0.55 ± 0.54	0.89 ± 2.24	<0.001
FIB-4 score	2.66 ± 3.00	3.31 ± 2.75	<0.001	1.86 ± 1.20	3.51 ± 3.66	<0.001	2.43 ± 2.22	4.24 ± 4.48	<0.001
BLR	0.02 ± 0.02	0.03 ± 0.06	<0.001	0.02 ± 0.02	0.02 ± 0.05	<0.001	0.02 ± 0.03	0.03 ± 0.04	<0.001
NLR	5.57 ± 5.27	10.78 ± 18.67	<0.001	5.18 ± 4.48	8.24 ± 14.32	<0.001	5.92 ± 10.64	11.43 ± 10.76	<0.001
PLR	220.1 ± 139.5	303.8 ± 315.0	<0.001	213.7 ± 126.5	264.6 ± 253.9	<0.001	230.8 ± 198.1	296.5 ± 225.0	<0.001
EBR	1.87 ± 4.31	1.06 ± 2.35	<0.001	1.61 ± 2.85	1.66 ± 4.58	0.800	1.89 ± 4.19	1.01 ± 2.47	<0.001
ELR	0.03 ± 0.10	0.02 ± 0.05	0.054	0.02 ± 0.04	0.03 ± 0.11	0.024	0.03 ± 0.09	0.02 ± 0.06	0.119
LMR	2.71 ± 2.07	2.33 ± 1.56	<0.001	2.82 ± 1.74	2.40 ± 1.70	<0.001	2.66 ± 1.83	2.43 ± 2.23	0.040

Values are expressed as means ± standard deviations. *p* values were calculated by Student's *t*-tests. Bold numbers indicate *p* value lower than 0.05. F: female; M: male; CCI: Charlson Comorbidity Index; CRP: C-reactive protein; LDH: lactate dehydrogenase; GGT: gamma glutamyl transferase; GOT: glutamic oxaloacetic transaminase; GPT: glutamate pyruvate transaminase; INR: international normalized ratio; AAR: AST/ALT ratio; APRI: AST to Platelet Ratio Index; FIB-4: Fibrosis-4 index; BLR: basophil-to-lymphocyte ratio; NLR: neutrophil-to-lymphocyte ratio; PLR: platelet-to-lymphocyte ratio; EBR: eosinophil-to-basophil ratio; ELR: eosinophil-to-lymphocyte ratio; LMR: lymphocyte-to-monocyte ratio.

Table 2. Clinical and phenotypical characteristics of COVID-19 patients based on median values of inflammatory and liver features.

Variable	CRS <73.67 (n = 933)	CRP ≥73.67 (n = 934)	p	Neutrophils <4.89 (n = 976)	Neutrophils ≥4.89 (n = 982)	p	FIB-4 <2.17 (n = 810)	FIB-4 ≥2.17 (n = 818)	p
Age	65.1 ± 17.2	69.9 ± 14.5	<0.001	65.2 ± 16.0	69.8 ± 15.7	<0.001	61.0 ± 15.8	74.3 ± 13.0	<0.001
Sex (F/M)	425/508	315/618	<0.001	416/560	363/618	0.003	350/460	281/537	<0.001
CCI	2.86 ± 2.42	3.42 ± 2.33	<0.001	2.87 ± 2.34	3.43 ± 2.46	<0.001	2.36 ± 2.28	4.01 ± 2.29	<0.001
Oxygen saturation (SO$_2$%)	94.4 ± 4.0	89.8 ± 4.4	<0.001	93.9 ± 4.5	90.3 ± 8.4	<0.001	93.1 ± 6.0	90.8 ± 8.0	<0.001
Leukocytes (×10^9/L)	6.58 ± 3.46	8.66 ± 5.11	<0.001	5.07 ± 2.98	10.20 ± 4.27	<0.001	8.15 ± 3.99	7.18 ± 4.99	<0.001
Lymphocytes (×10^9/L)	1.37 ± 1.61	0.99 ± 0.66	<0.001	1.18 ± 0.72	1.19 ± 1.62	0.172	1.28 ± 0.81	1.07 ± 1.70	0.002
Neutrophils (×10^9/L)	4.57 ± 2.71	7.01 ± 4.18	<0.001	3.31 ± 0.95	8.30 ± 3.80	<0.001	6.17 ± 3.76	5.51 ± 3.55	<0.001
Platelets (×10^9/L)	217.9 ± 94.9	231.7 ± 98.5	0.002	195.1 ± 80.1	254.2 ± 104.4	0.107	275.1 ± 102.8	177.0 ± 59.9	<0.001
Basophils (×10^9/L)	0.021 ± 0.022	0.022 ± 0.020	0.527	0.017 ± 0.018	0.024 ± 0.021	0.475	0.025 ± 0.021	0.017 ± 0.016	<0.001
Eosinophils (×10^9/L)	0.06 ± 0.28	0.03 ± 0.05	0.001	0.03 ± 0.07	0.04 ± 0.27	0.527	0.06 ± 0.30	0.02 ± 0.05	<0.001
Monocytes (×10^9/L)	0.56 ± 0.31	0.60 ± 2.34	0.548	0.52 ± 2.31	0.63 ± 0.41	0.241	0.60 ± 0.32	0.56 ± 2.50	0.692
CRP (mg/L)	31.2 ± 21.4	173.6 ± 97.4	<0.001	62.9 ± 61.1	142.3 ± 115.1	<0.001	95.8 ± 103.3	113.4 ± 98.6	<0.001
D-dimer (µg/mL)	1.66 ± 4.82	3.04 ± 9.60	0.001	1.37 ± 4.45	3.35 ± 9.79	<0.001	2.00 ± 5.59	2.76 ± 8.95	0.065
Fibrinogen (mg/dL)	553.4 ± 122.4	812.3 ± 240.8	<0.001	627.9 ± 187.0	725.7 ± 255.1	0.763	687.2 ± 254.6	692.3 ± 221.7	0.903
Ferritin (ng/mL)	724 ± 632	2011 ± 2566	<0.001	1046 ± 1474	1791 ± 2437	0.226	1414 ± 2243	1474 ± 1872	0.883
Procalcitonin (ng/mL)	0.09 ± 0.04	0.77 ± 1.40	0.100	0.10 ± 0.06	0.92 ± 1.52	0.142	0.51 ± 1.35	0.74 ± 1.10	0.547
Glucose (mg/dL)	199.8 ± 82.6	199.6 ± 126.5	0.117	194.1 ± 83.3	182.1 ± 110.2	0.117	177.4 ± 128.6	201.1 ± 79.7	0.670
Cholesterol (mg/dL)	162.5 ± 23.3	125.2 ± 28.8	0.997	127.5 ± 72.8	137.9 ± 99.4	0.971	137.6 ± 33.6	134.5 ± 16.3	0.980
LDH (U/L)	521.2 ± 311.0	714.8 ± 362.8	<0.001	554.4 ± 299.9	682.8 ± 389.4	<0.001	536.4 ± 218.7	712.2 ± 445.2	<0.001
GGT (U/L)	49.9 ± 48.7	101.9 ± 173.5	<0.001	56.6 ± 59.4	97.5 ± 177.5	0.978	81.5 ± 102.5	69.1 ± 157.6	0.404
GOT (U/L)	38.8 ± 30.2	55.7 ± 134.3	<0.001	41.1 ± 29.5	53.7 ± 135.5	0.265	34.3 ± 23.6	61.2 ± 137.2	<0.001
GPT (U/L)	36.1 ± 40.7	44.8 ± 96.5	0.020	34.5 ± 33.0	46.4 ± 99.4	0.108	38.0 ± 42.4	43.2 ± 96.9	0.159
INR ratio	1.34 ± 1.04	1.48 ± 1.44	0.050	1.34 ± 0.97	1.50 ± 1.56	<0.001	1.36 ± 1.34	1.47 ± 1.31	0.144
AAR ratio	1.40 ± 1.32	1.50 ± 0.67	0.054	1.45 ± 0.70	1.44 ± 1.27	<0.001	1.14 ± 0.51	1.76 ± 1.30	<0.001
APRI score	0.54 ± 0.53	0.70 ± 1.50	0.003	0.63 ± 0.65	0.61 ± 1.47	0.105	0.34 ± 0.22	0.92 ± 1.55	<0.001
FIB-4 score	2.52 ± 2.24	3.12 ± 3.29	<0.001	3.01 ± 2.66	2.67 ± 3.15	<0.001	1.37 ± 0.48	4.30 ± 3.54	<0.001
Bas/Lym ratio	0.02 ± 0.03	0.03 ± 0.04	<0.001	0.01 ± 0.02	0.02 ± 0.04	<0.001	0.02 ± 0.04	0.02 ± 0.03	0.027
Neu/Lym ratio	4.52 ± 5.45	9.64 ± 14.02	<0.001	3.54 ± 2.62	10.56 ± 14.18	<0.001	6.97 ± 14.29	7.52 ± 7.77	0.337
Plat/Lym ratio	199.8 ± 141.9	295.8 ± 255.8	<0.001	199.1 ± 128.4	293.6 ± 258.3	<0.001	274.3 ± 264.9	231.4 ± 165.1	<0.001
Eos/Bas ratio	2.21 ± 4.86	1.20 ± 2.34	<0.001	1.88 ± 3.29	1.54 ± 4.24	0.800	2.13 ± 4.69	1.24 ± 2.90	<0.001
Eos/Lym ratio	0.04 ± 0.11	0.03 ± 0.05	0.010	0.02 ± 0.05	0.03 ± 0.10	0.024	0.041 ± 0.114	0.020 ± 0.051	<0.001
Lym/Mon ratio	2.82 ± 1.76	2.44 ± 2.04	<0.001	3.04 ± 1.78	2.18 ± 1.93	<0.001	2.60 ± 1.84	2.65 ± 2.07	0.557

Values are expressed as means ± standard deviations. p values were calculated by Student's t-tests. Bold numbers indicate p value lower than 0.05. F: female; M: male; CCI: Charlson Comorbidity Index; CRP: C-reactive protein; LDH: lactate dehydrogenase; GGT: gamma glutamyl transferase; GOT: glutamic oxaloacetic transaminase; GPT: glutamate pyruvate transaminase; INR: international normalized ratio; AAR: AST/ALT ratio; APRI: AST to Platelet Ratio Index; FIB-4: Fibrosis-4 index; BLR: basophil-to-lymphocyte ratio; NLR: neutrophil-to-lymphocyte ratio; PLR: platelet-to-lymphocyte ratio; EBR: eosinophil-to-basophil ratio; ELR: eosinophil-to-lymphocyte ratio; LMR: lymphocyte-to-monocyte ratio.

Table 3. (a) Multiple logistic regression model using clinical, inflammatory and liver markers as important predictors of mortality plus ICU in COVID-19 patients: interaction between CCI and CRP. (b) Multiple logistic regression model using clinical, inflammatory and liver markers as important predictors of mortality plus ICU in COVID-19 patients: interaction between FIB-4 and CCI. (c) Multiple logistic regression model using clinical, inflammatory and liver markers as important predictors of mortality plus ICU in COVID-19 patients: interaction between FIB-4 and CRP. (d) Multiple logistic regression model using clinical, inflammatory and liver markers as important predictors of mortality plus ICU in COVID-19 patients: interaction between FIB-4 and NEU.

(a)		
Variable	**β Coefficients (CI 95%)**	***p***
Age (years)	0.0653 (0.0464, 0.0842)	**<0.001**
Sex (Female)	−0.5413 (−1.0090, −0.0735)	**0.023**
Neutrophils ($\times 10^9$/L)	0.0972 (0.0370, 0.1574)	**0.002**
D-dimer (μg/mL)	0.0218 (−0.0037, 0.0472)	0.093
Oxygen saturation (SO$_2$ < 92%)	0.6359 (0.1909, 1.0809)	**0.005**
FIB-4	0.2080 (0.1046, 0.3113)	**<0.001**
CCI * CRP	0.0013 (0.0007, 0.0018)	**<0.001**
R^2	0.3093	**<0.001**
(b)		
Variable	**β coefficients (CI 95%)**	***p***
Age (years)	0.0776 (0.0598, 0.0955)	**<0.001**
Sex (Female)	−0.6635 (−1.1213, −0.2056)	**0.005**
Neutrophils ($\times 10^9$/L)	0.0595 (−0.0026, 0.1216)	0.060
D-dimer (μg/mL)	0.0249 (−0.0009, 0.0507)	0.059
Oxygen saturation (SO$_2$ < 92%)	0.6374 (0.1976, 1.0772)	**0.005**
CRP (mg/L)	0.0039 (0.0017, 0.0061)	**<0.001**
FIB-4 * CCI (no age)	0.0307 (0.0137, 0.0477)	**<0.001**
R^2	0.2838	**<0.001**
(c)		
Age (years)	0.0655 (0.0471, 0.0839)	**<0.001**
Sex (Female)	−0.5982 (−1.0728, −0.1236)	**0.013**
Neutrophils ($\times 10^9$/L)	0.0763 (0.0205, 0.1321)	**0.007**
D-dimer (μg/mL)	0.0227 (−0.0027, 0.0482)	0.080
Oxygen saturation (SO$_2$ < 92%)	0.5183 (0.0658, 0.9709)	**0.025**
CCI (no age)	0.2094 (0.0962, 0.3226)	**<0.001**
FIB-4 * CRP	0.0014 (0.0009, 0.0020)	**<0.001**
R^2	0.3134	**<0.001**
(d)		
Age (years)	0.0601 (0.0408, 0.0793)	**<0.001**
Sex (Female)	−0.5279 (−1.0003, -0.0555)	**0.028**
CRP (mg/L)	0.0032 (0.0012, 0.0053)	**0.002**
D-dimer (μg/mL)	0.0225 (−0.0027, 0.0477)	0.080
Oxygen saturation (SO$_2$ < 92%)	0.5081 (0.0519, 0.9642)	**0.029**
CCI (no age)	0.2202 (0.1077, 0.3327)	**<0.001**
FIB-4 * NEU	0.0383 (0.0210, 0.0556)	**<0.001**
R^2	0.3151	**<0.001**

Bold numbers indicate $p < 0.05$.

The empirical frequencies and odds ratios (OR) of ICU plus death by the cutoffs (median) values of CRP, CCI index, FIB-4, neutrophils, platelets, and AAR ratio are depicted (Figure 1a–f). Compared to patients who did not enter to ICU and did not die, higher risks of ICU plus death were found when CRP levels were equal or higher than 73.67 mg/L (OR = 3.475, $p < 0.001$, Figure 1a); CCI index equal or higher than 3 (OR = 8.040, $p < 0.001$, Figure 1b); FIB-4 score equal or higher than 2.17 (OR = 3.590, $p < 0.001$, Figure 1c); neutrophils equal or higher than 4.89 × 10^9/L (OR = 2.539, $p < 0.001$, Figure 1d); and AAR ratio equal or higher than 1.29 (OR = 3.320, $p < 0.001$, Figure 1f). Instead, platelets equal or higher than 205×10^9/L protected for ICU pus death (OR = 0.723, $p = 0.013$, Figure 1e).

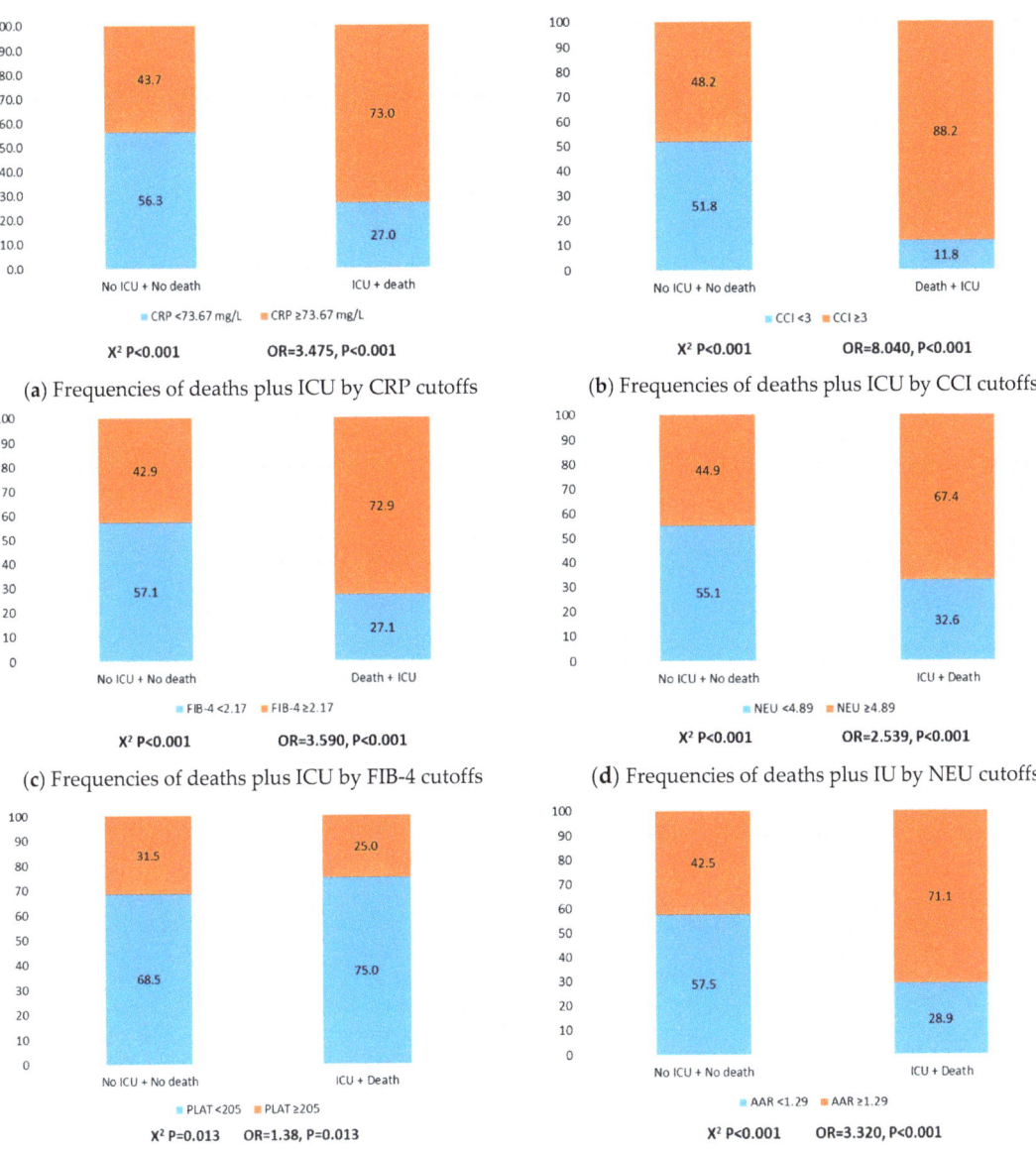

Figure 1. Frequencies and odds ratios (OR) of ICU plus death by the cutoffs (median) values of CRP, CCI index, FIB-4, neutrophils, platelets, and AAR ratio.

ROC curves were constructed to estimate and compare the predictive value of liver and proinflammatory markers concerning ICU plus death (Figure 2). The best predictor was FIB-4 (0.7339), followed by AAR (0.7107), CRP (0.7003), CCI index (0.6778), neutrophils (0.6772), and platelets (0.5618), all of them statistically significant ($p < 0.001$).

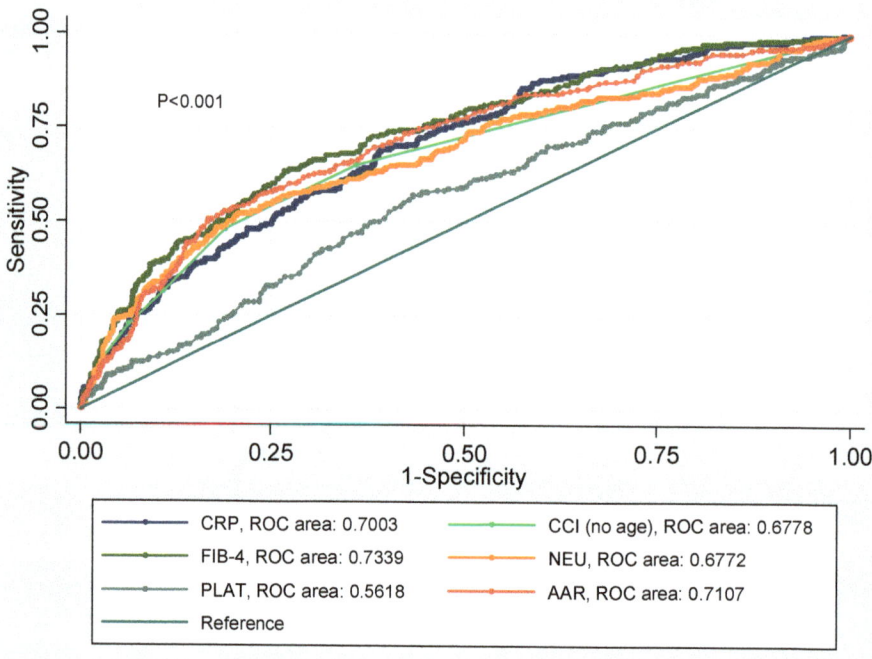

Figure 2. ROC curves showing the predictive value of CCI (no age), CRP, NEU, FIB-4, PLAT, and AAR concerning COVID-19 outcomes (ICU plus Death).

4. Discussion

As a result of the increased availability of data and collaborations between researchers, efforts have been made for the evaluation of laboratory tests and other phenotypical information as biomarkers related to COVID-19 disease severity [9]. This study should be considered a proof of concept, where biochemical and clinical variables significantly explained morbid and fatal outcomes in COVID-19 patients, including neutrophils, CRP, oxygen saturation < 92%, FIB-4, D-dimer and CCI index, which evidence the involvement of predominately liver and proinflammatory features in the evolution of this disease. These findings may enable early categorization of infected patients based on the risk of death or intensive care assistance, thus facilitating a more precise clinical management as well as the optimization of health resources and medical personnel [7].

In agreement with our results, neutrophils have been highlighted as essential effector cells in COVID-19 physiopathology through the stimulation of a hyperinflammation state in the lungs by enhanced degranulation of primary granules and the secretion of proinflammatory cytokines as well as the induction of oxidative stress via reactive oxygen species release [12]. In this context, bioinformatic analyses revealed that neutrophil activation is one of the most stimulated biological processes in the SARS-CoV infection [13]. Moreover, it has been reported the association of NLR with critical illness in COVID-19 patients [14].

Likewise, some investigations have confirmed the utility of CRP as prognostic factor in COVID-19 since it serves as an early marker of infection, inflammation, and tissue damage [15]. For example, CRP levels were independent discriminators of severe/critical illness on admission and a good predictor of adverse outcome in COVID-19 patients [16]. In hospitalized patients, median CRP values (206 mg/L) were significantly higher in the patients who died compared to those who survived, and increased linearly during the first week of hospitalization, which supports the utility of daily CRP monitoring in risk prognostication [17]. Accordingly, it has been documented that the risk of developing severe events in COVID-19 patients is increased by about 5% for every one-unit increase in CRP levels [18]. Interestingly, elevated levels of CRP (76.51 mg/L) correlated with lower oxygen saturation (<90%), indicating a relationship of these markers and a complementary utility in the prognosis of COVID-19 disease [19]. Indeed, oxygen saturation levels below 92% significantly contributed to predict ICU plus death in this sample. This hallmark is in agreement with the criteria for diagnosis of COVID-19-associated pneumonia and disease severity [20], as postulated in the guidelines of the World Health Organization for the Clinical Management of COVID-19 (https://apps.who.int/iris/handle/10665/332196 (accessed on 2 May 2021)). Certainly, 92% is under the current target oxygen saturation range (92–96%) for patients with COVID-19 recommended by the National Institutes of Health (https://www.covid19treatmentguidelines.nih.gov/critical-care/oxygenation-and-ventilation/ (accessed on 2 May 2021)).

Another important finding of this study was the interplay of FIB-4 in COVID-19 disease severity by interacting with proinflammatory and comorbid features. Thus, two statistical interactions were found concerning FIB-4 and inflammatory markers, where a higher FIB-4 score combined with increased levels of neutrophils and CRP were associated with more instances of ICU plus death (data not shown). These results suggest that an elevated FIB-4 score exacerbates the progression of the inflammatory process, and also suggests an organ-specific influence of inflammation as a prognostic marker. Besides, a significant interaction between CCI and FIB-4 in relation to death plus ICU was found in this research (data not shown), which suggest that when FIB-4 is low, the CCI dominates the entry to ICU admission and the risk of death; however, when FIB-4 is high (above 20), a preservative effect is found. This finding may be explained by the fact that the set of comorbidities (measured by CCI) has a greater influence on the outcomes of patients with COVID-19 than only liver fibrosis (measured by FIB-4). FIB-4 is not only an accurate marker of liver fibrosis, but it is also related to coagulation and oxidative stress since it takes into account age and the serum levels of transaminases (ALT and AST) and platelets, all of which have been consistently identified as potential risk factors of severe cases with COVID-19 in a recent meta-analysis [21]. Furthermore, elevation of this FIB-4 (equal or higher than 2.67) was associated with poor clinical outcomes in middle-aged patients with COVID-19, including required mechanical ventilation and ICU admission [22]. Moreover, FIB-4 was also related with increased risk of mortality in hospitalized patients with COVID-19 as well as with lower survival [23,24]. In addition, FIB-4 positively correlated to SARS-CoV-2 viral load and the levels of inflammatory cytokines [25]. Besides FIB-4, AAR was another liver marker also associated (equal or higher than 1.29) with an increased risk of ICU plus death in this research. Similarly, a retrospective study reported that AAR higher than 1 highly correlated with liver injury in conjunction with other proinflammatory variables [26]. Despite more investigation in this fled is necessary, these results evidence the involvement of liver damage in the evolution of COVID-19 and highlight the importance of evaluate liver status in the clinical setting. Although the role of liver disease in COVID-19 remains unclear, it has been hypothesized that liver injury is associated with innate immune dysfunction, which could enhance susceptibility to an acute proinflammatory response (cytokine storm) leading to severe outcomes in patients with COVID-19 by exacerbating the hyperinflammatory state [27,28]. Of note, although the presence of previous liver disease might artifact our findings, the low prevalence in the population (only 53 patients with liver disease) might reduce the confounding effect of this issue. In fact, no significant differences in the performance of the statistical models were found when patients with liver disease were removed.

In relation to the association of abnormal coagulation parameters with poor outcomes in COVID-19 patients, a meta-analysis evidenced that patients with a composite clinical end point, defined as all-cause mortality, ICU admission or ARDS, had elevated levels of D-dimer (standard mean difference of 1.67 µg/mL) than their counterparts [29]. In fact, results from another meta-analysis of 13 cohort studies revealed that severe COVID-19 infection was related to D-dimer higher than 0.5 µg/mL on admission [30].

Regarding comorbidity, in this study, the CCI index was included in the predictive models of ICU plus death mainly as an adjustment variable. The CCI has been commonly used in clinical research as a correction factor in a set of prognostic models due to proven consistency, validity, and reliability as supported by the results of several studies. In COVID-19, multivariate regression analysis showed that CCI was a prognostic factor for COVID-19-related mortality in patients hospitalized for pneumonia [31]. Additionally, CCI score above 0 was associated with an increased risk of severe outcome and death after controlled for age and sex [32]. In a meta-analysis, a 16% higher risk of mortality was attributed by each per point increase of CCI score [33].

On the one hand, the strengths of this investigation include a large sample screened and the use of robust statistical approaches for data depuration and the comparative predictive analyses. In this context, on the most important findings of this research is the integration of different predictors of COVID-19 outcomes including liver and pro-inflammatory features as well as the screening of potential interactions among these factors, which suggest that the prognostic value of these markers depends upon the behavior of concomitant variables influencing COVID-19 disease and that there is a mutual influence concerning the result. On the other hand, the fact that the population analyzed in this study has mainly European ancestry, the findings of this study could not be applied to groups with other ethnicity and exposed to diverse environmental factors. For instance, in Latin America, variables such as the high rates of obesity, the adoption of hepatopathogenic diets, and a sedentary lifestyle could exacerbate liver damage and a hyperinflammatory state in COVID-19 [34]. Moreover, the exploration of other variables influencing liver health and the immune response including the gut microbiota, genetic background, epigenetic signatures, metabolomic profiles, and interactions with specific lifestyle factors could be part of the scenario [35]. Additionally, although hyperinflammation worse COVID-19 infection, caution must be taken concerning the interpretation of the results since there can be wide fluctuations in levels of inflammatory markers during the time frame from admission to collection of labs.

In conclusion, the results of this research suggest that liver and proinflammatory features are important determinants of COVID-19 morbid and fatal outcomes. This information could contribute to improve the current comprehension of the COVID-19 physiopathology and the clinical management and therapy decision-making of this disease under a precision medicine approach [36]. Current results evidence that the hepatic responses may have a role in prognosis, treatment, and understanding of COVID-19.

Author Contributions: Conceptualization, O.R.-L. and J.A.M.; formal analysis, R.S.-C., G.C., V.M., L.D., D.M.-U. and P.V.-F.; investigation, O.R.-L., J.A.M., R.S.-C., G.C., V.M., L.D., D.M.-U., and P.V.-F.; data curation, R.S.-C. and V.M.; original draft preparation, O.R.-L., J.A.M.; supervision, D.M.-U. and P.V.-F. All authors have read and agreed to the published version of the manuscript.

Funding: R.S.-C. acknowledges financial support from the Juan de la Cierva Program Training Grants of the Spanish State Research Agency of the Spanish Ministerio de Ciencia e Innovación y Ministerio de Universidades (FJC2018-038168-I).

Institutional Review Board Statement: The study was conducted according to the guidelines of the Declaration of Helsinki, and approved by the Ethics Committee of the HM hospitals consortium (CEIm HM Hospitales Ref No. 20.05.1627-GHM).

Informed Consent Statement: Informed consent was obtained from all subjects involved in the study.

Data Availability Statement: The data presented in this study are available on request from the corresponding author.

Acknowledgments: Authors thank HM hospitals for access to the COVID-DATA-SAFE-LIFES database.

Conflicts of Interest: The authors declare that they have no conflict of interest concerning this investigation.

References

1. Tay, M.Z.; Poh, C.M.; Rénia, L.; MacAry, P.A.; Ng, L.F.P. The trinity of COVID-19: Immunity, inflammation and intervention. *Nat. Rev. Immunol.* **2020**, *20*, 363–374. [CrossRef]
2. Huang, C.; Wang, Y.; Li, X.; Ren, L.; Zhao, J.; Hu, Y.; Zhang, L.; Fan, G.; Xu, J.; Gu, X.; et al. Clinical features of patients infected with 2019 novel coronavirus in Wuhan, China. *Lancet* **2020**, *395*, 497–506. [CrossRef]
3. Lai, C.C.; Ko, W.C.; Lee, P.I.; Jean, S.S.; Hsueh, P.R. Extra-respiratory manifestations of COVID-19. *Int. J. Antimicrob. Agents* **2020**, *56*, 106024. [CrossRef]
4. Zhang, C.; Shi, L.; Wang, F.S. Liver injury in COVID-19: Management and challenges. *Lancet Gastroenterol. Hepatol.* **2020**, *5*, 428–430. [CrossRef]
5. Cha, M.H.; Regueiro, M.; Sandhu, D.S. Gastrointestinal and hepatic manifestations of COVID-19: A comprehensive review. *World J. Gastroenterol.* **2020**, *26*, 2323–2332. [CrossRef]
6. Rod, J.E.; Oviedo-Trespalacios, O.; Cortes-Ramirez, J. A brief-review of the risk factors for covid-19 severity. *Rev. Saude Publica* **2020**, *54*, 60. [CrossRef]
7. Ramos-Lopez, O.; Daimiel, L.; Ramírez de Molina, A.; Martínez-Urbistondo, D.; Vargas, J.A.; Martínez, J.A. Exploring Host Genetic Polymorphisms Involved in SARS-CoV Infection Outcomes: Implications for Personalized Medicine in COVID-19. *Int. J. Genom.* **2020**, *2020*, 6901217. [CrossRef] [PubMed]
8. Martinez-Urbistondo, M.; Mora-Vargas, A.; Expósito-Palomo, E.; Castejón, R.; Citores, M.J.; Rosado, S.; de Mendoza, C.; Baños, I.; Fernández-Cruz, A.; Daimiel, L.; et al. Inflammatory-Related Clinical and Metabolic Outcomes in COVID-19 Patients. *Mediat. Inflamm.* **2020**, *2020*, 2914275. [CrossRef] [PubMed]
9. Moradian, N.; Ochs, H.D.; Sedikies, C.; Hamblin, M.R.; Camargo, C.A., Jr.; Martinez, J.A.; Biamonte, J.D.; Abdollahi, M.; Torres, P.J.; Nieto, J.J.; et al. The urgent need for integrated science to fight COVID-19 pandemic and beyond. *J. Transl. Med.* **2020**, *18*, 205. [CrossRef] [PubMed]
10. Martinez-Urbistondo, D.; Suarez Del Villar, R.; Argemí, J.; Daimiel, L.; Ramos-López, O.; San-Cristobal, R.; Villares, P.; Martinez, J.A. Antioxidant Lifestyle, Co-Morbidities and Quality of Life Empowerment Concerning Liver Fibrosis. *Antioxidants* **2020**, *9*, 1125. [CrossRef] [PubMed]
11. Armstrong, R.A.; Kane, A.D.; Cook, T.M. Outcomes from intensive care in patients with COVID-19: A systematic review and meta-analysis of observational studies. *Anaesthesia* **2020**, *75*, 1340–1349. [CrossRef] [PubMed]
12. Cavalcante-Silva, L.H.A.; Carvalho, D.C.M.; Lima, É.A.; Galvão, J.G.F.M.; da Silva, J.S.F.; Sales-Neto, J.M.; Rodrigues-Mascarenhas, S. Neutrophils and COVID-19: The road so far. *Int. Immunopharmacol.* **2020**, *90*, 107233. [CrossRef]
13. Hemmat, N.; Derakhshani, A.; Bannazadeh Baghi, H.; Silvestris, N.; Baradaran, B.; De Summa, S. Neutrophils, Crucial, or Harmful Immune Cells Involved in Coronavirus Infection: A Bioinformatics Study. *Front. Genet.* **2020**, *11*, 641. [CrossRef] [PubMed]
14. Liu, J.; Liu, Y.; Xiang, P.; Pu, L.; Xiong, H.; Li, C.; Zhang, M.; Tan, J.; Xu, Y.; Song, R.; et al. Neutrophil-to-lymphocyte ratio predicts critical illness patients with 2019 coronavirus disease in the early stage. *J. Transl. Med.* **2020**, *18*, 206. [CrossRef] [PubMed]
15. Ali, N. Elevated level of C-reactive protein may be an early marker to predict risk for severity of COVID-19. *J. Med. Virol.* **2020**, *92*, 2409–2411. [CrossRef] [PubMed]
16. Luo, X.; Zhou, W.; Yan, X.; Guo, T.; Wang, B.; Xia, H.; Ye, L.; Xiong, J.; Jiang, Z.; Liu, Y.; et al. Prognostic Value of C-Reactive Protein in Patients with Coronavirus 2019. *Clin. Infect. Dis.* **2020**, *71*, 2174–2179. [CrossRef]
17. Sharifpour, M.; Rangaraju, S.; Liu, M.; Alabyad, D.; Nahab, F.B.; Creel-Bulos, C.M.; Jabaley, C.S.; Emory COVID-19 Quality & Clinical Research Collaborative. C-Reactive protein as a prognostic indicator in hospitalized patients with COVID-19. *PLoS ONE* **2020**, *15*, e0242400. [CrossRef]
18. Wang, G.; Wu, C.; Zhang, Q.; Wu, F.; Yu, B.; Lv, J.; Li, Y.; Li, T.; Zhang, S.; Wu, C.; et al. C-Reactive Protein Level May Predict the Risk of COVID-19 Aggravation. *Open Forum Infect. Dis.* **2020**, *7*, ofaa153. [CrossRef]
19. Xie, J.; Covassin, N.; Fan, Z.; Singh, P.; Gao, W.; Li, G.; Kara, T.; Somers, V.K. Association Between Hypoxemia and Mortality in Patients With COVID-19. *Mayo Clin. Proc.* **2020**, *95*, 1138–1147. [CrossRef]
20. Shenoy, N.; Luchtel, R.; Gulani, P. Considerations for target oxygen saturation in COVID-19 patients: Are we under-shooting? *BMC Med.* **2020**, *18*, 260. [CrossRef] [PubMed]
21. Ou, M.; Zhu, J.; Ji, P.; Li, H.; Zhong, Z.; Li, B.; Pang, J.; Zhang, J.; Zheng, X. Risk factors of severe cases with COVID-19: A meta-analysis. *Epidemiol. Infect.* **2020**, *148*, e175. [CrossRef] [PubMed]
22. Ibáñez-Samaniego, L.; Bighelli, F.; Usón, C.; Caravaca, C.; Carrillo, C.F.; Romero, M.; Barreales, M.; Perelló, C.; Madejón, A.; Marcos, A.C.; et al. Elevation of Liver Fibrosis Index FIB-4 Is Associated With Poor Clinical Outcomes in Patients With COVID-19. *J. Infect. Dis.* **2020**, *222*, 726–733. [CrossRef] [PubMed]
23. Sterling, R.K.; Oakes, T.; Gal, T.S.; Stevens, M.P.; deWit, M.; Sanyal, A.J. The Fibrosis-4 Index Is Associated With Need for Mechanical Ventilation and 30-Day Mortality in Patients Admitted With Coronavirus Disease 2019. *J. Infect. Dis.* **2020**, *222*, 1794–1797. [CrossRef]

24. Park, J.G.; Kang, M.K.; Lee, Y.R.; Song, J.E.; Kim, N.Y.; Kweon, Y.O.; Tak, W.Y.; Jang, S.Y.; Lee, C.; Kim, B.S.; et al. Daegu-Gyeongbuk Liver Study Group (DGLSG). Fibrosis-4 index as a predictor for mortality in hospitalised patients with COVID-19: A retrospective multicentre cohort study. *BMJ Open* **2020**, *10*, e041989. [CrossRef]
25. Li, Y.; Regan, J.; Fajnzylber, J.; Coxen, K.; Corry, H.; Wong, C.; Rosenthal, A.; Atyeo, C.; Fischinger, S.; Gillespie, E.; et al. Liver Fibrosis Index FIB-4 Is Associated With Mortality in COVID-19. *Hepatol. Commun.* **2021**, *5*, 434–445. [CrossRef]
26. Chen, F.; Chen, W.; Chen, J.; Xu, D.; Xie, W.; Wang, X.; Xie, Y. Clinical features and risk factors of COVID-19-associated liver injury and function: A retrospective analysis of 830 cases. *Ann. Hepatol.* **2020**, *21*, 100267. [CrossRef]
27. Xiang, F.; Sun, J.; Chen, P.-H.; Han, P.; Zheng, H.; Cai, S.; Kirk, G.D. Early Elevation of Fibrosis-4 Liver Fibrosis Score Is Associated With Adverse Outcomes Among Patients With Coronavirus Disease 2019. *Clin. Infect. Dis.* **2020**. [CrossRef]
28. Calapod, O.; Marin, A.; Onisai, M.; Tribus, L.; Pop, C.; Fierbinteanu-Braticevici, C. The Impact of Increased Fib-4 Score in Patients with Type II Diabetes Mellitus on COVID-19 Disease Prognosis. *Medicina* **2021**, *57*, 434. [CrossRef]
29. Bansal, A.; Singh, A.D.; Jain, V.; Aggarwal, M.; Gupta, S.; Padappayil, R.P.; Nadeem, M.; Joshi, S.; Mian, A.; Greathouse, T.; et al. The association of D-dimers with mortality, intensive care unit admission or acute respiratory distress syndrome in patients hospitalized with coronavirus disease 2019 (COVID-19): A systematic review and meta-analysis. *Heart Lung* **2021**, *50*, 9–12. [CrossRef]
30. Yu, H.H.; Qin, C.; Chen, M.; Wang, W.; Tian, D.S. D-dimer level is associated with the severity of COVID-19. *Thromb. Res.* **2020**, *195*, 219–225. [CrossRef] [PubMed]
31. Varol, Y.; Hakoglu, B.; Kadri Cirak, A.; Polat, G.; Komurcuoglu, B.; Akkol, B.; Atasoy, C.; Bayramic, E.; Balci, G.; Ataman, S.; et al. COVID Study Group. The impact of charlson comorbidity index on mortality from SARS-CoV-2 virus infection and A novel COVID-19 mortality index: CoLACD. *Int. J. Clin. Pract.* **2021**, *75*, e13858. [CrossRef]
32. Christensen, D.M.; Strange, J.E.; Gislason, G.; Torp-Pedersen, C.; Gerds, T.; Fosbøl, E.; Phelps, M. Charlson Comorbidity Index Score and Risk of Severe Outcome and Death in Danish COVID-19 Patients. *J. Gen. Intern. Med.* **2020**, *35*, 2801–2803. [CrossRef]
33. Tuty Kuswardhani, R.A.; Henrina, J.; Pranata, R.; Anthonius Lim, M.; Lawrensia, S.; Suastika, K. Charlson comorbidity index and a composite of poor outcomes in COVID-19 patients: A systematic review and meta-analysis. *Diabetes Metab. Syndr.* **2020**, *14*, 2103–2109. [CrossRef] [PubMed]
34. Buicu, A.L.; Cernea, S.; Benedek, I.; Buicu, C.F.; Benedek, T. Systemic Inflammation and COVID-19 Mortality in Patients with Major Noncommunicable Diseases: Chronic Coronary Syndromes, Diabetes and Obesity. *J. Clin. Med.* **2021**, *10*, 1545. [CrossRef] [PubMed]
35. Cuevas-Sierra, A.; Ramos-Lopez, O.; Riezu-Boj, J.I.; Milagro, F.I.; Martinez, J.A. Diet, Gut Microbiota, and Obesity: Links with Host Genetics and Epigenetics and Potential Applications. *Adv. Nutr.* **2019**, *10*, S17–S30. [CrossRef] [PubMed]
36. Omersel, J.; Karas Kuželički, N. Vaccinomics and Adversomics in the Era of Precision Medicine: A Review Based on HBV, MMR, HPV, and COVID-19 Vaccines. *J. Clin. Med.* **2020**, *9*, 3561. [CrossRef] [PubMed]

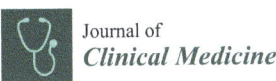

Journal of Clinical Medicine

Article

SARS-CoV-2 and Cytomegalovirus Co-Infections—A Case Series of Critically Ill Patients

Patrícia Moniz [1], Sérgio Brito [2] and Pedro Póvoa [1,3,4,*]

1. Polyvalent Intensive Care Unit, São Francisco Xavier Hospital, Centro Hospitalar de Lisboa Ocidental (CHLO), 449-005 Lisbon, Portugal; patricia.moniz25@gmail.com
2. Internal Medicine Department, São Francisco Xavier Hospital, Centro Hospitalar de Lisboa Ocidental (CHLO), 449-005 Lisbon, Portugal; sergioembrito@gmail.com
3. Nova Medical School, Comprehensive Health Research Centre (CHRC), New University of Lisbon, 449-005 Lisbon, Portugal
4. Center for Clinical Epidemiology and Research Unit of Clinical Epidemiology, Odense University Hospital (OUH), Odense University Hospital, 5000 Odense, Denmark
* Correspondence: pedrorpovoa@gmail.com; Tel.: +351-21-043-1000

Abstract: The SARS-CoV-2 pandemic has placed great strain on the most developed of health care systems, especially in the context of critical care. Although co-infections with cytomegalovirus (CMV) are frequent in the critically ill due to underlying immune suppression of multiple causes, the impact on COVID-19 patients remains unclear. Furthermore, severe COVID-19 has recently been associated with significant immune suppression, and this may in turn impact CMV reactivation, possibly contributing to clinical course. Nevertheless, multiple confounding factors in these patients will certainly challenge upcoming research. The authors present a case series of five patients admitted to the intensive care unit (ICU) in the context of respiratory failure due to severe COVID-19. All patients evolved with CMV reactivation during ICU stay.

Keywords: SARS-CoV-2; Cytomegalovirus; co-infections; critical care; COVID-19

1. Introduction

The current pandemic caused by SARS-CoV-2 virus infection has provoked an unprecedented health care burden worldwide with an abrupt demand for critical care provision and consequent strain on the intensive care unit (ICU) [1]. The experience and knowledge obtained during the past year have allowed the medical community to adapt and treat this emerging disease, but much uncertainty still prevails.

A history of cytomegalovirus (CMV) infection is very common among adults, the majority of which evolve with a period of latency characterized by a persistent control of viral replication [2]. Reactivation usually implies some type of weakened immunity which can be attributed to various etiologies [3]. Nevertheless, infection of immunocompetent patients in the ICU is well acknowledged, with the highest reactivation rates in septic patients. Furthermore, CMV reactivation is associated with higher ICU length of stay, longer need for invasive mechanical ventilation (IMV), increased risk of infections and mortality [4].

D'Ardes et al. were the first to report a case of CMV and SARS-CoV-2 co-infection [5]. Since then, the potentially adverse effects of CMV co-infection on COVID-19 outcome have been approached by recent publications [2]. However, case report publications of CMV co-infection remain relatively scarce [5–9], and the role of COVID-19 itself on CMV reactivation unclear.

The authors report a case series of five patients admitted to the ICU due to SARS-CoV-2 pneumonia who presented concomitant CMV infection/reactivation during ICU stay.

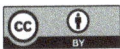

2. Case Presentation

2.1. Patient I

A 64-year-old male was admitted to the emergency department (ED) with a 7-day presentation of fever, dry cough, myalgia and chest pain. His past medical history (PMH) included stable human immunodeficiency virus 1 (HIV-1) infection (undetectable viral load; CD4+ cell count 321), diabetes mellitus (DM), hypertension (HT) and ischemic heart disease.

Initial diagnostic workup revealed a positive SARS-CoV-2 PCR assay, arterial blood gas examination (ABG) with hypoxemia (pO_2 71.1 mmHg with 3L/min of oxygen via nasal cannula) and chest X-ray with bilateral patchy lung infiltrates. He evolved with acute respiratory distress syndrome (ARDS) in the first 24 h and was transferred to the ICU, where he required invasive mechanical ventilation (IMV) for 22 days. Four days later, he presented respiratory distress and hemodynamic instability and was reintubated in the context of ventilator-associated pneumonia (VAP) due to Serratia. Laboratory reassessment revealed a lower CD4 count (114) and a positive CMV viral load (1012 UI/mL). The patient was extubated after 10 days of readmission and subsequently transferred to the medical ward. Hospital discharge occurred on day 67.

2.2. Patient II

A 61-year-old female presented to the ED with sustained fever and dyspnea within the last 24 h. She had a PMH of systemic lupus erythematosus with pulmonary, joint and renal involvement and chronic kidney disease (CKD) undergoing regular hemodialysis. Current medication included azathioprine and prednisolone (Table 1).

Table 1. Clinical characteristics of patients admitted to the ICU with SARS-CoV-2 infection due to respiratory failure who evolved with CMV infection/reactivation.

	Patient I	Patient II	Patient III	Patient IV	Patient V
Immunosuppression [a]	HIV [b], DM [c]	IS [d] therapy	IS therapy, DM	DM	HIV, DM
Time (days) (symptoms to ICU admission)	8	8	5	11	1
IMV [e] duration (days)	32	8	37	33	48
pO_2/FiO_2 (minimum)	169	105	88	105	113
First CMV [f] PCR [g] (date/result/sample)	D7 Positive Plasma	D2/D3 Positive Plasma/BAL [h]	D3 Negative Plasma	D37 Positive BAL	D2 ** Negative Plasma
Posterior CMV PCR (date/result/sample)	-	-	D16 Positive Plasma	-	D45 ** Positive BAL
Outcome (90 day)	Home discharge	Death	Rehabilitation Unit	Death	Rehabilitation Unit

[a] Immunosuppression besides critical illness; [b] HIV—human immunodeficiency virus infection; [c] DM—diabetes mellitus; [d] IS—immunosuppressive; [e] IMV—invasive mechanical ventilation; [f] CMV—cytomegalovirus; [g] PCR—polymerase chain reaction; [h] BAL—bronchoalveolar lavage; ** various plasma PCR assays remained negative throughout ICU stay. The only positive sample was obtained in BAL.

The patient presented hypotension responsive to fluid challenge and ABG with hypoxemia (pO_2 60.4 mmHg with 3L/min of oxygen via nasal cannula). The SARS-CoV-2 PCR assay was negative, and blood cultures were positive for *Enterococcus faecalis*. Antibiotics were started and the patient was transferred to the medical ward. Posteriorly, the PCR assay was repeated because of contact with a COVID-19 patient and turned out positive. She evolved with ARDS and was admitted to the ICU, where she initiated IMV. Plasma and bronchoalveolar lavage (BAL) CMV viral loads were positive (3528 UI/mL and 229 UI/mL, respectively). The patient died due to refractory circulatory shock on day 8.

2.3. Patient III

A 61-year-old male presented to the ED with a headache, fatigue and shortness of breath for the past 24 h. PMH included a heart transplant, DM, HT and CKD. Current medication included everolimus, mycophenolate mofetil, cyclosporine and prednisolone.

The patient had hypoxemia (ABG with pO_2 66.9 mmHg), the chest X-ray showed bilateral patchy pulmonary infiltrates and the SARS-CoV-2 PCR assay was positive. He was admitted to the medical ward, where he progressed with ARDS and therefore transferred to the ICU 2 days later. He underwent IMV for 37 days and the clinical course was complicated with septic shock in the context of a VAP due to *Proteus mirabillis* and *Klebsiella pneumoniae*, with the need for renal replacement therapy (RRT). Although CMV viral load upon admission had been negative, screening was repeated and viral load positive (518 UI/mL). A surgical tracheostomy was performed on day 35 due to ventilatory weaning failure. After readmission to the medical ward, he was discharged to a rehabilitation unit 87 days after admission.

2.4. Patient IV

A 77-year-old male was diagnosed with SARS-CoV-2 infection 10 days before presenting to the ED with dyspnea for the past 4 days. The patient's PMH included DM and HT.

The patient presented signs of respiratory distress and hypoxemia (ABG with pO_2 56.6 mmHg 6L/min of oxygen via facial mask). Chest X-ray showed patchy bilateral lung infiltrates. He was transferred to the medical ward with a Venturi Mask 35%, where he evolved with worsening hypoxemia and was therefore admitted to the ICU the next day. The patient evolved with circulatory shock and severe hypoxemia, which motivated the initiation of IMV, in the context of concomitant bacterial pneumonia due to *Klebsiella pneumoniae*. Clinical deterioration ensued in the context of candidemia. Bronchoalveolar lavage CMV viral load positive (170 UI/mL). On day 40 of admission, the patient evolved with refractory circulatory shock and died.

2.5. Patient V

A 78-year-old male presented to ED with anorexia, dry cough and shortness of breath for the past 2 days. He had contact with a COVID-19 patient 6 days before. The patient's PMH included HIV-1 infection (undetectable viral load and CD4+ cell count 743), DM with retinopathy and stage 3b CKD and HT.

The patient had hypoxemia (pO_2 50 mmHg with 4L/min of oxygen via nasal cannula), and a thoracic CT scan showed extensive bilateral pulmonary infiltrates. SARS-CoV-2 PCR screening was positive. He presented progressive clinical deterioration while in the ED and was transferred to the ICU. He required IMV for 48 days, and the clinical course was complicated with multiple respiratory infections and the need for RRT. CMV viral load upon admission was undetectable, but CMV viral load of bronchoalveolar lavage was positive on day 44 (108 copies/mL). A surgical tracheostomy was performed on day 24 due to a ventilatory weaning failure. He was subsequently transferred to the medical ward and discharged to a rehabilitation unit on day 83.

3. Discussion

We present five case reports of CMV reactivation in COVID-19 patients admitted to the ICU due to respiratory failure requiring IMV (Table 1). All patients were tested for CMV reactivation because of their respective underlying clinical severity and previous medical history of immune deficiency. The diagnosis was confirmed with CMV PCR testing (plasma or BAL), since antigen testing can be inaccurate in leukopenic patients [4]. Some patients had an initially negative CMV viral load, and therefore CMV reactivation occurred during ICU stay. All patients with the exception of patient IV, due to rapid clinical deterioration and death, began treatment with ganciclovir in the ICU. Although viral load was frequently low, given the positive PCR assay and underlying risk factors, curative therapy was initiated whenever possible. Patient III completed full-dose treatment for 3 weeks (5mg/kg IV q 12h), while all other patients began ganciclovir adjusted to renal function and RRT regimens.

It has been well acknowledged that critical illness itself can promote immune suppression, even in the absence of known immune deficiency states. This is due to an underlying complex immune system activation, composed of both pro- and anti-inflammatory responses. Recovery depends on the attainment of immunologic homeostasis, the lack of which can result in a type of secondary immune deficiency, compromising both innate and adaptive functions with a consequently increased risk of nosocomial infection [10,11]. Although CMV reactivation is quite common among the critically ill, debate still exists on whether such infection adversely affects the patient outcome or is merely an uneventful finding [4].

Recent findings associate severe COVID-19 with significant depletion of adaptive immune cells and increases in T-cell killing and immunosuppression. Critical care patients have demonstrated sustained T, NK and B cell lymphopenia and downregulation of HLA-DR expression, while increases in PD-1 have all been demonstrated in the first 7 days of ICU admission. These findings are not only worrisome but should reinforce careful evaluation of current therapeutic indications that can further hinder an effective immune response to SARS-CoV-2, such as glucocorticoids [12].

The role and the rate of CMV reactivation in SARS-CoV-2 patients are unclear. Clinical profiles that have been associated with worse outcomes in COVID-19 also prevail among patients with a higher risk of CMV reactivation. Characteristics such as older age, history of DM and cardiovascular diseases constitute such examples [2]. All five cases had ages older than 60 years, DM was highly prevalent and chronic immunosuppression either due to chronic illness or medication was also frequent.

Both HIV-infected patients presented recent negative viral loads previous to ICU admission, and significant HIV reactivation was excluded during ICU stay. Patient I had a very low viral load at the end of the ICU stay (35 copies), while patient V maintained a negative viral load.

CMV testing also occurred in patients without the aforementioned risk factors. However, these constituted a minority of ICU admissions, and CMV reactivation was not found in patients without comorbidities associated with immunosuppression. Consequently, this constitutes a limitation of our research, and the significance of SARS-CoV-2 infection in CMV reactivation cannot be clearly established based on our findings. The authors emphasize, however, that CMV reactivation can be overlooked, as can other nosocomial infections such as aspergillosis, characterized by unspecific clinical presentations. Considering the immunosuppression possibly associated with COVID-19, efforts should be made to prevent the underestimation of such infections in these patients.

4. Conclusions

The role of SARS-CoV-2 infection on CMV reactivation remains to be unraveled. Multiple confounding factors usually associated with immunosuppression, such as the clinical profile of older patients with multiple comorbidities, the secondary immune suppression of critical illness itself, underlying immunosuppressive treatments under investigation and probable immune suppression due to severe COVID-19 illness will certainly challenge further research.

Author Contributions: Conceptualization, P.M., P.P. and S.B.; methodology, P.M., P.P. and S.B.; validation, P.P.; writing—original draft preparation, P.M. and S.B.; writing—review and editing, P.M., P.P. and S.B.; visualization, P.M., P.P. and S.B.; supervision, P.P. All authors have read and agreed to the published version of the manuscript.

Funding: This research received no external funding.

Institutional Review Board Statement: Not applicable.

Informed Consent Statement: Patient consent was waived. Our institution's Health Ethics Committee authorizes such publications as long as data are provided anonymously.

Data Availability Statement: No new data were created or analyzed in this study. Data sharing is not applicable to this article.

Conflicts of Interest: The authors declare no conflict of interest.

References

1. Li, L.; Gong, S.; Yan, J. Covid-19 in China: Ten critical issues for intensive care medicine. *Crit. Care* **2020**, *24*, 1–3. [CrossRef] [PubMed]
2. Moss, P. "The ancient and the new": Is there an interaction between cytomegalovirus and SARS-CoV-2 infection? *Immun. Ageing* **2020**, *17*, 1–6. [CrossRef] [PubMed]
3. Li, X.; Huang, Y.; Xu, Z.; Zhang, R.; Liu, X.; Li, Y.; Mao, P. Cytomegalovirus infection and outcome in immunocompetent patients in the intensive care unit: A systematic review and meta-analysis. *BMC Infect. Dis.* **2018**, *18*, 289. [CrossRef]
4. Schildermans, J.; De Vlieger, G. Cytomegalovirus: A Troll in the ICU? Overview of the Literature and Perspectives for the Future. *Front. Med.* **2020**, *7*. [CrossRef] [PubMed]
5. D'Ardes, D.; Boccatonda, A.; Schiavone, C.; Santilli, F.; Guagnano, M.T.; Bucci, M.; Cipollone, F. A Case of Coinfection with SARS-COV-2 and Cytomegalovirus in the Era of COVID-19. *Eur. J. Case Rep. Intern. Med.* **2020**, *7*, 001652. [CrossRef]
6. Amaral, P.; Ferreira, B.; Roll, S.; Neves, P.; Pivetta, L.; Mohrbacher, S.; Dias, E.; Sato, V.; Oliveira, É.; Pereira, L.; et al. COVID-19 and Cytomegalovirus Co-infection: A Challenging Case of a Critically Ill Patient with Gastrointestinal Symptoms. *Eur. J. Case Rep. Intern. Med.* **2020**, *7*. [CrossRef]
7. Pitoyo, C.W.; Wijaya, I.P.E.K.; Wulani, V.; Wiraputri, A.K.; Romulo, M.A. Misleading Diagnosis of Radiological Imaging of COVID-19 Pneumonia During Pandemic Era: Risk on the Existence of CMV Infection. *Acta Med. Indones* **2020**, *52*, 375–382. [PubMed]
8. Oualim, S.; Elouarradi, A.; Hafid, S.; Naitelhou, A.; Sabry, M. A misleading CMV myocarditis during the COVID-19 pandemic: Case report. *Pan Afr. Med. J.* **2020**, *36*. [CrossRef] [PubMed]
9. Molaei, H.; Khedmat, L.; Nemati, E.; Rostami, Z.; Saadat, S.H. Iranian kidney transplant recipients with COVID-19 infection: Clinical outcomes and cytomegalovirus co-infection. *Transpl. Infect. Dis.* **2021**, *23*. [CrossRef] [PubMed]
10. Greathouse, K.C.; Hall, M.W. Critical Illness–Induced Immune Suppression: Current State of the Science. *Am. J. Crit. Care* **2016**, *25*, 85–92. [CrossRef] [PubMed]
11. Imlay, H.; Limaye, A.P. Current Understanding of Cytomegalovirus Reactivation in Critical Illness. *J. Infect. Dis.* **2020**, *221*, S94–S102. [CrossRef] [PubMed]
12. Jeannet, R.; Daix, T.; Formento, R.; Feuillard, J.; François, B. Severe COVID-19 is associated with deep and sustained multifaceted cellular immunosuppression. *Intensiv. Care Med.* **2020**, *46*, 1769–1771. [CrossRef] [PubMed]

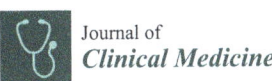

Article

Evaluation of Two Rapid Antigenic Tests for the Detection of SARS-CoV-2 in Nasopharyngeal Swabs

Ysaline Seynaeve [1,*], Justine Heylen [1], Corentin Fontaine [1], François Maclot [1], Cécile Meex [1], Anh Nguyet Diep [2], Anne-Françoise Donneau [2], Marie-Pierre Hayette [1] and Julie Descy [1]

1. Department of Clinical Microbiology, Center for Interdisciplinary Research on Medicines (CIRM), University of Liège, 4000 Liège, Belgium; jheylen@student.uliege.be (J.H.); c.fontaine@chuliege.be (C.F.); francois.maclot@chuliege.be (F.M.); c.meex@chuliege.be (C.M.); mphayette@chuliege.be (M.-P.H.); julie.descy@chuliege.be (J.D.)
2. Biostatistics Unit, Department of Public Health, University of Liège, 4000 Liège, Belgium; anhnguyet.diep@uliege.be (A.N.D.); afdonneau@uliege.be (A.-F.D.)
*   Correspondence: ysaline.seynaeve@chuliege.be

Abstract: (1) Background: In the current context of the COVID-19 crisis, there is a need for fast, easy-to-use, and sensitive diagnostic tools in addition to molecular methods. We have therefore decided to evaluate the performance of newly available antigen detection kits in "real-life" laboratory conditions. (2) Methods: The sensitivity and specificity of two rapid diagnostic tests (RDT)—the COVID-19 Ag Respi-Strip from Coris Bioconcept, Belgium (CoRDT), and the coronavirus antigen rapid test cassette from Healgen Scientific, LLC, USA (HeRDT)—were evaluated on 193 nasopharyngeal samples using RT-PCR as the gold standard. (3) Results: The sensitivity obtained for HeRDT was 88% for all collected samples and 91.1% for samples with Ct $\leq$ 31. For the CoRDT test, the sensitivity obtained was 62% for all collected samples and 68.9% for samples with Ct $\leq$ 31. (4) Conclusions: Despite the excellent specificity obtained for both kits, the poor sensitivity of the CoRDT did not allow for its use in the rapid diagnosis of COVID-19. HeRDT satisfied the World Health Organization's performance criteria for rapid antigen detection tests. Its high sensitivity, quick response, and ease of use allowed for the implementation of HeRDT at the laboratory of the University Hospital of Liège.

Keywords: rapid diagnostic test; antigen detection; SARS-CoV-2; COVID-19

1. Introduction

In December 2019, a new virus belonging to the *Betacoronavirus* genus from the *Coronaviridae* family appeared in the city of Wuhan in China. It was identified as the agent responsible for a severe respiratory syndrome, hence its name: SARS-CoV-2 for Severe Acute Respiratory Syndrome Coronavirus. The virus is responsible for coronavirus disease 19 (COVID-19), so named because it appeared in 2019. Other betacoronaviruses involved in human respiratory syndromes include SARS-CoV-1—the agent of the Severe Acute Respiratory Syndrome discovered in 2002—and MERS-CoV, responsible for the Middle East Respiratory Syndrome in 2012 [1,2]. Within a few months, SARS-CoV-2 spread rapidly, leading to the World Health Organization's (WHO) announcement of a COVID-19 pandemic on 11 March 2020 [3]. As of 3 June 2021, 171.3 million people have been infected and 3.7 million people have died worldwide [4]. This pandemic has caused microbiology labs to develop diagnostic methods based on antigen and RNA detection. The WHO defined a reverse transcription polymerase chain reaction (RT-PCR) assay on respiratory specimens as the reference method for the detection of SARS-CoV-2 [5]. This coronavirus is an enveloped virus with a positive-sense, single-stranded RNA genome of ~30 kb. Its genome encodes a minimum of 29 proteins. The ORF1a and ORF1b genes encode non-structural accessory proteins (nsps), while the S, M, E, and N genes encode structural proteins—namely, spike (S), membrane (M), envelope (E), and nucleocapsid

(N) proteins [6,7]. These genes are of particular interest for the diagnosis of COVID-19 by RT-PCR.

The real-time RT-PCR assay provides a semi-quantitative estimation of viral concentration expressed by the cycle threshold (Ct), which represents the number of amplification cycles required to detect a fluorescence signal above the threshold. The cycle threshold is correlated to the viral load and contagiousness [8,9]. Despite the very high specificity and sensitivity of molecular techniques, RT-PCR is time-consuming and requires specific laboratory equipment and experienced technical staff [10,11]. These limitations—combined with the shortage of PCR reagents and disposables—have led laboratories to investigate alternatives. In September 2020, the WHO reported the possible use of antigenic tests as a promising complement to RT-PCR. The WHO described rapid diagnostic tests (RDT) with a sensitivity $\geq$80% and a specificity $\geq$97% compared to the reference RT-PCR method that can be used when molecular tests are not available or when rapid screening is needed [8]. Confronted with the second wave of COVID-19, laboratories were under pressure to perform RT-PCR for the detection of SARS-CoV-2. The turnaround time was longer than the acceptable range of 24 h, which resulted in delays to diagnosis that compromised patients and epidemic management [12]. In addition, the emergency department of our hospital (CHU, Liège, Belgium) needed an early diagnosis of SARS-CoV-2 in order to manage patient hospitalization in COVID or non-COVID care units. Many companies have developed RDTs for the diagnosis of COVID-19 as point-of-care testing methods. Despite the high sensitivity announced by the manufacturers, the performance of these tests is varied and often lower than expected; therefore, their validation in real conditions is important [13–18]. A validation of two RDT kits for the detection of SARS-CoV-2 compared to RT-PCR was conducted at the microbiology laboratory of CHU Liège. The two kits are both membrane-based immunochromatographic assays that detect SARS-CoV-2 nucleocapsid proteins: (1) the coronavirus antigen rapid test cassette (Healgen Scientific, LLC, Houston, TX, USA), named hereafter HeRDT, and (2) the COVID-19 Ag Respi-Strip (Coris Bioconcept, Gembloux, Belgium), referred to as CoRDT.

2. Materials and Methods

2.1. Study Design

The diagnostic accuracy of HeRDT and CoRDT compared to RT-PCR (defined as the gold standard) was determined in a two-phase validation. The first phase—with nasopharyngeal (NP) swabs selected by convenience—aimed to verify that the minimum expected performance was achieved based on the recommendation of minimum sensitivities and specificities described by the WHO—i.e., a sensitivity $\geq$80% and a specificity $\geq$97% [8]. The second phase carried out on randomized NP samples aimed to validate the RDT in real diagnostic conditions.

2.2. Population and Study Period

Validation was conducted between 22 October 2020 and 11 November 2020 at CHU Liège, a tertiary hospital with 1038 beds in Belgium. We included NP-flocked swabs placed in 3 mL of transport media (Vacuette Virus Stabilization Tube (VST); Greiner Bio-One, Kremsmünster, Austria) containing phosphate-buffered saline. The samples were kept between 2 and 8 °C and tested within 24 h for both RT-PCR and RDT. The NP samples were collected from patients admitted to the emergency department and from the testing center of the CHU Liège.

Phase 1: Evaluation of samples based on the predefined Ct value. The sample selection took place from 22 October to 27 October 2020. The average SARS-CoV-2 prevalence at the CHU of Liège during the sample selection period was 43.7%. Following the RT-PCR analysis, 15 negative samples and 48 positive samples were selected based on convenience. Positive samples were chosen on the basis of Ct calculated for the N gene by Qiagen RT-PCR in triplicate for each Ct value ranging from 20 to 35.

Phase 1 bis: Evaluation of samples based on the predefined Ct value after methodology improvement. In order to improve the HeRDT sensitivity, 30 RT-PCR-positive samples were tested according to an adapted protocol between 28 October and 30 October 2020.

Phase 2: Evaluation of randomized samples. The validation was performed from 3 November to 11 November 2020. At the CHU Liège, the prevalence of SARS-CoV-2 positivity during this period averaged 29%. Following the Qiagen RT-PCR analysis, 50 negative and 50 positive samples were randomly selected.

2.3. Diagnostic Procedures

RT-PCR: The reference method used was the QIAprep&amp Viral RNA UM Kit (Qiagen, Hilden, Germany), combining liquid-based sample preparation with the one-step RT-qPCR detection of SARS-CoV-2 targets from human respiratory samples. Three different-colored channels (FAM™, HEX™, and Cy5) were used for the multiplex detection of SARS-CoV-2 (N1/N2 genes), human genetic material integrity (B2M and Rnase P), and inhibition control (synthetic transcript), respectively. RT-PCR detection was performed on a LC480 thermocycler (Roche, Basel, Switzerland) according to the following cycling conditions: 50 °C for 10 min, 95 °C for 2 min, 40 cycles at 95 °C for 5 s, 58 °C for 30 s. The quantification of the viral load was carried out using the calibrated standards provided by the Belgian National Reference Centre for Respiratory Viruses so that the virus concentrations could be estimated from the Qiagen Ct values (Table 1). Samples were considered negative when N1/N2 genes were not detected or they presented a Ct value >40.

Table 1. Correlation between Qiagen PCR Ct and standard viral quantification.

Interpretation	Viral Load (RNA Copies/mL)	Ct
Very strong positive	>10,000,000	<18.5
Very positive	100,000 to 10,000,000	18.5 to 25
Moderately positive	1000 to 100,000	25 to 31
Weakly positive	<1000	>31

Ct, cycle threshold.

RDTs: We evaluated the COVID-19 Ag Respi-Strip kit from Coris Bioconcept (CoRDT) and the coronavirus antigen rapid test cassette from Healgen Scientific, LLC (HeRDT). Both assays are qualitative membrane-based immunochromatographic tests that use monoclonal antibodies to detect nucleocapsid proteins from SARS-CoV-2 in direct nasopharyngeal swabs. For both tests, a nasopharyngeal specimen was taken using a sterile swab and the test was performed directly.

HeRDT manufacturer test procedure: The swab was dipped for 1 min in a dropper bottle containing 10 drops of buffer. After removing the swab from the bottle, 4 drops of the solution were placed in the well of the immunochromatographic test. The result was read 15 min later.

CoRDT manufacturer test procedure: The swab was dipped into a tube containing 8 drops of buffer and stirred thoroughly. After removing the swab, the immunochromatographic strip was placed in the tube. The result was read 30 min later.

Sample processing methods were modified from the manufacturer's instructions in order to perform the RDT from the same transport media as were used for the RT-PCR. We analyzed the transport medium containing the swab rather than the swab directly, as recommended by the manufacturer. As the tests were carried out in our laboratory, samples arrived in a virus stabilization tube containing phosphate-buffered saline solution. For both tests, 100 µL of transport fluid was added to the buffer.

In addition to the adapted sample use, we evaluated a second modification to the operating protocol to improve the sensitivity (by halving the lysis buffer) on thirty RT-PCR-positive samples. Instead of adding 10 drops of buffer, we added 5 drops for HeRDT and 4 for CoRDT instead of 8.

The results were read double blind and the technicians performing the RDT were also blinded to the RT-PCR results.

2.4. Clinical Data

We reviewed medical records to find clinical data regarding the presence of COVID-19 symptoms and, when present, the time from the onset of symptoms.

2.5. Statistics

The performance of both CoRDT and HeRDT was evaluated according to the criteria of sensitivity and specificity with a corresponding 95% confidence interval (95% CI). Qiagen RT-PCR was considered as the gold standard for this evaluation. Sensitivity was calculated for two groups: (1) on positive NP swabs including all Ct values and (2) in NP swabs with RT-PCR cycle threshold (Ct) values ≤31. This cut-off was used in the host laboratory to assist with the interpretation of Ct: a positive sample with a Ct value >31, equivalent to a viral load ≤1000 copies/mL, was considered to be a weakly positive result [8,9,15]. The agreement between the two techniques was evaluated using Cohen's kappa coefficient, κ, with a corresponding 95% CI. Analyses were performed using the R software [19].

3. Results

For the Phase 1 validation, 63 samples were selected from patients presenting at the COVID testing center of CHU Liège. This cohort included 15 negative (23.8%) and 48 positive NP swabs (76.2%). Positive samples presented RT-PCR Ct values between 20.2 and 35.9 Ct (median Ct = 28.3), corresponding to a SARS-CoV-2 viral load of between 1000 and 10,000,000 copies/mL. Of the 48 positive samples, 29 samples were detected as positive with HeRDT; the test was positive for each of the three specimens in triplicate, reaching a Ct value of 28. However, the results were increasingly inconsistent for those above this value. The sample with the lowest viral load detected with HeRDT presented a Ct value of 31.5 (corresponding to a weakly positive result ≤1000 copies/mL). All RT-PCR-negative samples were negative with both HeRDT and CoRDT, resulting in a specificity of 100%. As shown in Table 1, the sensitivity for HeRDT was 60.4% while CoRDT—which detected 18 positive samples out of the 48 RT-PCR-positive NP swabs—presented a sensitivity of 37.5%. Since the samples with positive RT-PCR presenting a Ct value >31 were usually considered to be weakly positive [15], the performance of both HeRDT and CoRDT was calculated for a subgroup of specimens. This subgroup included all negative samples ($n = 15$) and positive samples with a Ct value ≤31 in RT-PCR ($n = 39$). The improved sensitivity (84.9% for HeRDT and 54.5% for CoRDT) observed in this subgroup is also presented in Table 2.

By halving the volume of the lysis buffer (5 drops instead of 10, with 150 μL of sample) for HeRDT, we observed an improved sensitivity (73.3%). Of the 30 Qiagen RT-PCR-positive samples selected for this validation phase (Ct range: 24.1–33.8; median Ct 29.1), 22 samples were positive with HeRDT. The same specimens were also analyzed with CoRDT, which identified only four positive results out of the 30 RT-PCR-positive samples (leading to sensitivity of 13.3%). The results are shown in Table 3.

Table 2. Phase 1 performance of HeRDT and CoRDT compared to RT-PCR (P = positive, N = negative). The results for all Ct values ranging from 20.2 to 35.9 are presented in (**A**), and only Ct values ≤31.00 are presented in (**B**).

A.		RT-PCR		Sensitivity (%) (95% CI)	Specificity (%)	Lowest Viral Load (Ct)
		P (n = 48)	N (n = 15)			
HeRDT	P	29	0	60.4 (45.3–73.9)	100	31.51
	N	19	15			
CoRDT	P	18	0	37.5 (24.3–52.7)	100	27.16
	N	30	15			
B.		RT-PCR		Sensitivity (%) (95% CI)	Specificity (%)	Lowest Viral Load (Ct)
		P (n = 33)	N (n = 15)			
HeRDT	P	22	0	84.9 (68.1–94.9)	100	31.51
	N	8	15			
CoRDT	P	18	0	54.5 (36.4–71.9)	100	27.16
	N	15	15			

CI, confidence interval; CoRDT, COVID-19 Ag Respi-Strip from Coris Bioconcept; HeRDT, coronavirus antigen rapid test cassette from Healgen Scientific.

Table 3. Sensitivity of HeRDT and CoRDT compared to RT-PCR after the improvement of operating protocol (P = positive, N = negative). The results for all Ct values ranging from 24.1 to 33.8 are presented in (**A**).

A.		RT-PCR		Sensitivity (%) (95% CI)
		P (n = 30)	N (n = 0)	
HeRDT	P	22	/	73.3 (53.8–87.0)
	N	8	/	
CoRDT	P	4	/	13.3 (4.4–31.6)
	N	26	/	

Phase 2 validation was performed on 100 randomly selected routine NP swabs containing 50 negative and 50 positive Qiagen RT-PCR samples, with Ct values in the range of 16.7 to 37.3 (median Ct = 23.6); the viral load ranged from 1000 to >10,000,000 copies/mL (Figure 1). For NP swabs taken from patients admitted to the emergency department and from the testing center of the CHU Liège, 76% presented COVID-19 symptoms with a median duration of 3 days (from 0 to 11 days), and 86.8% of symptomatic patients had symptoms ≤5 days. As shown in Table 4, HeRDT identified 44/50 positive samples (88% sensitivity). The limit of detection was a sample with a Ct value of 33.8. The κ expressing the agreement between Qiagen RT-PCR and HeRDT was 0.880 (95% CI: 0.788–0.972), which indicated a strong agreement between the two techniques [20]. Thirty-one positive results out of the 50 RT-PCR-positive samples were detected with CoRDT (indicating 62% sensitivity), and the lowest viral load detected had a Ct value of 26.5 (corresponding to a positive result between 1000 and 100,000 RNA copies/mL). The agreement κ index between CoRDT and Qiagen RT-PCR was 0.620 (95% CI: 0.477–0.763), indicating a moderate agreement. All RT-PCR-negative samples were also negative with both HeRDT and CoRDT, leading to a 100% specificity. The performance of both assays was calculated for the subgroup, counting only negative (n = 50) and positive samples with a Ct value ≤31 in RT-PCR (n = 45). HeRDT showed a sensitivity of 91.1%. Cohen's kappa coefficient for this subgroup was 0.915 (CI: 0.833–0.997), indicating almost perfect agreement between HeRDT and RT-PCR. In this subgroup, the sensitivity of CoRDT was also improved (68.9%), but the κ expressing agreement between RT-PCR and CoRDT continued to indicate a moderate agreement (κ = 0.699 (CI: 0.560–0.837)).

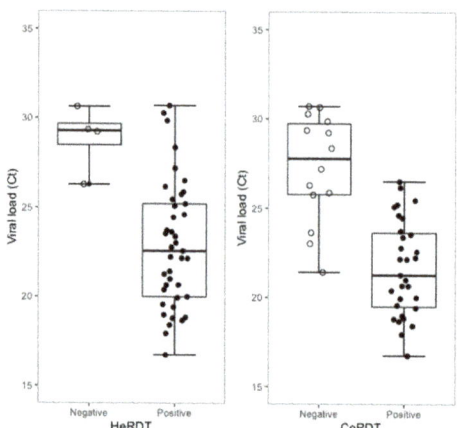

Figure 1. HeRDT and CoRDT results according to the viral load (Ct).

Table 4. Phase 2 performance of HeRDT and CoRDT compared to RT-PCR (P = positive, N = negative). The results for all Ct values ranging from 16.7 to 37.3 are presented in (**A**), and only Ct values ≤31.00 are presented in (**B**).

A.		RT-PCR		Sensitivity (%) (95% CI)	Specificity (%)	Lowest Viral Load (Ct)
		P (n = 50)	N (n = 50)			
HeRDT	P	44	0	88.0 (75.0–95.0)	100	33.77
	N	6	50			
CoRDT	P	31	0	62.0 (47.2–75.0)	100	26.5
	N	19	50			
B.		RT-PCR		Sensitivity (%) (95% CI)	Specificity (%)	Lowest Viral Load (Ct)
		P (n = 45)	N (n = 50)			
HeRDT	P	41	0	91.1 (78.8–97.5)	100	32.84
	N	4	50			
CoRDT	P	31	0	68.9 (53.4–81.8)	100	26.5
	N	14	50			

4. Discussion

Effective testing strategies combined with the good performance of diagnostic methods are essential for the control and management of COVID-19 patients, as well as for asymptomatic carriers [21]. Multiple manufacturers have proposed RDTs for the detection of SARS-CoV-2, with reported performances that should be confirmed by clinical validation to reach minimum performance requirements (sensitivity ≥80% and specificity ≥97%) [8]. In this study, we assessed the performance of two RDT kits (CoRDT and HeRDT) in comparison with RT-PCR, which is considered as the gold standard method. The present validation revealed a 100% specificity for both kits, while the sensitivity was, respectively, 88% and 62% for HeRDT and CoRDT. These results were applicable when considering all positive samples from the validation Phase 2. Moreover, we decided to determine the diagnostic accuracy of both RDTs in a subgroup of samples with RT-PCR-positive samples not exceeding 31 Ct. In accordance with the literature and the quantification of the viral load by calibrated standards, a SARS-CoV-2-positive individual with a value >31 Ct (corresponding to a viral load <1000 copies/mL) is considered to be weakly positive [22]. In this studied subgroup, the sensitivity was higher, with 68.9% for CoRDT and 91.1% for HeRDT. In October 2020, Sciensano (National Institute of Public Health in Belgium) updated the COVID-19 testing strategies: RDT can be used as a diagnostic method for

COVID-19 in symptomatic patients with symptoms ≤5 days consulting at the emergency department [21]. In fact, antigen detection methods are more effective in patients presenting high SARS-CoV-2 viral loads, most often corresponding to the recent onset of symptoms. As reported in other studies [14,23], a higher sensitivity of RDT was observed when testing patients at an early stage of the disease. Similar results were observed in our study: a predominant subgroup of patients presented COVID-19 symptoms with a symptom onset delay ≤5 days. Clinical data were missing in 24% of samples included in this validation step, while only 8% were taken from asymptomatic patients. Due to the high sensitivity of HeRDT and the updated recommendations from the Belgian authorities for the use of RDTs, we decided to implement HeRDT as a screening test for patients admitted to the emergency department at the CHU Liège. However, all negative antigenic test results had to be confirmed by RT-PCR.

In addition to the viral load and the number of days of post-symptoms, other factors may influence the performance of the RDT. Among these, our modified sample processing method may impact the results [14,23]. We chose to process RDTs directly from the transport medium, which was also used for RT-PCR, in order to compare results from the same sample. The adaptation led to a dilution of the NP swab that may partly explain the differences in the performance compared to those announced by the kit's manufacturers or described in other studies [13,24]. Carrying out the RDT directly using the NP swab transport medium—without diluting it in the kit buffer—may improve the sensitivity, as already demonstrated in other studies [14].

Rapid diagnostic tests (RDTs) can provide multiple advantages compared to PCR methods. They cost less and are easier to use (simpler equipment, requirement of basic skills compared to molecular tests). They present a shorter turnaround-time compared to RT-PCR and provide results at any hour in the day. However, RDTs may present a series of disadvantages, such as the immunochromatographic tests needing to be read by humans, the interpretation of the results possibly being subjective, and the manual encoding of data being a possible source of error in the Laboratory Information Management System (LIMS), especially in the case of decentralized point-of-care testing configurations. It is essential for laboratories to easily retrieve the results of these RDTs in the LIMS, which can be used for submission to authorities for pandemic monitoring or other purposes. However, the main disadvantage of RDTs is associated with their lower sensitivity compared to RT-PCR, often leading to the verification of negative results [9,25].

As previously described [23,24,26], the performance of an RDT depends on the viral load of SARS-CoV-2 in samples, the delay from the onset of symptoms, any adaptation of the testing protocol, and how the results are interpreted by the reader. Moreover, the performance of an RDT is also influenced by the SARS-CoV-2 infection rate; a higher prevalence of infection in the population corresponds to a higher positive predictive value (PPV). Conversely, as the disease prevalence decreases, PPV decreases and the risk of obtaining false positive results increases. During the beginning of the study period (22 October to 27 October 2020), the prevalence of SARS-CoV-2 at the host hospital was 43.7%, leading to a PPV of 100% and a negative predictive value (NPV) of 91.5% for HeRDT. For CoRDT, the calculated predictive values for the same period were 100% for PPV and 77.2% for NPV. For instance, in another context where the prevalence of COVID-19 is 5.0% (prevalence at CHU Liège in January 2021), HeRDT would show a PPV of 100% and an NPV of 99.4%. For CoRDT in the same situation, PPV and NPV would be 100% and 98%, respectively. Contrary to other studies [24], our specificity reached 100%; therefore, it was not possible to predict a PPV. It would be interesting to re-evaluate the specificity during a period with a lower prevalence of COVID-19. It should also be noted that the Phase 2 validation performed in our laboratory was carried out on only 100 samples (50 RT-PCR-positive and 50 RT-PCR-negative NP swabs). However, the European Centre for Disease Prevention and Control (ECDC) recommends testing at least 100 positive and 100 negative samples [25]. At the beginning of this validation study, these recommendations were not yet available. However, a routine daily verification was performed for several weeks and confirmed the sensitivity observed during the second phase of the validation of HeRDT. From 11 November to 31 December, 984 samples (971 negative and 13 positive) were analyzed in parallel using a HeRDT test and QIAGEN RT-PCR assay, revealing a 97% concordance between the two methods.

Increasing the number of sample tests and the examination of different prevalence conditions remain relevant for validating RDTs and precisely confirming the manufacturer's diagnostic accuracy in real-life conditions.

In conclusion, RDTs have a real role in the COVID-19 testing strategy thanks to their ease of use and capacity for mass screening and the rapid detection of SARS-CoV-2 24/7. This validation study showed that it is necessary to confirm the test performances announced by manufacturers before implementing RDTs, especially in the case of protocol adaptation. Although it is crucial to realize that RDT sensitivity is lower than RT-PCR, their use can be of benefit in cases of limited access to molecular methods or when the RT-PCR testing capacity is overburdened.

Author Contributions: Conceptualization: Y.S., C.F., M.-P.H., and J.D.; Data curation: Y.S., A.N.D., and A.-F.D.; Formal analysis: A.N.D. and A.-F.D.; Investigation: Y.S. and J.H.; Resources: C.M.; Supervision: M.-P.H.; Writing—original draft: Y.S. and J.D.; Writing—review and editing: Y.S., F.M., A.N.D., A.-F.D., M.-P.H., and J.D. All authors have read and agreed to the published version of the manuscript.

Funding: This research received no external funding.

Institutional Review Board Statement: Not applicable.

Informed Consent Statement: Not applicable.

Data Availability Statement: The data presented in this study are available on request from the corresponding author. The data are not publicly available due to privacy and ethical concerns.

Acknowledgments: The authors wish to thank Sebastien Bontems for his review of the manuscript and all microbiology laboratory staff for their assistance.

Conflicts of Interest: The authors declare no conflict of interest.

References

1. Zhu, N.; Zhang, D.; Wang, W.; Li, X.; Yang, B.; Song, J.; Zhao, X.; Huang, B.; Shi, W.; Lu, R.; et al. A Novel Coronavirus from Patients with Pneumonia in China, 2019. *N. Engl. J. Med.* **2020**, *382*, 727–733. [CrossRef] [PubMed]
2. Zheng, J. SARS-CoV-2: An Emerging Coronavirus that Causes a Global Threat. *Int. J. Biol. Sci.* **2020**, *16*, 1678–1685. [CrossRef] [PubMed]
3. WHO (World Health Organization). Coronavirus Disease (COVID-2019) Situation Report–51. 11 March 2020. Available online: https://www.who.int/docs/default-source/coronaviruse/situation-reports/20200311-sitrep-51-covid-19.pdf?sfvrsn=1ba62e57_10 (accessed on 22 March 2021).
4. WHO (World Health Organization). Coronavirus (COVID-19) Dashboard. Available online: https://covid19.who.int (accessed on 3 June 2021).
5. WHO (World Health Organization). Laboratory Testing Strategy Recommendations for COVID-19. Interim Guidance. 21 March 2020. Available online: https://apps.who.int/iris/bitstream/handle/10665/331509/WHO-COVID-19-lab_testing-2020.1-eng.pdf?sequence=1&isAllowed=y (accessed on 27 November 2020).
6. Yao, H.; Song, Y.; Chen, Y.; Wu, N.; Xu, J.; Sun, C.; Zhang, J.; Weng, T.; Zhang, Z.; Wu, Z.; et al. Molecular Architecture of the SARS-CoV-2 Virus. *Cell* **2020**, *183*, 730–738.e13. [CrossRef] [PubMed]
7. Kim, D.; Lee, J.-Y.; Yang, J.-S.; Kim, J.W.; Kim, V.N.; Chang, H. The Architecture of SARS-CoV-2 Transcriptome. *Cell* **2020**, *181*, 914–921.e10. [CrossRef] [PubMed]
8. WHO (World Health Organization). Antigen-Detection in the Diagnosis of SARS-CoV-2 Infection using Rapid ImmunoAssays. Interim Guidance. 20 September 2020. Available online: https://www.who.int/publications/i/item/antigen-detection-in-the-diagnosis-of-sars-cov-2infection-using-rapid-immunoassays (accessed on 27 November 2020).
9. CDC (US Centers for Disease Control and Prevention). Interim Guidance for Rapid Antigen Testing for SARS-CoV-2. 13 May 2021. Available online: https://www.cdc.gov/coronavirus/2019-ncov/lab/resources/antigen-tests-guidelines.html#previous (accessed on 21 May 2021).
10. D'Cruz, R.J.; Currier, A.W.; Sampson, V.B. Laboratory Testing Methods for Novel Severe Acute Respiratory Syndrome-Coronavirus-2 (SARS-CoV-2). *Front. Cell Dev. Biol.* **2020**, *8*, 468. [CrossRef] [PubMed]

11. Tang, Y.-W.; Schmitz, J.E.; Persing, D.H.; Stratton, C.W. Laboratory Diagnosis of COVID-19: Current Issues and Challenges. *J. Clin. Microbiol.* **2020**, *58*, e00512-20. [CrossRef] [PubMed]
12. Sciensano. Mise à Jour de la Stratégie de test, Utilisation de Tests Salivaires et de Tests Antigènes Rapides. 12 October 2020. Available online: https://covid-19.sciensano.be/sites/default/files/Covid19/20201012_Advice%20RAG_testing_update%20October_Fr.pdf (accessed on 27 November 2020).
13. Scohy, A.; Anantharajah, A.; Bodéus, M.; Kabamba-Mukadi, B.; Verroken, A.; Rodriguez-Villalobos, H. Low performance of rapid antigen detection test as frontline testing for COVID-19 diagnosis. *J. Clin. Virol.* **2020**, *129*, 104455. [CrossRef] [PubMed]
14. Mak, G.C.; Cheng, P.K.; Lau, S.S.; Wong, K.K.; Lau, C.S.; Lam, E.T.; Chan, R.C.; Tsang, D.N. Evaluation of Rapid Antigen Test for Detection of SARS-CoV-2 Virus. *J. Clin. Virol.* **2020**, *129*, 104500. [CrossRef] [PubMed]
15. CDC (US Centers for Disease Control and Prevention). Common Investigation Protocol for Investigating Suspected SARS-CoV-2 Reinfection. 27 October 2020. Available online: https://www.cdc.gov/coronavirus/2019-ncov/php/reinfection.html (accessed on 27 November 2020).
16. Osterman, A.; Baldauf, H.M.; Eletreby, M.; Wettengel, J.M.; Afridi, S.Q.; Fuchs, T.; Holzmann, E.; Maier, A.; Döring, J.; Grzimek-Koschewa, N.; et al. Evaluation of two rapid antigen tests to detect SARS-CoV-2 in a hospital setting. *Med. Microbiol Immunol.* **2021**, *210*, 65–72. [CrossRef] [PubMed]
17. Albert, E.; Torres, I.; Bueno, F.; Huntley, D.; Molla, E.; Fernández-Fuentes, M.Á.; Martínez, M.; Poujois, S.; Forqué, L.; Valdivia, A.; et al. Field evaluation of a rapid antigen test (Panbio™ COVID-19 Ag rapid test device) for COVID-19 diagnosis in primary healthcare centres. *Clin. Microbiol Infect.* **2021**, *27*, 472.e7–472.e10. [CrossRef] [PubMed]
18. Toptan, T.; Eckermann, L.; Pfeiffer, A.E.; Hoehl, S.; Ciesek, S.; Drosten, C.; Corman, V.M. Evaluation of a SARS-CoV-2 rapid antigen test: Potential to help reduce community spread? *J. Clin. Virol.* **2021**, *135*, 104713. [CrossRef]
19. R Core Team. *R: A Language and Environment for Statistical Computing*; R Foundation for Statistical Computing: Vienna, Austria. 2018. Available online: http://www.r-project.org/ (accessed on 14 December 2020).
20. McHugh, M.L. Interrater Reliability: The Kappa Statistic. *Biochem. Medica.* **2012**, *22*, 276–282. Available online: https://pubmed.ncbi.nlm.nih.gov/23092060 (accessed on 14 December 2020). [CrossRef]
21. Sciensano. Definition de cas, Indications de Demande d'un test et Déclaration Obligatoire de cas COVID-19. 31 December 2020. Available online: https://covid-19.sciensano.be/sites/default/files/Covid19/COVID-19_Case%20definition_Testing_FR.pdf (accessed on 22 March 2021).
22. Sciensano. RAG Interpretation and Reporting of SARS-CoV-2 PCR Results. 12 December 2020. Available online: https://covid-19.sciensano.be/sites/default/files/Covid19/20201208_Advice%20RAG%20Interpretation%20and%20reporting%20of%20COVID%20PCR%20results.pdf (accessed on 22 March 2021).
23. Porte, L.; Legarraga, P.; Vollrath, V.; Aguilera, X.; Munita, J.M.; Araos, R.; Pizarro, G.; Vial, P.; Iruretagoyena, M.; Dittrich, S.; et al. Evaluation of a Novel Antigen-Based Rapid Detection Test for the Diagnosis of SARS-CoV-2 in Respiratory Samples. *Int. J. Infect. Dis.* **2020**, *99*, 328–333. [CrossRef] [PubMed]
24. Favresse, J.; Gillot, C.; Oliveira, M.; Cadrobbi, J.; Elsen, M.; Eucher, C.; Laffineur, K.; Rosseels, C.; Van Eeckhoudt, S.; Nicolas, J.-B.; et al. Head-to-Head Comparison of Rapid and Automated Antigen Detection Tests for the Diagnosis of SARS-CoV-2 Infection. *J. Clin. Med.* **2021**, *10*, 265. [CrossRef] [PubMed]
25. ECDC (European Centre for Disease Prevention and Control). Technical Reports: Options for the Use of Rapid Antigen Tests for COVID-19 in the EU/EEA and the UK. 19 November 2020. Available online: https://www.ecdc.europa.eu/sites/default/files/documents/Options-use-of-rapid-antigen-tests-for-COVID-19_0.pdf (accessed on 27 November 2020).
26. Linares, M.; Pérez-Tanoira, R.; Carrero, A.; Romanyk, J.; Pérez-García, F.; Gómez-Herruz, P.; Arroyo, T.; Cuadros, J. Panbio Antigen Rapid Test is Reliable to Diagnose SARS-CoV-2 Infection in the First 7 Days After the Onset of Symptoms. *J. Clin. Virol.* **2020**, *133*, 104659. [CrossRef] [PubMed]

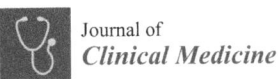

Article

Impact of Kidney Failure on the Severity of COVID-19

Dorota Zarębska-Michaluk [1,*], Jerzy Jaroszewicz [2], Magdalena Rogalska [3], Beata Lorenc [4], Marta Rorat [5,6], Anna Szymanek-Pasternak [5], Anna Piekarska [7], Aleksandra Berkan-Kawińska [7], Katarzyna Sikorska [8], Magdalena Tudrujek-Zdunek [9], Barbara Oczko-Grzesik [2], Beata Bolewska [10], Piotr Czupryna [11], Dorota Kozielewicz [12], Justyna Kowalska [13], Regina Podlasin [14], Krzysztof Kłos [15], Włodzimierz Mazur [16], Piotr Leszczyński [17,18], Bartosz Szetela [19], Katarzyna Reczko [1] and Robert Flisiak [3]

1. Department of Infectious Diseases, Jan Kochanowski University, 25-317 Kielce, Poland; reczko.katarzyna@poczta.fm
2. Department of Infectious Diseases and Hepatology, Medical University of Silesia, 40-055 Katowice, Poland; jjaroszewicz@sum.edu.pl (J.J.); bgrzesik@hoga.pl (B.O.-G.)
3. Department of Infectious Diseases and Hepatology, Medical University of Białystok, 15-089 Białystok, Poland; pmagdar@gmail.com (M.R.); robert.flisiak1@gmail.com (R.F.)
4. Pomeranian Center of Infectious Diseases, Department of Infectious Diseases, Medical University of Gdańsk, 80-210 Gdańsk, Poland; lormar@gumed.edu.pl
5. Department of Infectious Diseases and Hepatology, Wrocław Medical University, 50-367 Wrocław, Poland; marta.rorat@gmail.com (M.R.); aszymanek7@gmail.com (A.S.-P.)
6. Department of Forensic Medicine, Wrocław Medical University, 50-367 Wrocław, Poland
7. Department of Infectious Diseases and Hepatology, Medical University of Łódź, 90-549 Łódź, Poland; annapiekar@gmail.com (A.P.); aleksandra.berkan@gmail.com (A.B.-K.)
8. Department of Tropical and Parasitic Diseases, Medical University of Gdańsk, 80-210 Gdańsk, Poland; ksikorska@gumed.edu.pl
9. Department of Infectious Diseases and Hepatology, Medical University of Lublin, 20-059 Lublin, Poland; magdalena.tudrujek@gmail.com
10. Department of Infectious Diseases, University of Medical Sciences, 61-701 Poznań, Poland; bbolewska@ump.edu.pl
11. Department of the Infectious Diseases and Neuroinfections, Medical University in Białystok, 15-089 Białystok, Poland; avalon-5@wp.pl
12. Department of Infectious Diseases and Hepatology, Faculty of Medicine, Collegium Medicum in Bydgoszcz, Nicolaus Copernicus University, 87-100 Toruń, Poland; d.kozielewicz@wsoz.pl
13. Department of Adults Infectious Diseases, Medical University of Warsaw, 02-091 Warsaw, Poland; jdkowalska@gmail.com
14. Hospital of Infectious Diseases in Warsaw, 01-201 Warsaw, Poland; podlasin@zakazny.pl
15. Department of Infectious Diseases and Allergology, Military Institute of Medicine, 04-141 Warsaw, Poland; kklos@wim.mil.pl
16. Clinical Department of Infectious Diseases in Chorzów, Medical University of Silesia, 41-500 Katowice, Poland; wlodek.maz@gmail.com
17. Department of Rheumatology and Osteoporosis, Jozef Strus Hospital in Poznań, 61-285 Poznań, Poland; piotr_leszczynski@wp.pl
18. Department of Rheumatology, Rehabilitation and Internal Medicine, Poznan University of Medical Sciences, 61-701 Poznań, Poland
19. Department of Infectious Diseases, Liver Diseases and Acquired Immune Deficiencies, Wrocław Medical University, 50-367 Wrocław, Poland; bartoszetela@gmail.com
* Correspondence: dorota1010@tlen.pl; Tel.: +48-662441465; Fax: +48-41-3682262

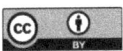

Abstract: Background: Patients with kidney failure are at an increased risk of progression to a severe form of coronavirus disease 2019 (COVID-19) with high mortality. The current analysis was aimed to assess the impact of renal failure on the severity of COVID-19 and identify the risk factors of the fatal outcome in this population. Methods: The analysis included patients from the SARSTer database, a national real-world study evaluating treatment for COVID-19 in 30 Polish centers. Data were completed retrospectively and submitted online. Results: A total of 2322 patients were included in the analysis. Kidney failure was diagnosed in 455 individuals (19.65%), of whom 373 presented moderate stage and 82 patients, including 14 dialysis individuals, presented severe renal failure. Patients with kidney failure were significantly older and demonstrated a more severe course of COVID-19. The age, baseline SpO$_2$, the ordinal scale of 4 and 5, neutrophil and platelet count, estimated glomerular filtration rate, and C-reactive protein concentration as well as malignancy and arterial hypertension were the independent predictors of 28-day mortality in logistic regression analysis. Conclusions: Underlying kidney disease in patients with COVID-19 is among the leading factors associated with a higher risk of severe clinical presentation and increased mortality rate.

Keywords: kidney failure; SARS-CoV-2; COVID-19; mortality

1. Introduction

Severe acute respiratory syndrome coronavirus 2 (SARS-CoV-2) has rapidly spread worldwide since it was first identified in December 2019 in Wuhan. Despite an unprecedented global public health effort, the outbreak became pandemic on 11 March 2020. After one year, more than 120 million affected people with nearly 3 million deaths globally due to coronavirus disease 2019 (COVID-19) were documented [1]. The clinical spectrum of SARS-CoV-2 infection ranges from asymptomatic through mild and moderate respiratory illness to critical life-threatening viral pneumonia with respiratory failure, septic shock, and multiple organ dysfunction. The higher risk of the severe clinical presentation of COVID-19 is associated with older age, immunosuppressive therapy, and underlying comorbidities including cardiovascular and chronic pulmonary illnesses, diabetes, cancers, and chronic kidney diseases (CKD) [2-4].

The progressive loss of renal function in CKD results in alterations of the innate and adaptive immune system, including decreased leukocyte phagocytic activity, dwindling dendritic cells responsible for presenting antigens, depletion and dysfunction of B lymphocytes, and impaired cell-mediated immunity through an accelerated T cell turnover and increased apoptosis of cluster of differentiation (CD) 4+ and CD8+ lymphocytes [5]. The impaired immune response is associated with higher incidence and more severe course of infections which appear to be responsible for a large part of the mortality, especially in patients with end-stage renal disease (ESRD). Alongside secondary immunodeficiency, the immune activation in patients with chronic kidney disease is observed [6]. The increased production and decreased clearance of pro-inflammatory cytokines lead to systemic inflammation and oxidative stress, which contribute to atherosclerotic cardiovascular disease and other conditions worsening the prognosis of patients with SARS-CoV-2 infection.

The current analysis was aimed to assess the impact of kidney failure on the severity of COVID-19 and to identify the risk factors of the fatal outcome of the disease in this population in the real-world setting.

2. Materials and Methods

The study population consisted of patients included in the national database SARSTer, which is an ongoing project supported by the Polish Association of Epidemiologists and Infectiologists and covers 2784 adult individuals treated for COVID-19 between 1 March and 31 December 2020 in 30 Polish centers. All the patients were diagnosed with COVID-19 based on positive results of the real-time reverse transcriptase-polymerase chain reaction (RT-PCR) from the nasopharyngeal swab specimen [7].

The therapeutic management decisions were taken at the discretion of the treating physician following the current medical knowledge and in line with the national recommendations [8-10]. The SARSTer study had the approval of the Ethical Committee of the Medical University of Białystok with a granted waiver of informed consent from study participants due to its retrospective design, and the local bioethics committees in case of the off-label use of medication in patients with COVID-19.

Patients' data were retrieved retrospectively from hospital files and completed online by a platform operated by "Tiba" sp. z o.o. The parameters gathered on admission included age, gender, body mass index (BMI), comorbidities and concomitant medications, clinical symptoms of SARS-CoV-2 infection, lung computed tomography scan, and selected lab values. The baseline laboratory data consisted of complete blood count, inflammatory indicators (C-reactive protein (CRP), procalcitonin (PCT), ferritin, and interleukin 6 (IL-6) concentration if tocilizumab (TCZ) prescription was considered), coagulation parameters such as D-dimer, international normalized ratio (INR), and fibrinogen, the activity of liver enzymes (aspartate and alanine aminotransferases, gamma-glutamyl transpeptidase, lactate dehydrogenase), and renal function tests. Estimated glomerular filtration rate (eGFR) was calculated with the MDRD Study equation and, using this measure, CKD was defined as eGFR < 60 mL/min/1.73 m^2 along with a history of kidney disease from medical records [11]. According to renal function on admission, patients were stratified into three groups: eGFR < 30 mL/min/1.73 m^2, eGFR 30–60 mL/min/1.73 m^2, and eGFR > 60 mL/min/1.73 m^2.

The COVID-19 severity on hospital admission was determined based on blood oxygen saturation (SpO$_2$) and clinical status was defined as symptomatic stable with SpO$_2$ > 95%, symptomatic unstable with two levels of baseline saturation SpO$_2$ 91–95% or SpO$_2$ $\leq$ 90%, and critical with acute respiratory distress syndrome (ARDS). The information on the medications applied for the treatment of COVID-19, including remdesivir (RDV), tocilizumab (TCZ), dexamethasone, convalescent plasma, low weight molecular heparin, and antibiotics, as well as drug-related adverse events, were collected during the hospitalization.

The patients were scored at baseline and then every 7 days during the following 28 days after admission on an ordinal scale, which includes eight categories: 1. unhospitalized, no activity restrictions; 2. unhospitalized, no activity restrictions and/or requiring oxygen supplementation at home; 3. hospitalized, does not require oxygen supplementation and does not require medical care; 4. hospitalized, requiring no oxygen supplementation, but requiring medical care; 5. hospitalized, requiring normal oxygen supplementation, low-flow by mask or nasal prongs; 6. hospitalized, on non-invasive ventilation with high-flow oxygen equipment; 7. hospitalized, for invasive mechanical ventilation or ECMO; 8. death.

The study outcomes included death, need for mechanical ventilation, and clinical improvement defined as at least a 2-point decrease in an ordinal scale classification from baseline to 14, 21, and 28 days of hospitalization.

To evaluate the impact of chronic kidney disease on the outcome of COVID-19, the analysis was performed concerning the eGFR at baseline.

Statistical Analysis

The results are expressed as mean ± standard deviation (SD) or n (%) and odds ratios with 95% confidence intervals. p values of <0.05 were considered to be statistically significant. The significance of difference was calculated by Fisher's exact test for nominal variables and by Mann–Whitney U and Kruskal–Wallis ANOVA for continuous and ordinal variables. Due to the highly variable group size, the Fisher's p-values were accompanied by OR as the sample size independent effect size measures. The association between variables was measured by Spearman's rank correlation coefficient and its significance test p-values. Survival analyses between patients with different eGFR ranges (Kaplan–Meier curves) were performed by Log-rank (Mantel–Cox) Test. Forward stepwise logistic regression models with Bayesian Information Criterion (BIC) as a model selection criterion were performed with death within 28-days after the start of hospitalization as the dependent variable. Among independent variables tested for the best model were age, sex, BMI, arterial hypertension, diabetes, coronary artery disease, chronic obstructive pulmonary disease, malignancy, GFR range, baseline levels of SpO2, CRP, procalcitonin, WBC, lymphocyte and neutrophil counts, platelets, D-dimer, ALT as well as therapy with dexamethasone, remdesivir, tocilizumab, and heparins. Logistic regression models were calculated by use of Statistica 13.0 (TIBCO Software Inc., Palo Alto, CA, USA).

3. Results

Among 2784 adult patients included in the SARSTer project, the data on kidney function were provided for 2322 individuals with a mean age of 60.4 ± 17.1 years and male predominance (53%). Among them, 455 individuals presented kidney impairment, a moderate stage of renal insufficiency was diagnosed in 373 patients with eGFR 30–60 mL/min/1.73 m^2, of which six underwent kidney transplantation, and 82 patients with eGFR < 30 mL/min/1.73 m^2 were diagnosed with severe renal failure (68 patients with non-dialysis dependent CKD) and ESRD (14 dialysis patients). Among patients with renal failure, 328 with moderate and 74 with severe stage had the diagnosis of chronic kidney disease based on the medical file, whereas in the remaining 53 individuals we were not able to confirm CKD due to incomplete records or disturbed communication with patients. Despite the lack of a previous diagnosis of CKD and no follow-up during three months after discharge from the hospital, we included these patients based on the depth-analysis of the available data concerning comorbidities and taking into account the age of patients as a risk factor of CKD and no improvement in the renal function after hydration. The detailed baseline characteristics of the patients according to kidney function on admission to the hospital are summarized in Table 1.

Table 1. Baseline characteristics of patients according to kidney function.

Characteristic	eGFR > 60 mL/min n = 1867	eGFR 30–60 mL/min n = 373	eGFR < 30 mL/min n = 82	p
Age				
Mean (SD)	57.1 (16.5)	73.4 (12.5)	76.5 (12.9)	<0.001
>70 years (%)	397 (21.3)	240 (64.3)	57 (69.5)	<0.001
Gender				
Female, n (%)	869 (46.5)	177 (47.5)	44 (53.7)	0.44
Male, n (%)	998 (53.5)	196 (52.5)	38 (46.3)	
Body mass index, mean (SD)	27.8 (5.1)	28.5 (5.3)	29.2 (6.9)	0.03
Disease severity at the baseline, n (%)				
Oxygen saturation 91–95%	596 (31.9)	129 (34.6)	24 (29.3)	0.51
Oxygen saturation ≤ 90%	526 (28.2)	169 (45.3)	43 (52.4)	<0.001
Score on ordinal scale, n (%)				
3. Hospitalized, does not require oxygen supplementation and does not require medical care	131 (7%)	3 (1.9%)	1 (1.2%)	<0.001
4. Hospitalized, requiring no oxygen supplementation, but requiring medical care	833 (44.6)	108 (29)	21 (25.6)	<0.001
5. Hospitalized, requiring normal oxygen supplementation	835 (44.7)	244 (65.4)	54 (65.9)	<0.001
6. Hospitalized, on non-invasive ventilation with high-flow oxygen equipment	61 (3.3)	14 (3.7)	3 (3.7)	0.88
7. Hospitalized, for invasive mechanical ventilation or ECMO	6 (0.3)	0	3 (3.7)	-
Concomitant medications, n (%)	1071 (57.4)	331 (88.7)	69 (84.1)	<0.001
Coexisting conditions, n (%)	1285 (68.9)	354 (94.9)	77 (93.9)	<0.001
Arterial hypertension	719 (38.5)	268 (71.8)	53 (64.6)	<0.001
Coronary artery disease	155 (8.3)	92 (24.7)	27 (32.9)	<0.001
Heart failure	58 (3.1)	51 (13.7)	20 (24.4)	<0.001
Atrial fibrillation	88 (4.7)	59 (15.8)	11 (13.4)	<0.001
Diabetes	268 (14.4)	53 (14.2)	30 (36.6)	<0.001
Cerebrovascular disease	48 (2.6)	23 (6.2)	4 (4.9)	0.001
Malignancy	99 (5.3)	42 (11.3)	9 (11)	<0.001
Chronic obstructive pulmonary disease	46 (2.5)	29 (7.8)	2 (2.4)	<0.001
Bronchial asthma	91 (4.9)	20 (5.4)	6 (7.3)	0.58
Chronic liver disease	49 (2.6)	7 (1.9)	1 (1.2)	0.53
Dementia	47 (2.5)	21 (5.6)	6 (7.3)	0.001
Hypothyroidism	136 (7.3)	28 (7.5)	1 (1.2)	0.10

eGRF, estimated glomerular filtration rate; SD, standard deviation; ECM, extracorporeal membrane oxygenation.

Patients with renal failure were significantly older and demonstrated a more severe course of COVID-19 on admission, defined by the higher rate of patients with an oxygen saturation ≤ 90% and a greater percentage of the more advanced categories on the ordinal scale. Patients with CKD more frequently suffered from diabetes and cardiovascular diseases including arterial hypertension, coronary artery disease, heart failure, and atrial fibrillation, and were more likely to be treated with insulin, oral antidiabetics, and antihypertensive drugs, compared to non-CKD individuals. Among medications reducing blood pressure, beta-blockers and diuretics were used predominantly in patients with renal failure (Supplementary Table S1).

Significantly higher values of inflammatory parameters including the concentration of CRP, PCT, and IL-6, as well as white blood cell and neutrophil counts, and lower platelet counts were documented in patients with CKD on admission (Table 2).

Table 2. Baseline laboratory indicators according to the baseline kidney function.

Characteristic	eGFR > 60 mL/min n = 1867	eGFR 30–60 mL/min n = 373	eGFR < 30 mL/min n = 82	p
CRP mg/L, mean (SD)	65.5 (73.8)	91.7 (85.2)	107 (85.2)	<0.001
Procalcitonin ng/mL, mean (SD)	0.28 (1.82)	1.30 (6.8)	2.83 (6.6)	<0.001
Leukocytes 1/µL, mean (SD)	6405 (3079)	8962 (15028)	8700 (4563)	<0.001
Lymphocytes 1/µL, mean (SD)	1311 (909)	1532 (4064)	1026 (630)	<0.001
Neutrocytes 1/µL, mean (SD)	4446 (2767)	5717 (4575)	7050 (4136)	<0.001
Platelets 1000/µL, mean (SD)	221 (90.5)	202 (96)	208.5 (125.1)	<0.001
IL-6 pg/mL, mean (SD)	47.0 (94.2)	108.7 (209.1)	211.2 (600.3)	<0.001
D-dimers ng/mL, mean (SD)	1638 (5448)	2127 (3628)	5113 (11612)	<0.001
ALT IU/L, mean (SD)	41 (39)	36 (29)	52 (223)	0.001

CRP, C-reactive protein; ALT, alanine aminotransferase.

Patients with CKD were more often treated for COVID-19 with IL-6 inhibitor tocilizumab (TCZ), dexamethasone, and low molecular weight heparin compared with patients without kidney abnormalities. The application of remdesivir (RDV) was significantly lower in CKD patients, and five individuals with severe renal failure received off-label RDV, four of them were concurrently treated with TCZ, and two with dexamethasone—all were scored on admission in category 5 on the ordinal scale. Antibiotics were administered more frequently in those with severe renal failure (Table 3).

Table 3. In-hospital treatment for COVID-19 according to the baseline kidney function.

Medications	eGFR > 60 mL/min n = 1867	eGFR 30–60 mL/min n = 373	eGFR < 30 mL/min n = 82	p
Related to COVID-19, n (%)				
Remdesivir	454 (24.3)	81 (21.7)	5 (6.1)	<0.001
Tocilizumab	186 (9.9)	79 (21.1)	14 (17.1)	<0.001
Dexamethason	492 (26.3)	137 (36.7)	35 (42.7)	<0.001
Convalescent plasma	216 (11.6)	44 (11.8)	16 (19.5)	0.09
Low molecular weight heparin	1306 (70) *	299 (80.2) **	69 (84.1) ***	<0.001

* 1208 patients received prophylactic dose and 98 therapeutic dose. ** 251 patients were on prophylactic dose only, 17 received prophylactic dose on admission and then therapeutic dose during hospitalization, and 31 patients were on therapeutic dose from admission. *** 55 patients were on prophylactic dose, 14 patients received prophylactic then therapeutic and remaining 8 were on therapeutic dose.

Continuous renal replacement therapy was continued only in 14 hemodialyzed patients, this therapy was not initiated by anyone else, and no patient was treated with hemoperfusion to remove cytokines.

As shown in Table 4, 28-day in-hospital mortality and the need for mechanical ventilation significantly increased in direct proportion to the degree of renal impairment. Moreover, clinical improvement was significantly slower in patients with advanced renal impairment.

Table 4. Outcome according to baseline kidney function.

	A eGFR > 60 mL/min	B eGFR 30–60 mL/min	C eGFR < 30 mL/min	Odds Ratio A vs. B	Odds Ratio B vs. C	Odds Ratio A vs. C
n	$n = 1867$	$n = 373$	$n = 82$			
Death, n (%)	132 (7.1)	82 (22)	35 (42.7)	0.27 (0.20–0.36) $p < 0.001$	0.38 (0.23–0.62) $p < 0.001$	0.10 (0.06–0.17) $p < 0.001$
Death time, mean (SD), days	14.4 (10.8)	10.8 (8.2)	8 (6.6)	<0.001	$p = 0.01$	$p = 0.48$
Mechanical ventilation, n (%)	86 (4.6)	35 (9.4)	10 (12.2)	0.47 (0.31–0.70) $p < 0.001$	0.74 (0.35–1.57) $p = 0.42$	0.35 (0.17–0.70) $p = 0.006$
Clinical improvement 14th day, n (%)	1068 (57.2)	158 (42.4)	21 (25.6)	1.81 (1.45–2.28) $p < 0.001$	2.13 (1.25–3.65) $p = 0.006$	3.89 (2.34–6.43) $p < 0.001$
Clinical improvement 21st day, n (%)	1467 (78.6)	222 (59.5)	34 (41.5)	2.45 (1.97–3.15) $p < 0.001$	2.07 (1.28–3.37) $p = 0.003$	5.18 (3.29–8.14) $p < 0.001$
Clinical improvement 28th day, n (%)	1601 (85.8)	262 (70.2)	40 (48.8)	2.55 (1.97–3.30) $p < 0.001$	2.47 (1.52–4.03) <0.001	6.32 (4.02–9.93) <0.001

The analysis of the outcome according to baseline kidney function that also takes into account the selected parameters at the admission is presented in the supplementary tables (Supplementary Tables S3–S5).

The analysis performed depending on the survival revealed that patients who died were significantly older, with a higher proportion of males, a greater percentage of baseline oxygen saturation $\leq 90\%$, more severe clinical presentation on admission in terms of oxygen demand, more frequent comorbidities and treatment with concomitant medications, with significantly higher values of inflammatory parameters and D-dimer level, and lower platelet count. Those patients were more likely to be treated with TCZ, dexamethasone, convalescent plasma, low molecular weight heparin, and antibiotics. Furthermore, higher rates of individuals with moderate and severe kidney failure were reported in this group of patients (Table 5).

Among patients with eGFR < 30 mL/min/1.73 m^2, no statistically significant differences were noticed between dialyzed and not dialyzed patients regarding baseline demographic and clinical measures as well as effectiveness outcomes (Supplementary Table S2). However, those who died were significantly older, with a higher proportion of baseline oxygen saturation $\leq 90\%$, were more likely to have coexisting conditions, with higher AST activity on admission, and were more frequently treated with antibiotics during hospitalizations (Table 6).

Table 5. Comparison of patients who died or survived regardless of kidney function.

Characteristic	Died N = 249	28-Day Survive N = 2073	p-Value
Age			
Mean (SD)	74.2 (11.9)	58.7 (16.9)	<0.001
>70 years (%)	158 (63.5)	536 (25.9)	<0.001
Gender			
Female, n (%)	95 (38.2)	995 (48)	0.04
Male, n (%)	154 (61.8)	1078 (52)	0.04
Body mass index, mean (SD)	27.9 (6.1)	28 (5.1)	0.47
Disease severity at the baseline, n (%)			
Oxygen saturation 91–95%	51 (20.5)	698 (33.7)	<0.001
Oxygen saturation ≤ 90%	169 (67.9)	569 (27.5)	<0.001
Score on ordinal scale, n (%)			
3. Hospitalized, does not require oxygen supplementation and does not require medical care	1 (0.4)	138 (6.7)	
4. Hospitalized, requiring no oxygen supplementation, but requiring medical care	36 (14.5)	926 (44.7)	<0.001
5. Hospitalized, requiring normal oxygen supplementation	174 (69.9)	959 (46.3)	
6. Hospitalized, on non-invasive ventilation with high-flow oxygen equipment	30 (12)	48 (2.3)	
7. Hospitalized, for invasive mechanical ventilation or ECMO	8 (3.2)	1 (0.05)	
Concomitant medications, n (%)	205 (82.3)	1266 (61.1)	<0.001
Coexisting conditions, n (%)	233 (93.6)	1483 (71.5)	<0.001
Medication related to COVID-19, n (%)			
Remdesivir	61 (24.5)	479 (23.1)	0.68
Tocilizumab	55 (22.1)	224 (10.8)	<0.001
Dexamethason	135 (54.2)	529 (25.5)	<0.001
Convalescent plasma	50 (20.1)	226 (10.9)	<0.001
Low molecular weight heparin	203 (81.5)	1471 (71)	<0.001
Antibiotics	183 (73.5)	1045 (50.4)	<0.001
CRP mg/L, mean (SD)	128.5 (91.7)	64.2 (72.1)	<0.001
Procalcitonin ng/mL, mean (SD)	2.0 (6.2)	0.36 (2.98)	<0.001
Leukocytes 1/µL, mean (SD)	10,622 (16,729)	6450 (3963)	<0.001
Lymphocytes 1/µL, mean (SD)	1186 (2122)	1354 (1798)	<0.001
Neutrocytes 1/µL, mean (SD)	7354 (5150)	4441 (2796)	<0.001
Platelets 1000/µL, mean (SD)	210 (109)	219 (91)	0.008
IL-6 pg/mL, mean (SD)	192.4 (399.7)	50.2 (107.4)	<0.001
D-dimers ng/mL, mean (SD)	4654 (9820)	1507 (4722)	<0.001
ALT IU/L, mean (SD)	51 (133)	39 (37)	0.06
eGFR < 30 mL/min/1,73 m^2, n(%)	35 (14.1)	47 (2.3)	
eGFR 30–60 mL/min/1,73 m^2, n(%)	82 (32.9)	291 (13.7)	<0.001
eGFR > 60 mL/min/1,73 m^2, n(%)	132 (53.0)	1735 (84.0)	

Table 6. Comparison of patients with eGFR < 30 mL/min who died or survived.

Characteristic	Died N = 35	28-Day Survive N = 47	p-Value
Age			
Mean (SD)	80.7 (9.4)	73.4 (14.2)	0.02
>70 years (%)	30 (85.7)	27 (57.4)	0.007
Gender			
Female, n (%)	19 (54.3)	25 (53.2)	1.00
Male, n (%)	16 (45.7)	22 (46.8)	1.00
Body mass index, mean (SD)	28.2 (7.7)	29.6 (6.5)	0.36
Disease severity at the baseline, n (%)			
Oxygen saturation 91–95%	7 (20)	17 (36.2)	0.14
Oxygen saturation ≤ 90%	24 (68.6)	19 (40.4)	0.01
Score on ordinal scale, n (%)			
3. Hospitalized, does not require oxygen supplementation and does not require medical care	0	1 (2.1)	1.00
4. Hospitalized, requiring no oxygen supplementation, but requiring medical care	7 (20)	14 (29.8)	0.44
5. Hospitalized, requiring normal oxygen supplementation	23 (65.7)	31 (66)	1.00
6. Hospitalized, on non-invasive ventilation with high-flow oxygen equipment	2 (5.7)	1 (2.1)	0.57
7. Hospitalized, for invasive mechanical ventilation or ECMO	3 (8.6)	0	0.07
Concomitant medications, n (%)	27 (77.1)	30 (63.8)	0.23
Coexisting conditions, n (%)	33 (94.3)	31 (66)	0.002
Medication related to COVID-19, n (%)			
Remdesivir	1 (2.9)	4 (8.5)	0.39
Tocilizumab	3 (8.6)	11 (23.4)	0.13
Dexamethason	15 (42.9)	20 (42.6)	1.00
Convalescent plasma	4 (11.4)	12 (25.6)	0.16
Low molecular weight heparin	28 (80)	41 (87.2)	0.54
Antibiotics	28 (65.1)	27 (57.5)	0.04
CRP mg/l, mean (SD)	120.1 (93)	97.3 (78.6)	0.28
Procalcitonin ng/mL, mean (SD)	4.75 (9.2)	1.45 (3.3)	0.07
Leukocytes 1/µL, mean (SD)	9351 (4540)	8214 (4568)	0.13
Lymphocytes 1/µL, mean (SD)	1042 (643)	1014 (628)	0.78
Neutrocytes 1/µL, mean (SD)	7803 (3871)	6527 (4274)	0.08
Platelets 1000/µL, mean (SD)	200 (103)	215 (141)	0.70
IL-6 pg/mL, mean (SD)	470.9 (1036.5)	95.8 (164.8)	0.24
D-dimers ng/mL, mean (SD)	4360 (4845)	5696 (14,940)	0.25
ALT IU/L, mean (SD)	86 (333)	26 (19)	0.43
AST IU/L, mean (SD)	72 (83)	38 (33)	0.03
GGTP IU/L, mean (SD)	33 (14)	69 (76)	0.60
LDH IU/L, mean (SD)	406 (205)	414 (192)	0.89
INR, mean (SD)	1.46 (0.83)	1.16 (0.14)	0.38
Fibrinogen mg/dL, mean (SD)	567 (150)	553.7 (216.1)	0.54
Ferritin mcg/L, mean (SD)	1828.2 (1507.3)	1244 (1533.7)	0.13

One of the five patients with eGFR < 30 mL/min/1.73 m^2 who received RDV died due to sepsis. In the remaining four, no safety issues were observed and no deterioration in renal function was documented, and in two of them clinical improvement—in one after 21 and in another after 28 days of hospitalization—was reported.

The independent predictors of 28-day mortality in logistic regression analyses were age, baseline SpO2, the ordinal scale of 4 and 5, neutrophil and platelet count, eGFR, and CRP concentration (Figure 1, Table 7).

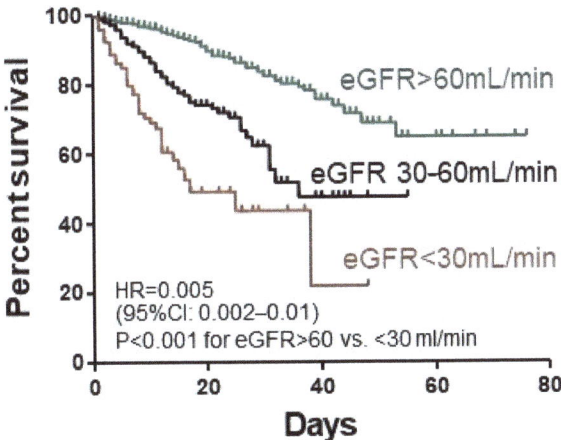

Figure 1. Kaplan–Meier survival curves of the CKD groups dependent on the eGFR.

Table 7. Baseline factors independently associated with 28-days mortality based on forward stepwise logistic regression model.

	Estimate of β	SE	tStat	p Value
(Intercept)			854,282	<0.001
Age (per year)	0.139	0.023	5991	<0.001
SpO2 (%)	−0.213	0.025	−8578	<0.001
Neutrophils	0.153	0.022	6915	<0.001
Platelets	−0.073	0.020	−3655	<0.001
CRP (mg/dL)	0.048	0.022	2123	0.034
Ordinal scale (2)	−0.038	0.044	−0.857	0.391
Ordinal scale (3)	−0.055	0.042	−1302	0.193
Ordinal scale (4)	−0.160	0.081	−1987	0.047
Ordinal scale (5)	−0.195	0.080	−2429	0.015
Ordinal scale (6)	0.027	0.033	0.821	0.411
Arterial hypertension (no)	0.069	0.021	3260	0.001
Iscehmic heart disease (no)	−0.053	0.020	−2637	0.008
Malignancy (No)	−0.120	0.019	−6384	<0.001
eGFR < 30 mL/min	0.195	0.034	5649	<0.001
eGFR 30–60 mL/min	−0.090	0.034	−2592	<0.001

p-value < 0.001.

Among comorbidities, most notably malignancy as well as arterial hypertension (HA) and ischemic heart diseases were associated with mortality, while diabetes mellitus (DM) and chronic obstructive pulmonary disease (COPD) were not. Interestingly, in this cohort of 2322 COVID-19 patients, we were not able to show an independent effect of therapies, BMI, and baseline D-dimers, ALT, or procalcitonin on overall 28-day mortality.

4. Discussion

Chronic kidney disease is an increasing public health issue affecting 8–16% of the population worldwide [12]. Patients with CKD are highly susceptible to COVID-19 and are at an increased risk of progression to a severe or critical form of the disease because of impaired immunity; additionally, they are at enhanced risk of SARS-CoV-2 infection due to frequent hospital attendance [2,13–18]. The prevalence of CKD in patients with COVID-19 has been reported in a wide range of approximately 1–47%; however, it is suggested that the lowest values result from underestimation [16,19–21]. Among patients with COVID-19 hospitalized in 30 Polish centers included in the current analysis, nearly 20% were diagnosed with CKD, of which 18% presented severe renal failure. In addition to the worse patient's status regarding the severity of COVID-19 when admitted to the hospital, we found the pre-existing renal disease to be independently associated with higher in-hospital mortality, especially in those with severe kidney failure, and our findings are in line with the results of previous studies [13,14,22–26]. The Global Burden of Disease (GBD) collaboration recently estimated the risk factors for severe COVID-19 worldwide using results from international databases and large multimorbidity studies from different countries, and determined that CKD is a condition conveying the highest risk for the severe presentation of the disease and COVID-19-related death [27]. In the current study, no difference in mortality was demonstrated between dialysis and non-dialysis dependent patients with severe renal failure, but it must be emphasized that the group of dialysis patients in the analyzed cohort was relatively small—only 14 patients. However, our findings of the comparable death risk regardless of the dialysis are consistent with observations from the study conducted by Flythe et al.

The reported death rates of 50% in 143 dialysis and 521 non-dialysis dependent individuals with CKD and 35% in 3600 non-CKD patients are higher than those noted in our analysis, but it is noteworthy that the abovementioned study included only critically ill patients with COVID-19 treated in intensive care units (ICU) [23]. The investigation performed by Yang et al. in 836 patients revealed in-hospital mortality rates of 9%, 50%, and 66.7% in non-CKD, non-dialysis dependent CKD, and dialysis patients, respectively. Of note, the proportions of individuals with the moderate presentation of COVID-19 were similar among those without and with non-dialysis dependent CKD (73.7% and 75%, respectively), and much lower in dialysis patients (40%), who were more frequently scored as severe cases on admission, which has had an impact on the fatal outcome [25].

The negative impact on the outcome was demonstrated for the baseline oxygen saturation corresponding to the severity of COVID-19 on admission—35.5% of patients with moderate and almost 56% with severe renal failure classified at baseline as $SpO_2 \leq 90\%$ died compared to a 16.5% mortality rate among non-CKD individuals. The category 5 in an ordinal scale on admission associated with the need for oxygen supplementation was an independent factor related to higher mortality, and our findings are consistent with the results of the other studies [28,29].

We confirmed older age as an independent strong predictor for in-hospital mortality, which is in line with previous reports and calculations performed by GBD collaboration in patients with CKD [2,3,15,22,23,27,30]. On the contrary, Cai et al., in a meta-analysis of 12 studies including CKD patients, documented a higher mortality rate in those below 70 years compared to older patients, explaining this finding by the more frequent rate of the other comorbidities with stronger than CKD association with increased risk of death among the elderly [14].

We did not demonstrate gender as a factor influencing the clinical status on admission and in-hospital mortality in CKD patients, and among those with severe renal failure, the death rate was nearly equal between females and males. Thus, the results of our study differ from other reports documenting a higher risk of severe course and COVID-19-related death rate in males [2,4,22,27,30,31].

In the current analysis, patients with CKD presented significantly increased baseline leukocyte and neutrophil counts, a higher level of inflammatory markers, including CRP, PCT, and IL-6 concentration, as well as D-dimer level compared to patients without CKD. Those parameters were increased in direct proportion to the degree of renal impairment and probably corresponded to a proinflammatory state. The high CRP concentration, the increased neutrophils, and the decreased platelet counts on admission were independently associated with a significantly higher in-hospital death rate in patients with CKD, which supported results from other studies [22,23,25,30,32,33]. Among comorbidities, arterial hypertension, ischemic heart disease, and malignancy were found to be independent negative predictors of 28-day survival and these findings, whereas diabetes and COPD were not. The impact of coexisting diseases was investigated in many studies and results are divergent depending on the analyzed population, sample size, and the nature of the study. Meta-analysis performed among Iranian patients by Merjalili et al. revealed that diabetes was associated with higher mortality, while arterial hypertension was not [26]. Park et al. analyzed the Korean population and found both diabetes and hypertension to be risk factors for death in the course of COVID-19 [34]. The same results were achieved by Gupta et al. among Indian patients [35]. Chen et al. demonstrated only ischemic heart disease and cerebrovascular disease to be independently associated with high mortality in Chinese patients [36]. According to the results of the meta-analysis conducted by Chaoqun et al., the presence of cerebrovascular disease, DM, COPD, malignancy, and hypertension was related to higher mortality in the course of COVID-19 [15]. Factors associated with an increased risk of death documented by Wiliamson et al. included ischemic heart disease, DM, and malignancy, especially hematological [2]. It should be pointed out that the percentage of diabetes among patients with severe renal failure was significantly higher compared to those with moderate kidney impairment and non-CKD individuals, which allows us to suppose that diabetic nephropathy is responsible for some cases of ESKD.

Of COVID-19-related medications, dexamethasone and tocilizumab were used more frequently in patients with CKD, probably as a result of more severe clinical presentation of the disease, so we were not able to show an independent effect of those therapies. According to the summary of product characteristics, the application of RDV was significantly lower in CKD patients; however, five individuals with severe renal failure scored at baseline in category 5 on an ordinal scale and received off-label RDV, and one of them died; however, it should be pointed out that in the remaining four patients no deterioration in renal function was documented [37]. Similar observations in a small series of 20 patients with ESKD treated with RDV were published by Pettit et al., where therapy appeared to be relatively safe and the potential benefit outweighed the theoretical risk of renal toxicity [38].

We are aware of several limitations of our study associated with its retrospective design—the analyses were based on the clinically available electronic captured data with possible entry errors, a lack of information about the causes of CKD, and in some cases a lack of confirmation of CKD due to incomplete records, and also missing laboratory tests in some patients, which did not allow us to assess the impact on the mortality of the selected parameters. As treatment with RDV and TCZ is not indicated in patients with eGFR <30 mL/min/1.73 m^2 and, in turn, the absence of such treatment may influence the investigated outcomes, we may overestimate the causal effect of CKD on study endpoints. Lastly, due to the lack of control laboratory tests during hospitalization in some patients, we performed analysis taking into consideration the baseline renal status of patients with CKD, not looking at the development of acute kidney injury (AKI) in the course of COVID-19 in those individuals, although the experience from previous reports showed that AKI is associated with higher mortality [24,39–41].

However, the strengths of our study include a large number of patients from the heterogeneous population, covering different parts of the country, which increases the generalizability of the findings—all of them had a laboratory-confirmed SARS-CoV-2 infection and the patients were followed up for 28 days.

Supplementary Materials: The following are available online at https://www.mdpi.com/article/10.3390/jcm10092042/s1, Table S1: Medications for the treatment of comorbidities, Table S2: Patients with eGFR < 30 mL/min according to dialysis, Table S3: Patients with baseline CRP ≥ 100 mg/L—outcome according to kidney function, Table S4: Patients with baseline SpO2 ≤ 90%—outcome according to kidney function, Table S5: Patients with baseline D-dimers ≥ 1000 ng/mL—outcome according to kidney function.

Author Contributions: Conceptualization—D.Z.-M., R.F., methodology—D.Z.-M., formal analysis—D.Z.-M., J.J., investigation—D.Z.-M., validation—R.F., writing—original draft preparation—D.Z.-M., writing—review and editing—R.F., supervision—R.F., project administration—R.F., funding acquisition—R.F., data collection—D.Z.-M., J.J., M.R. (Magdalena Rogalska), B.L., M.R. (Marta Rorat), A.S.-P., A.P., A.B.-K., K.S., M.T.-Z., B.O.-G., B.B., P.C., D.K., J.K., R.P., K.K., W.M., P.L., B.S., K.R., R.F. All authors have read and agreed to the published version of the manuscript.

Funding: This research was funded by the Medical Research Agency, grant number 2020/ABM/COVID19/PTEILCHZ, and the Polish Association of Epidemiologists and Infectiologists.

Institutional Review Board Statement: The study was conducted according to the guidelines of the Declaration of Helsinki. The SARSTer study had the approval of the Ethical Committee of the Medical University of Białystok (APK.002.303.2020).

Informed Consent Statement: Patient consent was waived due to the retrospective design of the study.

Data Availability Statement: Data supporting reported results can be provided upon request from the corresponding author.

Conflicts of Interest: D.Z.-M. reports personal fees from Gilead and Abbvie, outside the submitted work. R.F. reports grants from Abbvie, Gilead, Merck, personal fees from Gilead, Abbvie, Merck, Roche, and non-financial support from Abbvie, Gilead, and Merck outside the submitted work. J.J. reports personal fees from Gilead, Abbvie, Bausch Health, Merck, Promed, Roche, and non-financial support from Abbvie, Gilead, and Merck outside the submitted work. D.K. reports personal fees from Gilead and Abbvie outside the submitted work. J.K. reports personal fees from Gilead, Merck, ViiV, Janssen outside the submitted work. R.P. reports personal fees from Gilead outside the submitted work. W.M. reports grants and personal fees from Gilead, Abbvie, Abbott, Roche, Janssen outside the submitted work. P.L. reports grants and personal fees from Abbvie, Roche, UCB, Lilly, Novartis, BMS, Amgen, Janssen, Abivax, Viela-Bio outside the submitted work. BS reports grants from Abbvie, Gilead, Janssen, personal fees from Gilead, Abbvie, Janssen outside the submitted work. MRog, B.L., MRor, A.S.-P, A.P., A.B.-K., B.B., M.T.-Z., D.K., K.K., K.R., P.C., B.O.-G., K.S. declare no competing interests.

References

1. World Health Organization. Coronavirus Disease (COVID-19) Pandemic. Available online: https://www.who.int/emergencies/diseases/novel-coronavirus-2019/.WorldHealthOrganizationwebsite (accessed on 21 March 2021).
2. Williamson, E.J.; Walker, A.J.; Bhaskaran, K.; Bacon, S.; Bates, C.; Morton, C.E.; Curtis, H.J.; Mehrkar, A.; Evans, D.; Inglesby, P.; et al. Factors associated with COVID-19-related death using OpenSAFELY. *Nature* **2020**, *584*, 430–436. [CrossRef]
3. Du, R.H.; Liang, L.R.; Yang, C.Q.; Wang, W.; Cao, T.Z.; Li, M.; Guo, G.Y.; Du, J.; Zheng, C.L.; Zhu, Q.; et al. Predictors of mortality for patients with COVID-19 pneumonia caused by SARS-CoV-2: A prospective cohort study. *Eur. Respir. J.* **2020**, *55*, 2000524. [CrossRef] [PubMed]
4. Richardson, S.; Hirsch, J.S.; Narasimhan, M.; Crawford, J.M.; McGinn, T.; Davidson, K.W.; the Northwell COVID-19 Research Consortium; Barnaby, D.P.; Becker, L.B.; Chelico, J.D.; et al. Presenting Characteristics, Comorbidities, and Outcomes among 5700 Patients Hospitalized With COVID-19 in the New York City Area. *JAMA* **2020**, *323*, 2052–2059. [CrossRef] [PubMed]
5. Girndt, M.; Sester, M.; Sester, U.; Kaul, H.; Köhler, H. Molecular aspects of T- and B-cell function in uremia. *Kidney Int. Suppl.* **2001**, *78*, S206–S211. [CrossRef] [PubMed]
6. Syed-Ahmed, M.; Narayanan, M. Immune Dysfunction and Risk of Infection in Chronic Kidney Disease. *Adv. Chronic Kidney Dis.* **2019**, *26*, 8–15. [CrossRef]
7. World Health Organization. *Clinical Management of Severe Acute Respiratory Infection (SARI) When COVID-19 Disease Is Suspected: Interim Guidance*; Version 1.2; World Health Organization: Geneva, Switzerland, 13 March 2020.
8. Flisiak, R.; Horban, A.; Jaroszewicz, J.; Kozielewicz, D.; Pawłowska, M.; Parczewski, M.; Piekarska, A.; Simon, K.; Tomasiewicz, K.; Zarębska-Michaluk, D. Management of SARS-CoV-2 infection: Recommendations of the Polish Association of Epidemiologists and Infectiologists as of 31 March 2020. *Pol. Arch. Intern. Med.* **2020**, *130*, 352–357.
9. Flisiak, R.; Horban, A.; Jaroszewicz, J.; Kozielewicz, D.; Pawłowska, M.; Parczewski, M.; Piekarska, A.; Simon, K.; Tomasiewicz, K.; Zarębska-Michaluk, D. Management of SARS-CoV-2 infection: Recommendations of the Polish Association of Epidemiologists and Infectiologists. Annex no. 1 as of 8 June 2020. *Pol. Arch. Intern. Med.* **2020**, *130*, 557–558.
10. Flisiak, R.; Parczewski, M.; Horban, A.; Jaroszewicz, J.; Kozielewicz, D.; Pawłowska, M.; Piekarska, A.; Simon, K.; Tomasiewicz, K.; Zarębska-Michaluk, D. Management of SARS-CoV-2 infection: Recommendations of the Polish Association of Epidemiologists and Infectiologists. Annex no. 2 as of 13 October 2020. *Pol. Arch. Intern. Med.* **2020**, *130*, 915–918. [CrossRef]
11. Levey, A.S.; Stevens, L.A.; Schmid, C.H.; Zhang, Y.L.; Castro, A.F., 3rd; Feldman, H.I.; Kusek, J.W.; Eggers, P.; Van Lente, F.; Greene, T.; et al. A new equation to estimate glomerular filtration rate. *Ann. Intern Med.* **2009**, *150*, 604–612. [CrossRef]
12. Chen, T.K.; Knicely, D.H.; Grams, M.E. Chronic Kidney Disease Diagnosis and Management: A Review. *JAMA* **2019**, *322*, 1294–1304. [CrossRef]

13. Cheng, Y.; Luo, R.; Wang, K.; Zhang, M.; Wang, Z.; Dong, L.; Li, J.; Yao, Y.; Ge, S.; Xu, G. Kidney disease is associated with in-hospital death of patients with COVID-19. *Kidney Int.* **2020**, *97*, 829–838. [CrossRef]
14. Cai, R.; Zhang, J.; Zhu, Y.; Liu, L.; Liu, Y.; He, Q. Mortality in chronic kidney disease patients with COVID-19: A systematic review and meta-analysis. *Int. Urol. Nephrol.* **2021**, 1–7. [CrossRef]
15. Ma, C.; Gu, J.; Hou, P.; Zhang, L.; Bai, Y.; Guo, Z.; Wu, H.; Zhang, B.; Li, P.; Zhao, X. Incidence, clinical characteristics and prognostic factor of patients with COVID-19: A systematic review and meta-analysis. *medRxiv* **2020**. [CrossRef]
16. ERA-EDTA Council; ERACODA Working Group. Chronic kidney disease is a key risk factor for severe COVID-19: A call to action by the ERA-EDTA. *Nephrol. Dial. Transplant.* **2021**, *36*, 87–94. [CrossRef]
17. Singh, A.K.; Gillies, C.L.; Singh, R.; Singh, A.; Chudasama, Y.; Coles, B.; Seidu, S.; Zaccardi, F.; Davies, M.J.; Khunti, K. Prevalence of co-morbidities and their association with mortality in patients with COVID-19: A systematic review and meta-analysis. *Diabetes Obes. Metab.* **2020**, *22*, 1915–1924. [CrossRef] [PubMed]
18. Henry, B.M.; Lippi, G. Chronic kidney disease is associated with severe coronavirus disease 2019 (COVID-19) infection. *Int. Urol. Nephrol.* **2020**, *52*, 1193–1194. [CrossRef]
19. Russo, E.; Esposito, P.; Taramasso, L.; Magnasco, L.; Saio, M.; Briano, F.; Russo, C.; Dettori, S.; Vena, A.; Di Biagio, A.; et al. GECOVID working group. Kidney disease and all-cause mortality in patients with COVID-19 hospitalized in Genoa, Northern Italy. *J. Nephrol.* **2021**, *34*, 173–183. [CrossRef] [PubMed]
20. Askari, H.; Sanadgol, N.; Azarnezhad, A.; Tajbakhsh, A.; Rafiei, H.; Safarpour, A.R.; Gheibihayat, S.M.; Raeis-Abdollahi, E.; Savardashtaki, A.; Ghanbariasad, A.; et al. Kidney diseases and COVID-19 infection: Causes and effect, supportive therapeutics and nutritional perspectives. *Heliyon* **2021**, *7*, e06008. [CrossRef] [PubMed]
21. Emami, A.; Javanmardi, F.; Pirbonyeh, N.; Akbari, A. Prevalence of Underlying Diseases in Hospitalized Patients with COVID-19: A Systematic Review and Meta-Analysis. *Arch. Acad. Emerg. Med.* **2020**, *8*, e35.
22. Ozturk, S.; Turgutalp, K.; Arici, M.; Odabas, A.R.; Altiparmak, M.R.; Aydin, Z.; Cebeci, E.; Basturk, T.; Soypacaci, Z.; Sahin, G.; et al. Mortality analysis of COVID-19 infection in chronic kidney disease, haemodialysis and renal transplant patients compared with patients without kidney disease: A nationwide analysis from Turkey. *Nephrol. Dial. Transplant.* **2020**, *35*, 2083–2095. [CrossRef]
23. Flythe, J.E.; Assimon, M.M.; Tugman, M.J.; Chang, E.H.; Gupta, S.; Shah, J.; Sosa, M.A.; Renaghan, A.D.; Melamed, M.L.; Wilson, F.P.; et al. STOP-COVID Investigators. Characteristics and Outcomes of Individuals With Pre-existing Kidney Disease and COVID-19 Admitted to Intensive Care Units in the United States. *Am. J. Kidney Dis.* **2021**, *77*, 190–203.e1. [CrossRef] [PubMed]
24. Coca, A.; Burballa, C.; Centellas-Pérez, F.J.; Pérez-Sáez, M.J.; Bustamante-Munguira, E.; Ortega, A.; Dueñas, C.; Arenas, M.D.; Pérez-Martínez, J.; Ruiz, G.; et al. Outcomes of COVID-19 among Hospitalized Patients with Non-dialysis CKD. *Front. Med.* **2020**, *7*, 615312. [CrossRef]
25. Yang, D.; Xiao, Y.; Chen, J.; Chen, Y.; Luo, P.; Liu, Q.; Yang, C.; Xiong, M.; Zhang, Y.; Liu, X.; et al. COVID-19 and chronic renal disease: Clinical characteristics and prognosis. *QJM* **2020**, *113*, 799–805. [CrossRef] [PubMed]
26. Mirjalili, H.; Dastgheib, S.A.; Shaker, S.H.; Bahrami, R.; Mazaheri, M.; Sadr-Bafghi, S.M.H.; Sadeghizadeh-Yazdi, J.; Neamatzadeh, H. Proportion and mortality of Iranian diabetes mellitus, chronic kidney disease, hypertension and cardiovascular disease patients with COVID-19: A meta-analysis. *J. Diabetes Metab. Disord.* **2021**, 1–13. [CrossRef]
27. Clark, A.; Jit, M.; Warren-Gash, C.; Guthrie, B.; Wang, H.H.X.; Mercer, S.W.; Sanderson, C.; McKee, M.; Troeger, C.; Ong, K.L.; et al. Centre for the Mathematical Modelling of Infectious Diseases COVID-19 working group. Global, regional, and national estimates of the population at increased risk of severe COVID-19 due to underlying health conditions in 2020: A modelling study. *Lancet Glob. Health.* **2020**, *8*, e1003–e1017. [CrossRef]
28. Xie, J.; Covassin, N.; Fan, Z.; Singh, P.; Gao, W.; Li, G.; Kara, T.; Somers, V.K. Association between Hypoxemia and Mortality in Patients with COVID-19. *Mayo Clin Proc.* **2020**, *95*, 1138–1147. [CrossRef] [PubMed]
29. Pan, F.; Yang, L.; Li, Y.; Liang, B.; Li, L.; Ye, T.; Li, L.; Liu, D.; Gui, S.; Hu, Y.; et al. Factors associated with death outcome in patients with severe coronavirus disease-19 (COVID-19): A case-control study. *Int. J. Med. Sci.* **2020**, *17*, 1281–1292. [CrossRef]
30. Hsu, C.M.; Weiner, D.E.; Aweh, G.; Miskulin, D.C.; Manley, H.J.; Stewart, C.; Ladik, V.; Hosford, J.; Lacson, E.C.; Johnson, D.S.; et al. COVID-19 Infection among US Dialysis Patients: Risk Factors and Outcomes from a National Dialysis Provider. *Am. J. Kidney Dis.* **2021**, *77*, 748–756. [CrossRef]
31. Gebhard, C.; Regitz-Zagrosek, V.; Neuhauser, H.K.; Morgan, R.; Klein, S.L. Impact of sex and gender on COVID-19 outcomes in Europe. *Biol. Sex Differ.* **2020**, *11*, 29. [CrossRef]
32. Liu, W.; Tao, Z.W.; Wang, L.; Yuan, M.L.; Liu, K.; Zhou, L.; Wei, S.; Deng, Y.; Liu, J.; Liu, H.G.; et al. Analysis of factors associated with disease outcomes in hospitalized patients with 2019 novel coronavirus disease. *Chin. Med. J.* **2020**, *133*, 1032–1038. [CrossRef]
33. Valeri, A.M.; Robbins-Juarez, S.Y.; Stevens, J.S.; Ahn, W.; Rao, M.K.; Radhakrishnan, J.; Gharavi, A.G.; Mohan, S.; Husain, S.A. Presentation and Outcomes of Patients with ESKD and COVID-19. *J. Am. Soc. Nephrol.* **2020**, *31*, 1409–1415. [CrossRef]
34. Park, B.E.; Lee, J.H.; Park, H.K.; Kim, H.N.; Jang, S.Y.; Bae, M.H.; Yang, D.H.; Park, H.S.; Cho, Y.; Lee, B.Y.; et al. Daegu COVID-19 Research Project. Impact of Cardiovascular Risk Factors and Cardiovascular Diseases on Outcomes in Patients Hospitalized with COVID-19 in Daegu Metropolitan City. *J. Korean Med. Sci.* **2021**, *36*, e15. [CrossRef] [PubMed]
35. Gupta, A.; Nayan, N.; Nair, R.; Kumar, K.; Joshi, A.; Sharma, S.; Singh, J.; Kapoor, R. Diabetes Mellitus and Hypertension Increase Risk of Death in Novel Corona Virus Patients Irrespective of Age: A Prospective Observational Study of Co-morbidities and COVID-19 from India. *SN Compr. Clin. Med.* **2021**, *3*, 937–944. [CrossRef]

36. Chen, R.; Liang, W.; Jiang, M.; Guan, W.; Zhan, C.; Wang, T.; Tang, C.; Sang, L.; Liu, J.; Ni, Z.; et al. Medical Treatment Expert Group for COVID-19. Risk Factors of Fatal Outcome in Hospitalized Subjects with Coronavirus Disease 2019 from a Nationwide Analysis in China. *Chest* **2020**, *158*, 97–105. [CrossRef]
37. Veklury—Summary of Product Characteristics. Available online: https://www.ema.europa.eu/en/documents/product-information/veklury-epar-product-information_pl.pdf (accessed on 21 March 2021).
38. Pettit, N.N.; Pisano, J.; Nguyen, C.T.; Lew, A.K.; Hazra, A.; Sherer, R.; Mullane, K. Remdesivir Use in the Setting of Severe Renal Impairment: A Theoretical Concern or Real Risk? *Clin. Infect. Dis.* **2020**, ciaa1851. [CrossRef] [PubMed]
39. Kant, S.; Menez, S.P.; Hanouneh, M.; Fine, D.M.; Crews, D.C.; Brennan, D.C.; Sperati, C.J.; Jaar, B.G. The COVID-19 nephrology compendium: AKI, CKD, ESKD and transplantation. *BMC Nephrol.* **2020**, *21*, 449. [CrossRef] [PubMed]
40. Adapa, S.; Chenna, A.; Balla, M.; Merugu, G.P.; Koduri, N.M.; Daggubati, S.R.; Gayam, V.; Naramala, S.; Konala, V.M. COVID-19 Pandemic Causing Acute Kidney Injury and Impact on Patients with Chronic Kidney Disease and Renal Transplantation. *J. Clin. Med. Res.* **2020**, *12*, 352–361. [CrossRef] [PubMed]
41. Egbi, O.G.; Adejumo, O.A.; Akinbodewa, A.A. Coronavirus infection and kidney disease: A review of current and emerging evidence. *Pan Afr. Med. J.* **2020**, *37*, 149. [CrossRef]

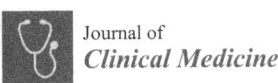

Article

HGF, IL-1α, and IL-27 Are Robust Biomarkers in Early Severity Stratification of COVID-19 Patients

Álvaro Tamayo-Velasco [1,†], Pedro Martínez-Paz [2,3,†], María Jesús Peñarrubia-Ponce [1], Ignacio de la Fuente [1], Sonia Pérez-González [1], Itziar Fernández [4], Carlos Dueñas [5], Esther Gómez-Sánchez [2,3,6,*,‡], Mario Lorenzo-López [2,3,6], Estefanía Gómez-Pesquera [2,3,6], María Heredia-Rodríguez [2,3,7,‡], Irene Carnicero-Frutos [8,9], María Fe Muñoz-Moreno [8], David Bernardo [10], Francisco Javier Álvarez [3,11], Eduardo Tamayo [2,3,6,§] and Hugo Gonzalo-Benito [3,8,9,§]

1. Department of Hematology, University Clinical Hospital, 47003 Valladolid, Spain; alvarotv1993@gmail.com (Á.T.-V.); mpenarrubia@saludcastillayleon.es (M.J.P.-P.); ifuentegr@saludcastillayleon.es (I.d.l.F.); sperezgon@saludcastillayleon.es (S.P.-G.)
2. Department of Surgery, Faculty of Medicine, University of Valladolid, 47005 Valladolid, Spain; pedrojose.martinez@uva.es (P.M.-P.); mlorenzol@saludcastillayleon.es (M.L.-L.); egomezp@saludcastillayleon.es (E.G.-P.); maria_her_05@hotmail.com (M.H.-R.); tamayo@med.uva.es (E.T.)
3. BioCritic (Group for Biomedical Research in Critical Care Medicine), University of Valladolid, 47005 Valladolid, Spain; alvarez@med.uva.es (F.J.Á.); hgonzalob@saludcastillayleon.es (H.G.-B.)
4. IOBA (Institute of Applied Ophthalmobiology), University of Valladolid, 47011 Valladolid, Spain; itziar.fernandez@uva.es
5. Department of Internal Medicine, University Clinical Hospital, 47003 Valladolid, Spain; jduenas@saludcastillayleon.es
6. Department of Anaesthesiology & Critical Care, University Clinical Hospital, 47003 Valladolid, Spain
7. Department of Anaesthesiology & Critical Care, University Hospital, 37007 Salamanca, Spain
8. Research Unit, University Clinical Hospital, 47003 Valladolid, Spain; icarnicerof@saludcastillayleon.es (I.C.-F.); mfmunozm@saludcastillayleon.es (M.F.M.-M.)
9. Institute of Health Sciences of Castile and Leon (IECSCYL), 47003 Valladolid, Spain
10. Mucosal Immunology Laboratory, Institute of Biology and Molecular Genetics (IBGM), University of Valladolid, 47005 Valladolid, Spain; d.bernardo.ordiz@gmail.com
11. Pharmacological Big Data Laboratory, Pharmacology, Faculty of Medicine, University of Valladolid, 47005 Valladolid, Spain
* Correspondence: esthergzam@hotmail.com
† Equal contribution.
‡ Equal contribution.
§ Equal contribution.

Abstract: Pneumonia is the leading cause of hospital admission and mortality in coronavirus disease 2019 (COVID-19). We aimed to identify the cytokines responsible for lung damage and mortality. We prospectively recruited 108 COVID-19 patients between March and April 2020 and divided them into four groups according to the severity of respiratory symptoms. Twenty-eight healthy volunteers were used for normalization of the results. Multiple cytokines showed statistically significant differences between mild and critical patients. High HGF levels were associated with the critical group (OR = 3.51; $p < 0.001$; 95%CI = 1.95–6.33). Moreover, high IL-1α (OR = 1.36; $p = 0.01$; 95%CI = 1.07–1.73) and low IL-27 (OR = 0.58; $p < 0.005$; 95%CI = 0.39–0.85) greatly increased the risk of ending up in the severe group. This model was especially sensitive in order to predict critical status (AUC = 0.794; specificity = 69.74%; sensitivity = 81.25%). Furthermore, high levels of HGF and IL-1α showed significant results in the survival analysis ($p = 0.033$ and $p = 0.011$, respectively). HGF, IL-1α, and IL 27 at hospital admission were strongly associated with severe/critical COVID-19 patients and therefore are excellent predictors of bad prognosis. HGF and IL-1α were also mortality biomarkers.

Keywords: coronavirus disease 2019; cytokines; severity; prognosis; mortality

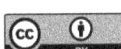

1. Introduction

In December 2019, a new strain of coronavirus, severe acute respiratory syndrome coronavirus 2 (SARS-CoV-2), was recognized to have emerged in Wuhan, China. Along with SARS-CoV [1] and Middle East respiratory syndrome-coronavirus (MERS-CoV), SARS-CoV-2 is the third coronavirus that causes severe respiratory disease in humans, called coronavirus disease 2019 (COVID-19) [2]. The epidemiology of the disease is not completely understood [3]. After a median incubation period of approximately 5 days, around half of patients present mild or no symptoms [4]. The others present moderate or severe respiratory disease including 20% of them who present serious illness with high fever and pneumonia [5], leading to acute respiratory distress syndrome (ARDS) [6].

Although its pathophysiology has not been fully understood [7], it is clear now that COVID-19 pathology arises from a primary deficit in type I interferon production followed by a dysregulated monocyte/macrophage infiltration which, in turn, drive an exacerbated adaptive immune response [8]. Viral infection leads to rapid activation of innate immune cells, especially in patients who develop severe disease. The infection induces lymphocytopenia that primarily affects $CD4^+$ T cells, including effector, memory, and regulatory T cells 3 [9,10]. Some biomarkers are related to moderate and severe COVID-19 infection like low lymphocytes absolute numbers [11] or increased levels of serum C-reactive protein (CRP), hypoalbuminemia, alanine aminotransferase, lactate dehydrogenase, ferritin, and/or D-dimer [12,13]. Indeed, these patients display increased levels of proinflammatory cytokines in serum like IL-1B, IL-6, IL-12, IFNγ, IP10, or MCP1/CCL2 [14,15] which are related to T helper 1 (Th1) cell responses. Moreover, the more severe patients (including those which require ICU admission) display higher plasma levels of GCSF, IP10, MCP1, MIP1A, and TNFα suggesting an association with the severity degree [16–18].

Based on this background, studies attribute the systemic impact of COVID-19 disease to a cytokine storm; a kind of ARDS induced by cytokine release syndrome (SRC) [19] or hemophagocytic lymphohistiocytosis (SHLH) [20], similar to that described in SARS-CoV and MERS-CoV patients. In this regard, and in order to confirm this point, most studies focused on the characterization of the cytokine response in COVID-19 patients are retrospective, present small series of patients, and/or are focused on a limited number of cytokines making them not suitable to understand the pathogenesis characterizing the cytokine release syndrome [5,12,16,18]. Moreover, the identification of prognosis biomarkers remains an urgent need.

In this regard, here we aimed to perform a cytokine array in plasma samples from a prospective COVID-19 cohort, aiming not just to characterize the cytokine storm but also to identify the early biomarkers of severity as well as mortality outcome.

2. Material and Methods

2.1. Patient Selection

A total of 108 adult patients, over 18 years, who were diagnosed with COVID-19 and admitted at the "Hospital Clínico Universitario" (Valladolid, Spain) were prospectively recruited between 24th of March and 11th of April 2020. Positive result in severe acute respiratory syndrome coronavirus 2 (SARS-CoV-2) infection was confirmed in all patients by polymerase chain reaction on nasopharyngeal samples. Patients with of other acute diseases, infections, or chronic terminal illness were not included. In addition, we also included 28 age- and gender-matched healthy volunteers for the normalization of the analytical data of the cytokines. The study was approved by the Hospital's Clinical Ethics Committee (CEIm) and the approval was obtained from all study participants (cod: PI 20-1717). This study followed the code of ethics of the World Medical Association (Declaration of Helsinki).

2.2. Biological Samples

We prospectively recruited plasma samples from each patient at 9 am immediately after their first night in the hospital in order to prevent circadian variations. Blood was collected in 3.2% sodium citrate tubes and centrifuged at 2000× g for 20 min at room temperature. The resulting plasma was aliquoted and directly frozen at −80 °C until used.

2.3. Degrees of Severity

Patients were divided into four groups based on their subsequent clinical outcome according to the severity of the respiratory symptoms: (i) Mild (n = 34): pneumonia—Adolescent or adult with clinical signs of pneumonia (fever, cough, dyspnea, fast breathing) but no signs of severe pneumonia, including SpO2 ≥ 90% on room air; (ii) moderate (n = 26): adolescent or adult with clinical signs of pneumonia (fever, cough, dyspnea, fast breathing) plus one of the following: respiratory rate > 30 breaths/min; severe respiratory distress; or SpO2 < 90% on room air- [200 mmHg < PaO2/FiO2a ≤ 300 mmHg (with PEEP or CPAP ≥ 5 cmH2O, or non-ventilated]; (iii) severe (n = 16): adolescent or adult with clinical signs of pneumonia (fever, cough, dyspnea, fast breathing) plus one of the following: respiratory rate > 30 breaths/min; severe respiratory distress; or SpO2 < 90% on room air [100 mmHg < PaO2/FiO2 ≤ 200 mmHg (with PEEP ≥ 5 cmH2O, or non-ventilated]; (iv) critical (n = 32): adolescent or adult with clinical signs of pneumonia (fever, cough, dyspnea, fast breathing) plus one of the following: respiratory rate >30 breaths/min; severe respiratory distress; or SpO2 < 90% on room air [100 mmHg < PaO2/FiO2 ≤ 200 mmHg (with PEEP ≥ 5 cmH2O] and mechanical ventilation. This classification is based on the WHO guide [21].

2.4. Cytokines and Chemokines Analysis

Plasma aliquots at hospital admission were analyzed, in duplicate, for the quantification of soluble mediators by the kit 45-plex Human XL Cytokine Luminex Performance Panel (R&D) following the manufacturer's guidelines and recommendations. Cytokines or chemokines included in the Panel were BDNF, EGF, Eotaxin (also known as CCL11), FGF-2, GM-CSF, GRO-α (CXCL1), HGF, IFN-α, IFN-γ, IL-1α, IL-1β, IL-10, IL-12 p70, IL-13, IL-15, IL-17a (CTLA-18), IL-18, IL-1RA, IL-2, IL-21, IL-22, IL-23, IL-27, IL-31, IL-4, IL-5, IL-6, IL-7, IL-8 (CXCL8), IL-9, IP-1 beta (CCL4), IP-10 (CXCL10), LIF, MCP-1 (CCL2), MIP-1α (CCL3), NGF-β, PDGF-BB, PIGF-1, RANTES (CCL5), SCF, SDF-1α, TNF-α, TNF-β, VEGF-A, VEGF-D.

2.5. Variables

Demographic, clinical and analytical data (leukocytes, lymphocytes, neutrophils, platelets, bilirubin, creatinine, glucose, troponin Ths, C-reactive protein (CRP), lactate dehydrogenase (LDH), ferritin, procalcitonin, and D-dimer) of each patient were also recorded to describe the clinical phenotype.

2.6. Statistical Analysis

Statistical analysis was performed by a PhD-licensed statistician (co-author IF) using the R statistical package version 4.0.2 (R Core Team; Foundation for Statistical Computing, Vienna, Austria; URL: https://www.R-project.org/, accessed on 5 April 2021). Statistical significance was set at $p \leq 0.05$.

To impute cytokine values below the assay detection limit, robust regression on order statistics was used: this method performs a regression to impute low values assuming log-normal quantiles for samples with a detection rate of at least 20%, after checking that the data follow a log-normal distribution. To accomplish this, the non-detects and data analysis (NADA) R package was used [Lopaka, 2017] [22]. Molecules detected in less than 20% of the samples were not statistically analyzed any further. Cytokine expression data were transformed using the logarithmic base 2 scale. Continuous variables are represented as [median, (interquartile range, IQR)], while categorical variables are represented as [%, (n)].

The strength of each biomarkers was evaluated at the individual level to determine the pulmonary severity of the patient. The main variable was severity, which is an ordinal variable with four levels. The first model to be fitted was an ordinal logistic regression model or proportional odds model [Hosmer & Lemeshow, 2000]. To confirm this, the proportional odds model was compared with a multinomial logistic regression one through the likelihood ratio test. However, in none of the cases was it possible to assume this hypothesis, so multinomial models were fitted.

Biomarkers associated with the severity at the 10% significance level were identified as potential biomarkers and they were evaluated simultaneously to fit a multivariable model.

The leave-one-out-cross-validation (LOOCV) procedure was used to estimate the prediction accuracy of the final fitted models, and receiver operation characteristic (ROC) curve analysis was used to assess their discriminate ability. The final models were evaluated according to the area under the ROC curve (AUC). In addition, sensitivity and specificity were obtained by setting an optimal threshold.

A survival analysis was also performed with the final panel of cytokines identified by the multivariable models. The outcome was tested related to T2 (time since the hospitalization until death/end of the survey). For survivals, the days of follow-up were hospitalization time or 28 days in outpatients after leaving the hospital. The Kaplan-Meier survival function was used by the log-rank test to determine differences in survival rates, considered different when $p < 0.05$. The cut-off point is established in each cytokine selecting the one with the greatest area under the ROC curve (AUC) in the individual model.

3. Results

Our cohort had a median age of 67 years, mostly male (63.26%). The control group of healthy volunteers had a median age of 61 years and most of them (57.1%) were also male. Patients were divided into four severity degrees based on the subsequent outcome during their hospital stay: (i) mild [$n = 34$, 31.5%, IC 95% (23.07–41.23)], (ii) moderate [$n = 26$, 24.1%, IC 95% (16.59–33.43)], (iii) severe [$n = 16$, 14.8%, IC 95% (8.96–23.24)], and (iv) critical [$n = 32$, 29.6%, IC 95% (21.43–39.3)] defined by their need of oxygen supplementation.

Patient clinical and analytical profile at hospital admission are shown in Table 1. Patient's group did not differ regarding age, gender, or comorbidities. However, ferritin, D-dimer, leukocytes, neutrophils, procalcitonin, and glycaemia displayed higher levels with the greater severity. On the other hand, lymphocytes, platelets, and PaO2/FiO2 were decreased in critical patients. Length of hospital stay was also increased according to the severity (8 days, 8 days, 13.5 days and 26.5 days respectively). Mortality was also higher in severe [50% (8 patients)] and critical [43.8% (14 patients)] patients compared with moderate [3.8% (1 patients)] and mild [2.9% (1 patients)].

To impute low values assuming log-normal quantiles for samples, a detection rate of at least 20% is required. Under these conditions, eight cytokines (FGF-2, IL-12, IL-21, IL-23, IL-31, IL-9, NGF-β, and TNF-β) were therefore excluded from the analysis (Supplement Table S1). Median values of each cytokine according to the severity degree are shown in Supplement Table S2. Based on a likelihood ratio test (Supplement Table S3), the most plausible model in all cases is the multinomial one. Hence, we performed individual multinomial models using the mild group as a reference (Figure 1a–c).

The comparison of mild with moderate (Figure 1a) or severe (Figure 1b) patients was not statistically significant for any of the studied cytokines although Eotaxin, IL1-α, Il-27, IL-5, and PIGF1 were borderline in the latter. Nevertheless, the comparison of mild with patients who ended up critical displayed statistical differences for several cytokines. Hence, HGF, PDGFBB, PIGF1, IL-1α, MCP1, and VEGFA were over-expressed at hospital admission in the critical group by 3.83, 1.38, 1.15, 1.13, 1.5, 1.31 times respectively. On the contrary, IL-15 and IL-2 were under-expressed in the critical patients at hospital admission by 1.56 (1/0.64) and 1.47 (1/0.68).

The best multivariable model based on these molecules is the one with four cytokines: HGF, IL1a, IL2, and IL27 (Table 2). The sex- and age-adjusted odds ratios are shown in Table 3. This analysis revealed an association between high levels of HGF and IL-1α coupled with low levels of IL-27 at hospital admission as bad prognosis predictors as these patients ended up in the severe or the critical group. In this regard, patients with twice the expression of HGF at admission had 3.51 times more chances of being critical than mild [OR: 3.51; $p < 0.001$; CI 95% (1.95–6.33)]. In a similar manner, if IL-1α [OR: 1.36; $p = 0.01$; CI 95% (1.07–1.73)] or IL-27 [OR: 0.58; $p < 0.005$; CI 95% (0.39–0.85)] were over- or under-expressed at admission, the risk of being in the severe group was 1.36 and 1.74 respectively (1/0.5753) referred to as the mild group.

Table 1. Clinical characteristics of the patients.

	Mild ($n = 34$)	Moderate ($n = 26$)	Severe ($n = 16$)	Critical ($n = 32$)	p Value
Age [median (IQR)]	68 (18)	65 (17)	75 (14)	70 (16)	0.121
Male [%(n)]	45.2% (14)	61.5% (16)	62.5% (10)	54.8% (17)	0.568
-Comorbidities, [%(n)]					
Use of tobacco	8.80% (3)	3.80% (1)	6.3% (1)	12.5% (4)	0.679
Use of alcohol	5.90% (2)	0% (0)	0% (0)	3.1% (1)	0.488
Coronary cardiopathy	8.8% (3)	11.5% (3)	12.5% (2)	6.30% (2)	0.870
Valvular disease	5.90% (2)	0% (0)	12.5% (2)	0% (0)	0.104
Atrial fibrillation	17.6% (6)	3.80% (1)	18.8% (3)	6.3% (2)	0.206
Diabetes	11.8% (4)	11.5% (3)	18.8% (3)	25% (8)	0.435
Hypertension	50% (17)	34.6% (9)	56.3% (9)	46.9% (15)	0.521
Liver disease	0% (0)	0% (0)	0% (0)	6.3% (2)	-
COPD	0% (0)	7.7% (2)	18.8% (3)	6.3% (2)	0.094
Kidney disease	2.90% (1)	0% (0)	0% (0)	6.3% (2)	0.452
Asthma	11.8% (4)	3.80% (1)	0% (0)	3.1% (1)	0.268
-Laboratory, [median (IQR)]					
Glucemia (mg/dL)	90 (13)	109 (56)	120 (59)	209 (99)	<0.001
Leukocytes (n°/mL)	4620 (2880)	6990 (3020)	6630 (3480)	7900 (8680)	<0.001
Lymphocytes (n°/mL)	1000 (430)	1000 (1000)	1120 (531)	440 (455)	<0.001
Neutrophil (n°/mL)	3215 (2420)	4945 (2380)	5315 (3450)	7045 (7800)	<0.001
Procalcitonin (ng/mL)	0.06 (0)	0.05 (0)	0.15 (1)	0.24 (0)	<0.001
CRP (mg/L)	76.5 (88)	73.5 (106)	127.0 (113)	97.0 (153)	0.250
Creatinine (mg/dL)	0.81 (0)	0.78 (0)	0.88 (0)	0.89 (1)	0.242
Total bilirubin (mg/dL)	0.40 (0)	0.5 (0)	0.65 (0)	0.50 (1)	0.187
Platelet (cell/mm^3)	(82,000)	232,500 (171,000)	198,500 (108,500)	216,500 (108,000)	0.005
Ferritin (ng/mL)	587 (600)	674 (906)	1025 (938)	1700 (1093)	<0.001
D-dimer (ng/mL)	547 (333)	693 (702)	1083 (1398)	1847 (1823)	<0.001
PaO2/FiO2	371 (48)	304 (94)	238 (102)	127 (44)	<0.001
-Hospital meters, [median (IQR)]					
Length of hospital stay (days)	8 (4)	8 (6)	13.5 (10)	26.5 (39)	<0.001
Length of ICU stay (days)	0 (0)	0 (0)	0 (0)	18.5 (14)	0.172
Intubation time (days)	0 (0)	0 (0)	0 (0)	14 (12)	0.172
-Mortality, [%(n)]					
90-days mortality	2.9% (1)	3.8% (1)	50% (8)	43.8% (14)	<0.001
28-days mortality	0% (0)	3.8% (1)	43.8% (7)	37.5% (12)	<0.001

Continuous variables are represented as [median, (interquartile range, IQR)]; categorical variables are represented as [%, (n)]; COPD, chronic obstructive pulmonary disease; CRP, C-reactive protein.

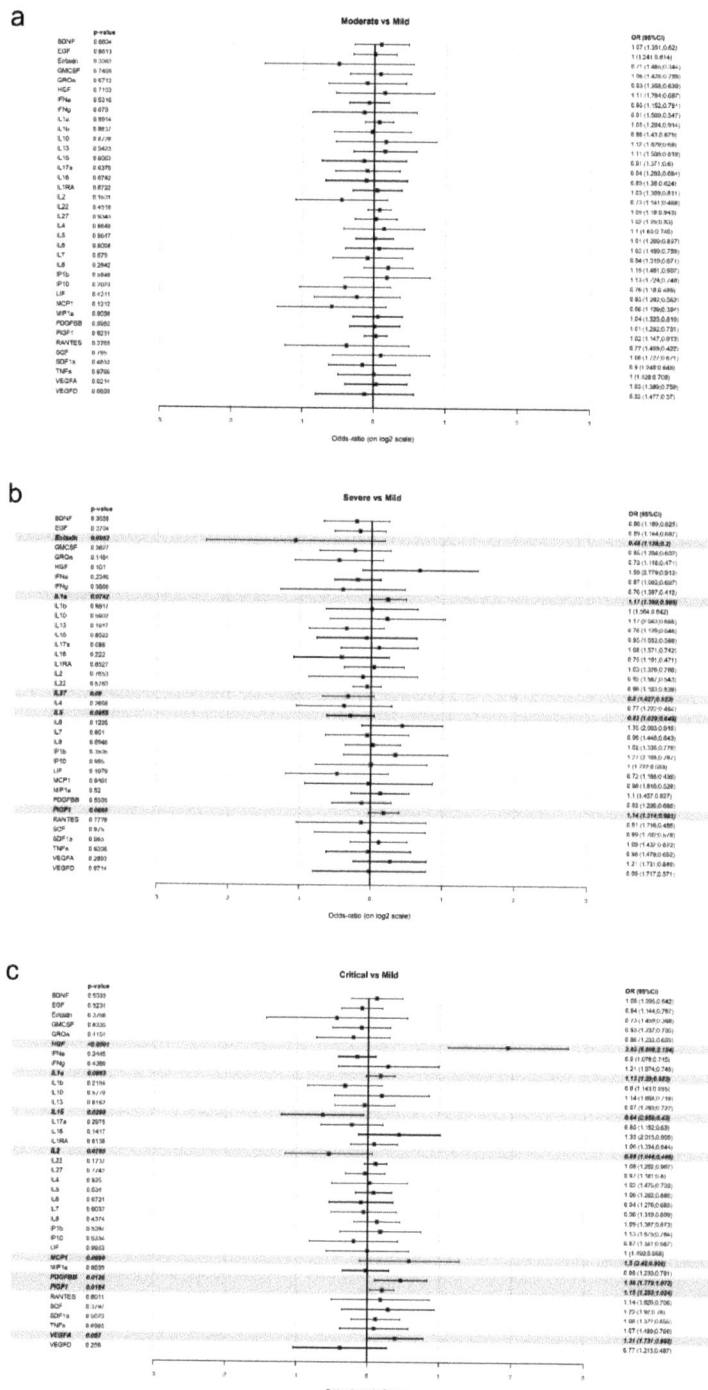

Figure 1. Individual multinomial models using the mild group as a reference. (**a**) Moderate. (**b**) Severe. (**c**) Critical.

Table 2. Identification of the best multivariable model following AIC ("Akaike's Information Criterion").

	Int.	Age	Sex	HGF	IL-1α	IL-15	IL-2	IL-27	IL-5	MCP1	PDGFBB	PlGF1	VEGFA	AIC
M0	√	√	√											301.7077
M1	√	√	√	√										268.1021
M2	√	√	√	√					√					268.3859
M3	√	√	√	√			√		√					265.8642
M4	√	√	√	√	√		√	√						264.8347
M5	√	√	√	√		√	√	√			√	√		265.6192
M6	√	√	√	√	√	√	√	√			√	√		267.9954
M7	√	√	√	√	√	√	√	√		√	√	√		271.669
M8	√	√	√	√	√	√	√	√			√	√	√	274.8803
M9	√	√	√	√	√	√	√	√	√	√	√	√	√	278.3977
M10	√	√	√	√	√	√	√	√	√	√	√	√	√	282.1787

Int, intercept.

Table 3. Different multivariable models according to the degrees of severity.

Severity	Effect	p Value	OR	CI 95% Low	CI 95% High
Moderate	Age	0.573	0.9883	0.9486	1.0296
	Sex = Female	0.1648	0.4618	0.1553	1.3735
	HGF	0.7528	1.0853	0.652	1.8066
	IL1a	0.4346	1.081	0.8891	1.3144
	IL2	0.067	0.57	0.3124	1.0401
	IL27	0.487	1.1148	0.8206	1.5144
Severe	Age	0.0452	1.0687	1.0014	1.1405
	Sex = Female	0.1504	0.3517	0.0847	1.4611
	HGF	0.2144	1.5301	0.7818	2.9946
	IL1a	0.0109	1.3634	1.0741	1.7308
	IL2	0.4125	1.4144	0.6172	3.2414
	IL27	0.0057	0.5753	0.3888	0.8511
Critical	Age	0.13	0.9615	0.9139	1.0116
	Sex = Female	0.758	0.8242	0.241	2.8192
	HGF	<0.0001	3.5122	1.9495	6.3276
	IL1a	0.1977	1.134	0.9365	1.3731
	IL2	0.1105	0.5776	0.2943	1.1334
	IL27	0.8571	0.9677	0.6772	1.383

CI, confidence interval; OR, odds ratio.

The fitted models are used to estimate the predicted probabilities and their associated confidence bands of severity group. These estimated probabilities are visualized as effect plots in Figure 2a–c. We clearly see how the chances of ending up in a critical condition were directly related to higher HGF levels at admission. Hence, HGF levels above 128 pg/mL (2^7) imply a 25% chance of being critical while levels above 223 pg/mL increase that critical risk up to 50%. On the contrary, patients with HGF levels below 64 pg/mL (2^6) have no risk (practically 0%) of ending up critical. In the same manner, low IL-1α levels at admission had a probability over 37% of being mild, while IL-1alpha levels over 1024 pg/mL (2^{10}) had 50% chances of being in the severe group. Last, but not least, lower levels of IL-27 at admission were also associated with the severe group since level under 1 are reflected in a 50% chance of belonging to the severe group while IL-27 levels over 64 pg/mL (2^6) decrease that risk to practically 0%.

Internal validation by the LOOCV procedure shows that AUC is significantly greater than 0.5 in all severity groups (Table 4), especially in severe group (AUC 0.730) and critical group (0.794). This model is especially sensitive in order to classify patients who end up critical (sensitivity = 81.25%). Last, but not least, the survival analysis taking into account the three statistically significance cytokines included in the multivariable model was significant for HGF and IL-1α (Figure 3a,b) but not IL-27 (Figure 3c).

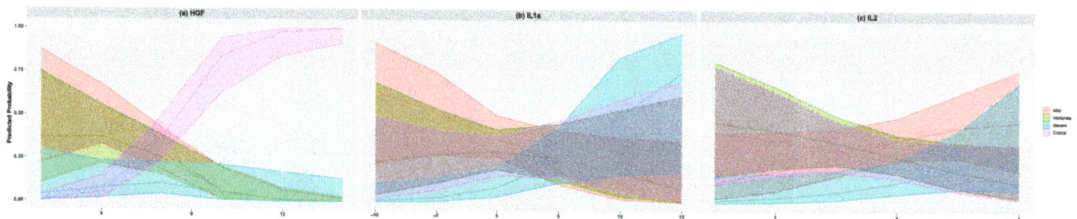

Figure 2. Effect plots of the estimated probabilities of belonging to each severity group according to the level of HGF (**a**), IL-1α (**b**), and IL-27 (**c**). The log2 level of each cytokine is measured in pg/mL.

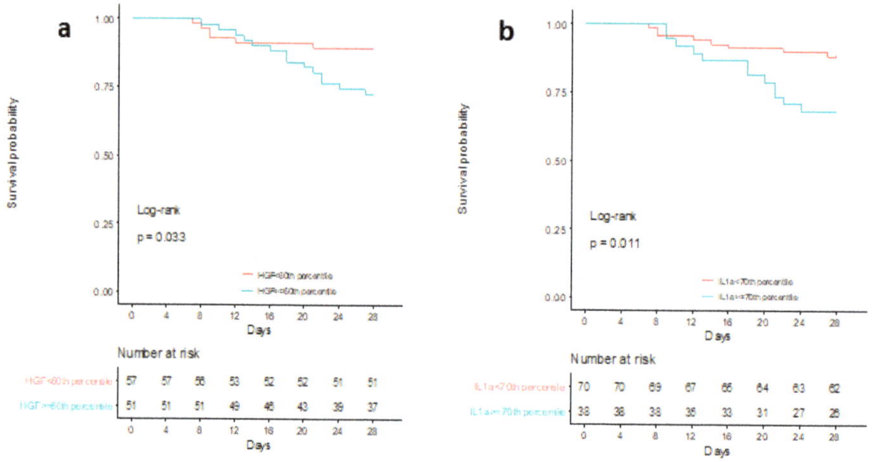

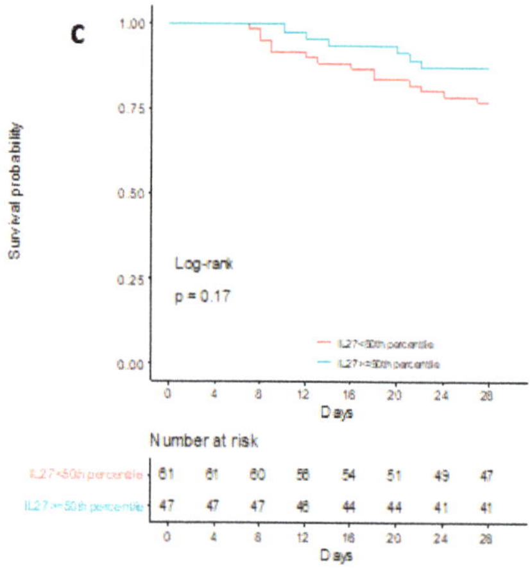

Figure 3. Kaplan-Meier survival curves for HGF (**a**), IL-1α (**b**), IL-27 (**c**).

Cytokine	Cut-off point	AUC
HGF	$P_{60} = 178.70$	0.667
IL1a	$P_{70} = 5.57$	0.648
IL27	$P_{50} = 24.35$	0.563

Table 4. Internal validation in each degree of severity using the AUC (area under the ROC curve).

	Mild Threshold: 0.3597126			Moderate Threshold: 0.2513263			Severe Threshold: 0.1438022			Critical Threshold: 0.2084408		
	Value	CI 95%		Value	CI 95%		Value	CI 95%		Value	CI 95%	
		Lower	Higher		Lower	Higher		Lower	Higher		Lower	Higher
AUC	0.647	0.535	0.759	0.602	0.477	0.727	0.730	0.624	0.837	0.794	0.701	0.888
Sensitivity (%)	58.82	42.28	75.37	53.85	34.68	73.01	62.5	38.78	86.22	81.25	67.73	94.77
Specificity (%)	70.27	59.86	80.68	65.85	55.59	76.12	73.91	64.94	82.89	69.74	59.41	80.07
Accuracy (%)	66.67	57.78	75.56	62.96	53.86	72.07	72.22	63.77	80.67	73.15	64.79	81.51

CI, confident interval.

4. Discussion

Here we have described, after performing a 45-plex cytokine array on plasma samples from 108 patients at hospital admission, that five cytokines are statistically significantly different according to the degrees of severity in COVID-19. Indeed, high levels of HGF and IL-1α coupled with low levels of IL-27 at admission can predict bad clinical outcome referred to the patient subset with better prognosis, being especially important the high level of HGF as predictors of admission in intensive care units. Moreover, this multivariate model was especially sensitive in order to identify those patients who end up in a critical status (AUC = 0.794; specificity 69.74%; sensitivity = 81.25%) following hospital admission. Last, but not the least, we have also described how the combination of high levels of HGF IL-1 α at admission can predict mortality, showing significant results in the survival analysis ($p = 0.033$ and $p = 0.011$ respectively).

During the last months, several studies have tried to understand the cytokine profile in patients with COVID-19. Most of them relate severity of lung disease to high levels of multiple cytokines in blood, according to what has been defined as a cytokine storm. Indeed, even some authors describe three different clinical phenotypes of COVID-19 based on cytokines levels [23]. In this regard, Huang et al. suggest that the cytokine storm is associated with severity after analyzing 27 cytokines in 41 patients as ICU patients had higher plasma levels of IL-2, IL-7, IL-10, GSCF, IP10, MCP1, MIP1A, and TNFα [18]. In a similar manner, Liu et al. studied 40 patients, 13 of them severe, and found increased plasma levels of IL-6, IL-10, IL-2, and IFN-γ levels in severe compared to mild cases [24]. Zhao et al. included 71 patients, (53 mild and 18 severe) referred 18 healthy volunteers describing that IL-1RA and IL-10 correlated with disease severity, while Zhang et al. analyzed in 326 patients finding higher levels of IL-6 and IL-8 in severe or critical patients [25]. Nevertheless, these studies display several limitations like small sample sizes, the study of few numbers of cytokines, and the lack of well-defined severity degrees. Moreover, patients who required mechanical ventilation were not usually differentiated from patients with severe disease despite this aggressive intervention increases cytokine levels. Last, but not least, these studies usually applied basic statistical approaches. Therefore, and in order to overcome these limitations, we hereby have analyzed in duplicate the plasma levels of 45 cytokines from an extremely well-categorized cohort of 108 COVID-19 patients which were classified into severity groups based on their clinical evolution defined by objective criteria, at the time that we also performed an exhaustive statistical analysis. Hence, we have considered all confounders by using both univariate and multivariate regression analysis showing, at least, an internal validation.

Other studies have performed a similar approach to the one here described, like the one by Han et al. that classified 102 patients into moderate, severe, and critical groups according to their symptoms. It also presented a control group of healthy volunteers. Such study showed higher serum levels of TNF-α, IFN-γ, IL-2, IL-4, IL-6, IL-10, and CRP referred to controls. Using a logistic regression analysis, IL-6 and IL-10 were found to predict disease severity and the internal validation could further confirm this result [26]. However, they only analyzed six cytokines and a duplicate analysis was not performed on each sample. In a similar manner, Meizlish et al. analyzed a cohort with 49 adult patients (40 in the medical intensive care unit (ICU) and 9 in non-ICU units), as well as 13 non-COVID-19 healthy volunteers. They analyzed 78 circulating proteins with immunologic functions. Their study identified a neutrophil activation signature composed of neutrophil activators (G-CSF, IL-8) and effectors (resistin (RETN), lipocalin-2 (LCN2) and hepatocyte growth factor (HGF)), which had the greater power to identify critically ill patients [27]. As default, the small number of patients and the different degrees of pulmonary severity do not differ in non-ICU patients.

Based on the results displayed by these two studies, and in agreement with ours, we can conclude that there is no specific cytokine pattern correlating with the disease severity. On the one hand, high levels of HGF were associated with a risk of up to 3.5 times of being critical with mechanical ventilation. This growth factor, that has already been related to severity in other studies, primarily elicits its effects on epithelial cells. In a similar manner, IL-1α, which is a pro-inflammatory cytokine from the innate immune system mainly produced by macrophages but also epithelial cells, can also predict a bad prognosis and disease outcome. Hence, both cytokines could be reflecting the tissue damage elicited by the macrophage infiltration to the lungs [28,29]. Indeed, these findings suggest the implication of non-immune cells in COVID-19 in agreement with the results from Lucas et al. [30] who proved how increased stromal growth factors involved in tissue repairing were associated with a favorable immune signature. Hence, it seems obvious now that the crosstalk between immune and stromal cells in the lungs may shape the fate of the immune response and, with that, the outcome of the patient evolution.

We have also found how low level of IL-27, which belongs to the IL-12 family and is therefore involved in Th1 differentiation, is a good prognosis biomarker in COVID-19 patients. Together, these results suggest that, although in our hands the cytokine storm may not be the trigger of the bilateral pneumonia, there is certainly a mixed and altered cytokine profile which drives disease progression and inflammation as highlighted by the fact that high HGF levels combined with low IL-27 levels are revealed as early mortality markers. We are nevertheless aware that we have not found increased levels of IL-6 levels to be relevant in our cohort as many studies have already reported [31,32]. One possible explanation is that, in our case, we simultaneously determined the levels of 45 cytokines in a large cohort and performed a multivariate analysis. Hence, the single effect of IL-6 may be diluted in favor of the combined of several other cytokines. Nevertheless, the moment when the samples were obtained may also provide an explanation. Indeed, our cohort was recruited during the worst days of the pandemics in Spain between March and April 2020, when some patients were immediately transferred into the ICU after arriving to the hospital. Hence, given that our cohort also displayed high levels of CRP (a downstream mediator of IL-6), we cannot discard the possibility that IL-6 was higher and driving inflammation in previous stages of the disease before the patients were admitted to the hospital and therefore recruited.

Since the beginning of this health crisis, treatment strategies in the most severe cases were aimed at blocking interleukins like IL-6 (Tocilizumab), IL-1 (Anakinra), and TNFα (Infliximab, Adalimumab, etc.,) [33]. The REMAP-CAP and RECOVERY studies show modest but significant improvement in mortality [34,35] and these findings were confirmed in the Cochrane review showing high certainty of improvement in 28 day mortality in patients who received IL-6 blockade (RR 0.89, 95% CI 0.82–0.97). The use of dexamethasone at two drops for 10 days decreased mortality at day 28 in patients who were receiving invasive mechanical ventilation [36]. Nevertheless, and as a corticosteroid, this approach did not identify the key immune components involved in this process. According to this, and the results hereby reported, it is to be expected that these strategies entail a modest reduction in mortality since increased levels of IL-6, IL-1, or TNFα are not directly responsible to drive disease severity in these patients. Therefore, and although the increased levels of plasma cytokines in COVID-19 patients has been largely reported, the identification of disease progression and severity biomarkers remains an urgent need. In this regard, we hereby report that HGF, IL1α, and IL27 contribute to the deterioration of the disease and the adverse outcome of COVID-19 revealing these three compounds as novel biomarkers but as future therapeutic targets in COVID-19.

We are aware of the main limitations of our study. (i) Our study did not include a large sample size. Perhaps, we should have performed previously a statistical power analysis. Nevertheless, our sample size is consistent with previous reports [18,24,25,30]. We were very careful with the recruitment and analysis of plasma samples, at the same time each day and with a duplicate analysis, in order to avoid circadian variations. Therefore, we intended to get samples as homogeneous as possible. (ii) Lack of external validation. Therefore, we consider that validating the model in a different cohort of patients in the future would be essential to give consistency to the results. (iii) The most relevant buffering system in the COVID-cytokine storm is the IL-6: sIL-6R:sgp130 system in trans signaling, which has been described in recent publications [37,38]. Thus, an inherent limitation of these multi-PLEX cytokine studies is that they typically only measure the cytokine itself, whereas there are other aspects of these cytokine signaling pathways that are omitted.

Our study characterized the plasma cytokine profile of COVID-19 patients at hospital admission, based on their subsequent clinical evolution into four well-defined degrees of severity, revealing that HGF, IL-1α, and IL27 were strongly associated with disease severity and could be used as excellent predictors of bad prognosis. Indeed, HGF and IL-1α are also mortality biomarkers. Therefore, the early detection of HGF, IL-1α, and IL27 plasma levels in patients in COVID-19 patients can provide useful information for getting quickly intensive treatment as well as providing possible therapeutic targets.

Supplementary Materials: The following are available online at https://www.mdpi.com/article/10.3390/jcm10092017/s1, Table S1: Cytokine/chemokine detection percentage. Table S2: Comparison between the value of cytokines according to their degree of severity. Table S3: Likelihood-ratio test (LRT) to check the assumption of proportional odds by comparing the proportional odds model with a multinomial model.

Author Contributions: Conceptualization: E.T., Á.T.-V.; methodology: E.G.-S., P.M.-P., Á.T.-V., E.T.; software: I.F., M.F.M.-M.; validation: M.J.P.-P., I.d.l.F., S.P.-G.; formal analysis: M.F.M.-M., Á.T.-V., E.T.; investigation: E.G.-S., C.D., M.L.-L., E.G.-P.; resources: H.G.-B., E.T., D.B.; data curation: E.G.-S., M.L.-L., E.G.-P., M.H.-R., I.C.-F.; writing: Á.T.-V., E.T., F.J.Á.; original draft preparation: Á.T.-V., E.T., E.G.-S.; writing—review and editing: Á.T.-V., M.H.-R., E.G.-S.; visualization: I.F., M.F.M.-M.; supervision: E.T.; project administration: E.T., Á.T.-V.; funding acquisition: E.T. All authors have read and agreed to the published version of the manuscript.

Funding: This work was supported by the Carlos III Health Institute (Grant COV20/00491).

Institutional Review Board Statement: The study was approved by the Hospital's Clinical Ethics Committee (CEIm) and the approval was obtained from all study participants (cod: PI 20-1717). This study followed the code of ethics of the World Medical Association (Declaration of Helsinki).

Informed Consent Statement: Informed consent was obtained from all subjects involved in the study.

Data Availability Statement: The datasets generated during and/or analyzed during the current study are available from the corresponding author on reasonable request.

Acknowledgments: We appreciate the collaboration of the nursing staff and the Research Unit of the University Clinical Hospital, Valladolid, Spain.

Conflicts of Interest: The authors declare no conflict of interest. All authors have read the journal's authorship agreement and policy on disclosure of potential conflicts of interest.

References

1. Yang, Y.; Peng, F.; Wang, R.; Guan, K.; Jiang, T.; Xu, G.; Sun, J.; Chang, C. The Deadly Coronaviruses: The 2003 SARS Pandemic and the 2020 Novel Coronavirus Epidemic in China. *J. Autoimmun.* **2020**, *109*, 102434. [CrossRef] [PubMed]
2. Zhu, N.; Zhang, D.; Wang, W.; Li, X.; Yang, B.; Song, J.; Zhao, X.; Huang, B.; Shi, W.; Lu, R.; et al. A Novel Coronavirus from Patients with Pneumonia in China, 2019. *N. Engl. J. Med.* **2020**. [CrossRef]
3. Li, R.; Pei, S.; Chen, B.; Song, Y.; Zhang, T.; Yang, W.; Shaman, J. Substantial Undocumented Infection Facilitates the Rapid Dissemination of Novel Coronavirus (SARS-CoV2). *Science* **2020**. [CrossRef]

4. Lauer, S.A.; Grantz, K.H.; Bi, Q.; Jones, F.K.; Zheng, Q.; Meredith, H.R.; Azman, A.S.; Reich, N.G.; Lessler, J. The Incubation Period of Coronavirus Disease 2019 (COVID-19) From Publicly Reported Confirmed Cases: Estimation and Application. *Ann. Intern. Med.* **2020**. [CrossRef] [PubMed]
5. Yang, X.; Yu, Y.; Xu, J.; Shu, H.; Xia, J.; Liu, H.; Wu, Y.; Zhang, L.; Yu, Z.; Fang, M.; et al. Clinical Course and Outcomes of Critically Ill Patients with SARS-CoV-2 Pneumonia in Wuhan, China: A Single-Centered, Retrospective, Observational Study. *Lancet Respir. Med.* **2020**. [CrossRef]
6. Clinical Management of Severe Acute Respiratory Infection When COVID-19 Is Suspected. Available online: https://www.who.int/publications-detail/clinical-management-of-severe-acute-respiratory-infection-when-novel-coronavirus-(ncov)-infection-is-suspected (accessed on 26 April 2020).
7. Li, G.; Fan, Y.; Lai, Y.; Han, T.; Li, Z.; Zhou, P.; Pan, P.; Wang, W.; Hu, D.; Liu, X.; et al. Coronavirus Infections and Immune Responses. *J. Med. Virol.* **2020**, *92*, 424–432. [CrossRef] [PubMed]
8. Schultze, J.L.; Aschenbrenner, A.C. COVID-19 and the Human Innate Immune System. *Cell* **2021**, *184*, 1671–1692. [CrossRef]
9. Schett, G.; Sticherling, M.; Neurath, M.F. COVID-19: Risk for Cytokine Targeting in Chronic Inflammatory Diseases? *Nat. Rev. Immunol.* **2020**. [CrossRef] [PubMed]
10. Qin, C.; Zhou, L.; Hu, Z.; Zhang, S.; Yang, S.; Tao, Y.; Xie, C.; Ma, K.; Shang, K.; Wang, W.; et al. Dysregulation of Immune Response in Patients with COVID-19 in Wuhan, China. *Clin. Infect. Dis.* **2020**. [CrossRef]
11. Li, Y.X.; Wu, W.; Yang, T.; Zhou, W.; Fu, Y.M.; Feng, Q.M.; Ye, J.M. Characteristics of peripheral blood leukocyte differential counts in patients with COVID-19. *Zhonghua Nei Ke Za Zhi* **2020**, *59*, E003. [CrossRef]
12. Chen, G.; Wu, D.; Guo, W.; Cao, Y.; Huang, D.; Wang, H.; Wang, T.; Zhang, X.; Chen, H.; Yu, H.; et al. Clinical and Immunological Features of Severe and Moderate Coronavirus Disease 2019. *J. Clin. Investig.* **2020**. [CrossRef] [PubMed]
13. Ruan, Q.; Yang, K.; Wang, W.; Jiang, L.; Song, J. Clinical Predictors of Mortality Due to COVID-19 Based on an Analysis of Data of 150 Patients from Wuhan, China. *Intensive Care Med.* **2020**, 1–3. [CrossRef] [PubMed]
14. Induction of Pro-Inflammatory Cytokines (IL-1 and IL-6) and Lung Inflammation by Coronavirus-19 (COVI-19 or SARS-CoV-2): Anti-Inflammatory Strategies. Available online: https://www.ncbi.nlm.nih.gov/pubmed/?term=Induction+of+pro-inflammatory+cytokines+(IL-1+and+IL-6)+and+lung+inflammation+by+COVID-19%3A+anti-inflammatory+strategies (accessed on 26 April 2020).
15. Bizzarri, M.; Laganà, A.S.; Aragona, D.; Unfer, V. Inositol and Pulmonary Function. Could Myo-Inositol Treatment Downregulate Inflammation and Cytokine Release Syndrome in SARS-CoV-2? *Eur. Rev. Med. Pharmacol. Sci.* **2020**, *24*, 3426–3432. [CrossRef]
16. Chen, L.; Liu, H.G.; Liu, W.; Liu, J.; Liu, K.; Shang, J.; Deng, Y.; Wei, S. Analysis of clinical features of 29 patients with 2019 novel coronavirus pneumonia. *Zhonghua Jie He He Hu Xi Za Zhi* **2020**, *43*, E005. [CrossRef] [PubMed]
17. Wan, S.; Yi, Q.; Fan, S.; Lv, J.; Zhang, X.; Guo, L.; Lang, C.; Xiao, Q.; Xiao, K.; Yi, Z.; et al. Relationships among Lymphocyte Subsets, Cytokines, and the Pulmonary Inflammation Index in Coronavirus (COVID-19) Infected Patients. *Br. J. Haematol.* **2020**. [CrossRef] [PubMed]
18. Huang, C.; Wang, Y.; Li, X.; Ren, L.; Zhao, J.; Hu, Y.; Zhang, L.; Fan, G.; Xu, J.; Gu, X.; et al. Clinical Features of Patients Infected with 2019 Novel Coronavirus in Wuhan, China. *Lancet* **2020**, *395*, 497–506. [CrossRef]
19. Moore, B.J.B.; June, C.H. Cytokine Release Syndrome in Severe COVID-19. *Science* **2020**. [CrossRef]
20. Karakike, E.; Giamarellos-Bourboulis, E.J. Macrophage Activation-Like Syndrome: A Distinct Entity Leading to Early Death in Sepsis. *Front. Immunol.* **2019**, *10*. [CrossRef]
21. WHO-2019-NCoV-Clinical-2021. Available online: https://apps.who.int/iris/bitstream/handle/10665/338882/WHO-2019-nCoV-clinical-2021.1-eng.pdf?sequence=1&isAllowed=y (accessed on 25 January 2021).
22. Lee, L. NADA: Nondetects and Data Analysis for Environmental Data. 2020. Available online: https://cran.r-project.org/web/packages/NADA/NADA.pdf (accessed on 25 January 2021).
23. Bindoli, S.; Felicetti, M.; Sfriso, P.; Doria, A. The Amount of Cytokine-Release Defines Different Shades of Sars-Cov2 Infection. *Exp. Biol. Med.* **2020**, *245*, 970–976. [CrossRef]
24. Liu, J.; Li, S.; Liu, J.; Liang, B.; Wang, X.; Wang, H.; Li, W.; Tong, Q.; Yi, J.; Zhao, L.; et al. Longitudinal Characteristics of Lymphocyte Responses and Cytokine Profiles in the Peripheral Blood of SARS-CoV-2 Infected Patients. *EBioMedicine* **2020**, *55*, 102763. [CrossRef]
25. Zhang, X.; Tan, Y.; Ling, Y.; Lu, G.; Liu, F.; Yi, Z.; Jia, X.; Wu, M.; Shi, B.; Xu, S.; et al. Viral and Host Factors Related to the Clinical Outcome of COVID-19. *Nature* **2020**, *583*, 437–440. [CrossRef]
26. Han, H.; Ma, Q.; Li, C.; Liu, R.; Zhao, L.; Wang, W.; Zhang, P.; Liu, X.; Gao, G.; Liu, F.; et al. Profiling Serum Cytokines in COVID-19 Patients Reveals IL-6 and IL-10 Are Disease Severity Predictors. *Emerg. Microbes. Infect.* **2020**, *9*, 1123–1130. [CrossRef]
27. Meizlish, M.L.; Pine, A.B.; Bishai, J.D.; Goshua, G.; Nadelmann, E.R.; Simonov, M.; Chang, C.-H.; Zhang, H.; Shallow, M.; Bahel, P.; et al. A Neutrophil Activation Signature Predicts Critical Illness and Mortality in COVID-19. *medRxiv* **2020**. [CrossRef]
28. Wang, C.; Xie, J.; Zhao, L.; Fei, X.; Zhang, H.; Tan, Y.; Nie, X.; Zhou, L.; Liu, Z.; Ren, Y.; et al. Alveolar Macrophage Dysfunction and Cytokine Storm in the Pathogenesis of Two Severe COVID-19 Patients. *EBioMedicine* **2020**, *57*. [CrossRef] [PubMed]
29. Abassi, Z.; Knaney, Y.; Karram, T.; Heyman, S.N. The Lung Macrophage in SARS-CoV-2 Infection: A Friend or a Foe? *Front. Immunol.* **2020**, *11*. [CrossRef] [PubMed]
30. Lucas, C.; Wong, P.; Klein, J.; Castro, T.B.R.; Silva, J.; Sundaram, M.; Ellingson, M.K.; Mao, T.; Oh, J.E.; Israelow, B.; et al. Longitudinal Analyses Reveal Immunological Misfiring in Severe COVID-19. *Nature* **2020**, *584*, 463–469. [CrossRef] [PubMed]

31. Galván-Román, J.M.; Rodríguez-García, S.C.; Roy-Vallejo, E.; Marcos-Jiménez, A.; Sánchez-Alonso, S.; Fernández-Díaz, C.; Alcaraz-Serna, A.; Mateu-Albero, T.; Rodríguez-Cortes, P.; Sánchez-Cerrillo, I.; et al. IL-6 Serum Levels Predict Severity and Response to Tocilizumab in COVID-19: An Observational Study. *J. Allergy Clin. Immunol.* **2021**, *147*, 72–80.e8. [CrossRef] [PubMed]
32. Utrero-Rico, A.; Ruiz-Hornillos, J.; González-Cuadrado, C.; Rita, C.G.; Almoguera, B.; Minguez, P.; Herrero-González, A.; Fernández-Ruiz, M.; Carretero, O.; Taracido-Fernández, J.C.; et al. IL-6-Based Mortality Prediction Model for COVID-19: Validation and Update in Multicenter and Second Wave Cohorts. *J. Allergy Clin. Immunol.* **2021**. [CrossRef]
33. Stone, J.H.; Frigault, M.J.; Serling-Boyd, N.J.; Fernandes, A.D.; Harvey, L.; Foulkes, A.S.; Horick, N.K.; Healy, B.C.; Shah, R.; Bensaci, A.M.; et al. Efficacy of Tocilizumab in Patients Hospitalized with Covid-19. *N. Engl. J. Med.* **2020**. [CrossRef]
34. REMAP-CAP Investigators; Gordon, A.C.; Mouncey, P.R.; Al-Beidh, F.; Rowan, K.M.; Nichol, A.D.; Arabi, Y.M.; Annane, D.; Beane, A.; van Bentum-Puijk, W.; et al. Interleukin-6 Receptor Antagonists in Critically Ill Patients with Covid-19. *N. Engl. J. Med.* **2021**, *384*, 1491–1502. [CrossRef]
35. Group, R.C.; Horby, P.W.; Pessoa-Amorim, G.; Peto, L.; Brightling, C.E.; Sarkar, R.; Thomas, K.; Jeebun, V.; Ashish, A.; Tully, R.; et al. Tocilizumab in Patients Admitted to Hospital with COVID-19 (RECOVERY): Preliminary Results of a Randomised, Controlled, Open-Label, Platform Trial. *MedRxiv* **2021**. [CrossRef]
36. RECOVERY Collaborative, Group; Horby, P.; Lim, W.S.; Emberson, J.R.; Mafham, M.; Bell, J.L.; Linsell, L.; Staplin, N.; Brightling, C.; Ustianowski, A.; et al. Dexamethasone in Hospitalized Patients with Covid-19—Preliminary Report. *N. Engl. J. Med.* **2020**. [CrossRef]
37. McElvaney, O.J.; Curley, G.F.; Rose-John, S.; McElvaney, N.G. Interleukin-6: Obstacles to Targeting a Complex Cytokine in Critical Illness. *Lancet Respir. Med.* **2021**. [CrossRef]
38. Chen, L.Y.C.; Biggs, C.M.; Jamal, S.; Stukas, S.; Wellington, C.L.; Sekhon, M.S. Soluble Interleukin-6 Receptor in the COVID-19 Cytokine Storm Syndrome. *Cell Rep. Med.* **2021**, 100269. [CrossRef] [PubMed]

Article

Tocilizumab Improves the Prognosis of COVID-19 in Patients with High IL-6

Robert Flisiak [1,*], Jerzy Jaroszewicz [2], Magdalena Rogalska [1], Tadeusz Łapiński [1], Aleksandra Berkan-Kawińska [3], Beata Bolewska [4], Magdalena Tudrujek-Zdunek [5], Dorota Kozielewicz [6], Marta Rorat [7,8], Piotr Leszczyński [9,10], Krzysztof Kłos [11], Justyna Kowalska [12], Paweł Pabjan [13], Anna Piekarska [3], Iwona Mozer-Lisewska [4], Krzysztof Tomasiewicz [5], Małgorzata Pawłowska [6], Krzysztof Simon [14], Joanna Polanska [15] and Dorota Zarębska-Michaluk [13]

1. Department of Infectious Diseases and Hepatology, Medical University of Białystok, 15-089 Białystok, Poland; pmagdar@gmail.com (M.R.); twlapinski@gmail.com (T.Ł.)
2. Department of Infectious Diseases and Hepatology, Medical University of Silesia, 40-055 Katowice, Poland; jerzy.jr@gmail.com
3. Department of Infectious Diseases and Hepatology, Medical University of Łódź, 90-549 Łódź, Poland; aleksandra.berkan@gmail.com (A.B.-K.); annapiekar@gmail.com (A.P.)
4. Department of Infectious Diseases, University of Medical Sciences, 61-701 Poznań, Poland; bbolewska@ump.edu.pl (B.B.); iwonalisewska@poczta.onet.pl (I.M.-L.)
5. Department of Infectious Diseases and Hepatology, Medical University of Lublin, 20-059 Lublin, Poland; magdalena.tudrujek@gmail.com (M.T.-Z.); tomaskdr@poczta.fm (K.T.)
6. Department of Infectious Diseases and Hepatology, Faculty of Medicine, Collegium Medicum in Bydgoszcz, Nicolaus Copernicus University, 87-100 Toruń, Poland; d.kozielewicz@wsoz.pl (D.K.); mpawlowska@cm.umk.pl (M.P.)
7. Department of Forensic Medicine, Wrocław Medical University, 50-367 Wrocław, Poland; marta.rorat@gmail.com
8. First Infectious Diseases Ward, Gromkowski Regional Specialist Hospital in Wrocław, 51-149 Wrocław, Poland
9. Department of Rheumatology, Rehabilitation and Internal Medicine, Poznan University of Medical Sciences, 61-701 Poznań, Poland; piotr_leszczynski@wp.pl
10. Department of Rheumatology and Osteoporosis, Szpital im. J. Strusia w Poznaniu, Szpital im. J. Strusia, 61-285 Poznań, Poland
11. Department of Infectious Diseases and Allergology, Military Institute of Medicine, 04-141 Warsaw, Poland; kklos@wim.mil.pl
12. Department of Adults' Infectious Diseases, Medical University of Warsaw, 02-091 Warsaw, Poland; jdkowalska@gmail.com
13. Department of Infectious Diseases, Jan Kochanowski University, 25-369 Kielce, Poland; pabjan3@tlen.pl (P.P.); dorota1010@tlen.pl (D.Z.-M.)
14. Department of Infectious Diseases and Hepatology, Wrocław Medical University, 50-367 Wrocław, Poland; krzysimon@gmail.com
15. Department of Data Science and Engineering, Silesian University of Technology, 44-100 Gliwice, Poland; Joanna.Polanska@polsl.pl
* Correspondence: robert.flisiak1@gmail.com

Abstract: Despite direct viral effect, the pathogenesis of coronavirus disease 2019 (COVID-19) includes an overproduction of cytokines including interleukin 6 (IL-6). Therefore, tocilizumab (TOC), a monoclonal antibody against IL-6 receptors, was considered as a possible therapeutic option. Patients were selected from the SARSTer database, containing 2332 individuals with COVID-19. Current study included 825 adult patients with moderate to severe course. Analysis was performed in 170 patients treated with TOC and 655 with an alternative medication. The end-points of treatment effectiveness were death rate, need for mechanical ventilation, and clinical improvement. Patients treated with TOC were balanced compared to non-TOC regarding gender, age, BMI, and prevalence of coexisting conditions. Significant effect of TOC on death was demonstrated in patients with baseline IL-6 > 100 pg/mL (hazard ratio [HR]: 0.21, 95% confidence interval [CI]: 0.08–0.57). The best effectiveness of TOC was achieved in patients with a combination of baseline IL-6 > 100 pg/mL and either SpO2 ≤ 90% (HR: 0.07) or requiring oxygen supplementation (HR: 0.18). Tocilizumab administration in COVID-19 reduces mortality and speeds up clinical improvement in patients with a baseline concentration of IL-6 > 100 pg/mL, particularly if they need oxygen supplementation owing to the lower value of SpO2 $\leq$ 90%.

Keywords: COVID-19; SARS-CoV-2; interleukin-6; tocilizumab; therapy

1. Introduction

A novel coronavirus named severe acute respiratory syndrome coronavirus 2 (SARS-CoV-2) was identified in December 2019 and found to be responsible for an outbreak of respiratory tract infections discovered in Wuhan, China. The outbreak of the disease known as a coronavirus disease 2019 (COVID-19) was announced as a global pandemic by the World Health Organization (WHO) in March 2020. The search for effective therapy focused on repurposing of approved drugs with confirmed activity against other viruses, that included, for example, remdesivir (RDV), which was previously studied for the treatment of Ebola virus disease as well as SARS-CoV-1 and middle east respiratory syndrome (MERS) coronaviruses [1,2]. Based on findings from phase III clinical trials and real-world experience study, RDV received both American and European authorization [3–5]. Recommendations were also given to low-molecular-weight heparin and dexamethasone [6,7]. However, the pathogenesis of COVID-19 is complicated and includes, in addition to direct viral effect and coagulopathy, an overproduction of proinflammatory cytokines termed a cytokine storm, which is responsible for organ damage and is considered a major reason for death due to COVID-19 [8]. Unfortunately, standard anti-inflammatory treatments appear to be insufficient for controlling the cytokine storm. Concentrations of several proinflammatory cytokines, including interleukin (IL)-6, are substantially increased in patients with severe COVID-19 [9]. Higher concentrations of IL-6 was shown to be associated with faster progression of the disease and worse prognosis. Therefore, tocilizumab (TOC), an inhibitor of the IL-6 receptors, was considered as a possible therapeutic option [9–11]. Data from several studies have been contradictory mostly because of the difficulties in the selection of optimal population and finding the proper stage of the disease for administration [12–14]. Although the most recent randomized, double-blind, placebo-controlled trial by Stone et al. was not able to confirm the effectiveness of TOC, authors did not exclude the possible benefit from interleukin-6 receptor blockade in some patient populations because of wide confidence intervals for efficacy comparisons [14].

The purpose of the study is to search for the population of patients with severe COVID-19, which could obtain maximal benefit from the administration of tocilizumab, and identify the predictors of response to the treatment with this drug.

2. Materials and Methods

Patients were selected from the SARSTer national database, which included 2332 patients treated between 1 March and 31 October 2020 in 30 Polish centers. This ongoing project, supported by the Polish Association of Epidemiologists and Infectiologists, is a national real-world experience study assessing treatment in patients with COVID-19. The decision about the treatment regimen was taken entirely by the treating physician concerning current knowledge and recommendations of the Polish Association of Epidemiologists and Infectiologists [15–17]. The SARSTer study was approved by the Ethical Committee of the Medical University of Białystok. If necessary, the local bioethics committees approved experimental use of drugs in patients with COVID-19. Patients aged below 18 years, those with oxygen saturation >95%, or acute respiratory distress syndrome (ARDS) at baseline were excluded from the database of 2332 patients. As a result, the current study included 825 adult patients with moderate to severe course of the disease.

Among those 825 patients, the retrospective analysis was carried out in 170 patients treated with tocilizumab (RoActemra, Roche Pharma AG) and 655 patients who did not receive this medication as well as any other monoclonal antibody directed against cytokine receptors. Tocilizumab was administered intravenously at 8 mg/kg (maximum dose: 800 mg) in a single dose (1-h infusion) after exclusion of severe bacterial and HBV infection. If no improvement was observed, the second dose was considered after 8 to 12 h (administered in 42% patients) according to the national recommendations [15–17]. Data were entered retrospectively and submitted online by a web-based platform operated by Tiba sp. z o.o. Parameters collected at baseline included age, gender, body mass index (BMI), coexisting conditions, other medication-related to COVID-19, clinical status at admission, and adverse events. Baseline clinical status at hospital admission was classified according to oxygen saturation (SpO2) 91–95%, or SpO2 $\leq$ 90%, as well as based on the score on an ordinal scale.

The end-points of treatment effectiveness were rate of death, need for mechanical ventilation, and clinical improvement in the ordinal scale based on WHO recommendations modified to fit the specificity of the national health care system. Clinical improvement was defined as at least a 2-point decrease from baseline to 14, 21, and 28 days of hospitalization. The ordinal scale was scored as follows: (1) unhospitalized, no activity restrictions; (2) unhospitalized, no activity restrictions and/or requiring oxygen supplementation at home; (3) hospitalized, does not require oxygen supplementation and does not require medical care; (4) hospitalized, requiring no oxygen supplementation, but requiring medical care; (5) hospitalized, requiring normal oxygen supplementation; (6) hospitalized, on non-invasive ventilation with high-flow oxygen equipment; (7) hospitalized, for invasive mechanical ventilation or extracorporeal membrane oxygenation (ECMO); (8) death.

To identify possible predictors of response to the treatment with TOC, we compared rates of achieved end-points in patients receiving versus not receiving TOC. The following baseline predictors were included: age above 70 years, the need for oxygen high flow (ordinal scale 6 points) at baseline, clinical worsening during 7 days of hospitalization in patients with regular oxygen supplementation at baseline (5 points in original scale), SpO2 < 90% at baseline, and several laboratory measures at baseline, such as IL-6 > 100 pg/mL, C-reactive protein (CRP) > 200 mg/L, neutrophils > 7500/μL, lymphocytes > 1200/μL, D-dimer > 1000 μg/L, and procalcitonin > 0.1 ng/mL.

Statistical Analysis

The results are expressed as mean $\pm$ standard deviation (SD) or n (%). p values of <0.05 were considered to be statistically significant. The significance of difference was calculated by Fisher's exact test for nominal variables and by Mann–Whitney U and Kruskal Wallis ANOVA for continuous and ordinal variables. Due to the highly variable group size, the Fisher's p-values were accompanied by odds ratio (OR) as the effect size measure independent of the sample size. The association between variables was measured by Spearman's rank correlation coefficient and its significance test p-values. Survival analyses were performed by log-rank (Mantel–Cox) test supported by the Mantel–Haenszel hazard ratio (MH HR) and its 95% confidence interval as the effect size measure and depicted as Kaplan–Meier (KM) plots. The threshold value of IL-6, splitting between the low and the high IL-6 level groups, was found as maximizing the non-TOC vs. TOC hazard ratio value in the high IL-6 group providing the significant differences between the IL-6 group-specific KM survival functions (as measured by log-rank test p-value). Univariable comparisons were calculated by GraphPad Prism 5.1 (GraphPad Software, Inc., La Jolla, CA, USA).

3. Results

Among 825 patients included in the study, 170 received therapy with TOC and 655 did not receive TOC. As shown in Table 1, groups were balanced based on gender, age, and BMI, but there was a predominance of males in both arms. Patients treated with TOC more frequently demonstrated a course of the disease with SpO2 $\leq$ 90% at admission to the hospital (65.9%) compared to those without TOC (37.7%). Moreover, patients treated with TOC more often required normal or high flow oxygen supplementation (93.6%) compared to the non-TOC group (76.8%). The prevalence of coexisting conditions was similar in both groups, but patients treated with TOC more frequently received other medications related to COVID-19 (Table 1).

Table 1. Baseline demographic and clinical characteristics of included patients.

Characteristic	All Patients n = 825	Tocilizumab n = 170	No Tocilizumab n = 655	p
Age				
Mean (SD)	63.1 (15.1)	63.2 (13.8)	63.0 (15.4)	0.94
>70 years (%)	267 (32.4)	53 (31.2)	214 (32.7)	0.78
Gender				
Female, n (%)	337 (40.8)	60 (35.3)	277 (42.3)	0.11
Male, n (%)	488 (59.2)	110 (64.7)	378 (57.7)	0.11
Body mas index, mean (SD)	28.8 (4.9)	29.7 (4.8)	28.5 (5.0)	0.01
Disease severity at the baseline, n (%)				
Oxygen saturation 91–95%	466 (56.5)	58 (34.1)	408 (62.3)	<0.001
Oxygen saturation ≤90%	359 (43.5)	112 (65.9)	247 (37.7)	<0.001
Score on ordinal scale, n (%)				
4. Hospitalized, requiring no oxygen supplementation, but requiring medical care	163 (19.8)	11 (6.5)	152 (23.2)	<0.001
5. Hospitalized, requiring normal oxygen supplementation	615 (74.5)	147 (86.5)	468 (71.5)	<0.001
6. Hospitalized, on non-invasive ventilation with high-flow oxygen equipment	47 (5.7)	12 (7.1)	35 (5.3)	0.36
Coexisting conditions, n (%)	638 (77.3)	131 (77.1)	507 (77.4)	0.91
Other medications related to COVID-19, n (%)				
Remdesivir	284 (34.4)	67 (39.4)	217 (33.1)	0.15
Dexamethason	272 (33.0)	83 (48.8)	189 (28.9)	<0.001
Covalescent plasma	103 (12.5)	29 (17.1)	74 (11.3)	0.05
Low molecular weight heparin	713 (86.5)	170 (100.0)	543 (82.9)	<0.001

As shown in Table 2, the rate of clinical improvement after 21 and 28 days was significantly better in patients who did not receive TOC. However, a statistically significant effect of TOC on rates of death was demonstrated in patients with baseline IL-6 exceeding 100 pg/mL or those needing oxygen supplementation at baseline whose condition worsened within the initial 7 days of hospitalization (Table 2, Figure 1). As shown with the Kaplan–Meier analysis, there were no significant differences between TOC and non-TOC arms when the analysis was carried out in all patients or those with baseline IL-6 concentration below 100 pg/mL. Further analysis included the correlation between IL-6 concentration and several possible clinical and laboratory indices associated with the course of the disease. Among patients with baseline SpO2 ≤ 90%, who are potential TOC recipients, significant correlation was demonstrated among serum concentrations of IL-6 and SpO2, levels of C-reactive protein, procalcitonin D-dimers, as well as white blood cell and neutrophil counts (Table 3).

Table 2. Tocilizumab effect on rates of death, need for mechanical ventilation, and clinical improvement depending on possible outcomes predictors.

Outcomes	Tocilizumab	No Tocilizumab	p	OR (95%CI)
	Overall			
n	170	655		
Death, n (%)	19 (11.2)	70 (10.7)	0.89	1.05 (0.61–1.80)
Mechanical ventilation, n (%)	11 (6.5)	39 (6.0)	0.86	1.09 (0.55–2.18)

Table 2. Cont.

Outcomes	Tocilizumab	No Tocilizumab	p	OR (95%CI)
	Overall			
Clinical improvement after 14 days, n (%)	70 (41.2)	351 (53.6)	0.004	0.61 (0.43–0.85)
Clinical improvement after 21 days, n (%)	112 (65.9)	492 (75.1)	0.02	0.64 (0.44–0.92)
Clinical improvement after 28 days, n (%)	134 (78.8)	531 (81.1)	0.51	0.87 (0.57–1.32)
	Age > 70 years			
n	53	215		
Death, n (%)	11 (20.8)	49 (22.8)	0.85	0.89 (0.42–1.85)
Mechanical ventillation, n (%)	5 (9.4)	20 (9.3)	1.00	1.02 (0.36–2.84)
Clinical improvement after 14 days, n (%)	16 (30.2)	77 (35.8)	0.52	0.83 (0.43–1.59)
Clinical improvement after 21 days, n (%)	28 (52.8)	124 (57.7)	0.54	0.82 (0.45–1.50)
Clinical improvement after 28 days, n (%)	35 (66.0)	141 (65.6)	1.00	1.02 (0.54–1.92)
	The need for oxygen high flow (score 6 in ordinal scale) at baseline			
n	14	35		
Death, n (%)	4 (28.6)	12 (34.3)	1.00	0.77 (0.20–2.97)
Mechanical ventillation, n (%)	4 (28.6)	8 (22.9)	0.72	1.35 (0.33–5.50)
Clinical improvement after 14 days, n (%)	6 (42.9)	9 (25.7)	0.31	2.17 (0.59–7.97)
Clinical improvement after 21 days, n (%)	9 (64.3)	15 (42.9)	0.21	2.40 (0.67–8.65)
Clinical improvement after 28 days, n (%)	9 (64.3)	17 (48.6)	0.36	1.91 (0.53–6.85)
	Clinical worsening during 7 days of hospitalization in patients with regular oxygen supplementation at baseline (5 points in original scale)			
n	41	55		
Death, n (%)	18 (43.9)	37 (67.3)	0.04	0.38 (0.16–0.88)
Mechanical ventillation, n (%)	20 (48.8)	23 (41.8)	0.54	1.32 (0.59–3.00)
Clinical improvement after 14 days, n (%)	0	2 (3.6)	0.51	-
Clinical improvement after 21 days, n (%)	1 (2.4)	8 (14.5)	0.07	0.15 (0.01–1.23)
Clinical improvement after 28 days, n (%)	14 (34.1)	12 (21.8)	0.24	1.85 (0.75–4.61)

Table 2. Cont.

Outcomes	Tocilizumab	No Tocilizumab	p	OR (95%CI)
SpO2 ≤ 90% at the baseline				
n	125	247		
Death, n (%)	23 (17.6)	52 (21.1)	0.59	0.84 (0.49–1.46)
Mechanical ventillation, n (%)	23 (17.6)	30 (11.7)	0.12	1.63 (0.90–2.95)
Clinical improvement after 14 days, n (%)	41 (32.8)	106 (42.5)	0.07	0.65 (0.41–1.10)
Clinical improvement after 21 days, n (%)	66 (52.8)	156 (62.8)	0.06	0.65 (0.42–1.01)
Clinical improvement after 28 days, n (%)	83 (66.4)	173 (69.6)	0.47	0.84 (0.53–1.34)
IL-6 > 100 pg/mL at baseline				
n	56	42		
Death, n (%)	6 (10.7)	13 (31.0)	0.02	0.27 (0.10–0.78)
Mechanical ventillation, n (%)	7 (12.5)	7 (16.7)	0.57	0.71 (0.23–2.20)
Clinical improvement after 14 days, n (%)	22 (39.3)	14 (33.3)	0.67	1.29 (0.56–2.99)
Clinical improvement after 21 days, n (%)	35 (62.5)	19 (45.2)	0.10	2.02 (0.89–4.55)
Clinical improvement after 28 days, n (%)	41 (73.2)	23 (54.8)	0.08	2.26 (0.97–5.27)
CRP > 200 mg/L at the baseline				
n	39	61		
Death, n (%)	6 (15.4)	13 (21.3)	0.60	0.74 (0.25–2.17)
Mechanical ventillation, n (%)	6 (15.4)	10 (16.4)	1.00	0.92 (0.31–2.79)
Clinical improvement after 14 days, n (%)	12 (30.8)	17 (27.9)	0.82	1.15 (0.48–2.78)
Clinical improvement after 21 days, n (%)	20 (51.3)	35 (57.4)	0.68	0.78 (0.35–1.75)
Clinical improvement after 28 days, n (%)	27 (69.2)	39 (63.9)	0.67	1.27 (0.54–2.99)
Neutrophils > 7500/µL at the baseline				
n	39	90		
Death, n (%)	7 (17.9)	23 (25.6)	0.49	0.63 (0.25–1.64)
Mechanical ventillation, n (%)	2 (5.1)	8 (8.9)	1.00	0.55 (0.11–2.73)
Clinical improvement after 14 days, n (%)	15 (38.5)	33 (36.7)	0.84	1.08 (0.50–2.34)
Clinical improvement after 21 days, n (%)	23 (59.0)	51 (56.7)	0.84	1.10 (0.51–2.35)
Clinical improvement after 28 days, n (%)	28 (71.8)	59 (65.6)	0.54	1.34 (0.59–3.04)

Table 2. Cont.

Outcomes	Tocilizumab	No Tocilizumab	p	OR (95%CI)
Lymphocytes > 1200/µL at the baseline				
n	47	239		
Death, n (%)	1 (2.1)	20 (8.4)	0.22	0.24 (0.03–1.82)
Mechanical ventilation, n (%)	0	8 (3.3)	0.36	-
Clinical improvement after 14 days, n (%)	28 (59.6)	142 (59.4)	1.00	1.01 (0.53–1.90)
Clinical improvement after 21 days, n (%)	36 (76.6)	192 (80.3)	0.55	0.80 (0.38–1.69)
Clinical improvement after 28 days, n (%)	43 (91.5)	201 (84.1)	0.26	2.03 (0.69–6.00)
D-dimers > 1000 µg/L at the baseline				
n	75	221		
Death, n (%)	12 (16.0)	45 (20.4)	0.50	0.74 (0.37–1.50)
Mechanical ventilation, n (%)	7 (9.3)	21 (9.5)	1.00	0.98 (0.40–2.41)
Clinical improvement after 14 days, n (%)	25 (33.3)	101 (45.7)	0.08	0.59 (0.34–1.03)
Clinical improvement after 21 days, n (%)	43 (57.3)	143 (64.7)	0.27	0.73 (0.43–1.25)
Clinical improvement after 28 days, n (%)	54 (72.0)	158 (71.5)	1.00	1.02 (0.57–1.84)
Procalcitonin > 0.1 ng/mL at the baseline				
n	92	193		
Death, n (%)	18 (19.6)	44 (22.8)	0.64	0.82 (0.44–1.52)
Mechanical ventilation, n (%)	10 (10.9)	25 (13.0)	0.70	0.82 (0.37–1.79)
Clinical improvement after 14 days, n (%)	34 (37.0)	74 (38.3)	0.89	0.94 (0.56–1.57)
Clinical improvement after 21 days, n (%)	53 (57.6)	117 (60.6)	0.70	0.88 (0.53–1.46)
Clinical improvement after 28 days, n (%)	68 (73.9)	128 (66.3)	0.22	1.44 (0.83–2.50)

Bold: statistical significance.

To improve the predictive value, a combination of several measures was also analyzed. As shown in Table 4, the best effectiveness of TOC administration can be achieved in patients with serum IL-6 > 100 pg/mL and either SpO2 ≤ 90% or requiring normal or high-flow oxygen supplementation. Statistically significant effectiveness was achieved regarding the risk of death, the need for mechanical ventilation, as well as clinical improvement after 21 and 28 days (Table 4). Significantly better survival among such patients treated with TOC was also demonstrated with a Kaplan–Meier analysis (Figure 2).

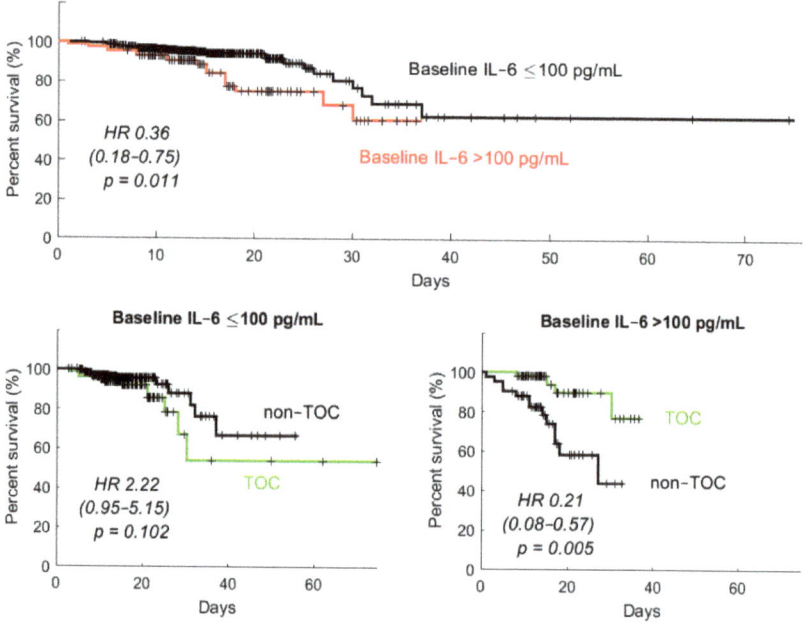

Figure 1. Kaplan–Meier graphs demonstrating the effect of tocilizumab versus no tocilizumab administration on patients' survival depending on the obtained optimal threshold baseline serum concentration of interleukin 6. The hazard ratios (HR) and their 95% confidence intervals are provided as well as the log-rank test p-values.

Table 3. Correlations between baseline serum IL-6 vs. selected clinical and laboratory indices.

IL-6 Versus	All Patients (n = 825)		SpO2 ≤ 90% (n = 372)		SpO2 91–95% (n = 453)	
	r_s	p	r_s	p	r_s	p
Age	0.15	<0.001	0.07	0.32	0.18	0.002
BMI	0.01	0.86	−0.03	0.63	0.01	0.89
SpO$_2$	−0.33	<0.001	−0.19	0.003	−0.31	<0.001
CRP	0.58	<0.001	0.44	<0.001	0.68	<0.001
Procalcitonin	0.40	<0.001	0.37	<0.001	0.36	<0.001
WBC	0.26	<0.001	0.22	<0.001	0.25	<0.001
Lymphocytes	−0.21	<0.001	−0.05	0.42	−0.28	<0.001
Neutrophils	0.32	<0.001	0.23	<0.001	0.37	<0.001
Platelets	−0.10	0.04	−0.10	0.14	−0.13	0.03
D-dimers	0.28	<0.001	0.20	0.003	0.27	<0.001
ALT	0.13	0.03	0.10	0.13	0.10	0.09

Table 4. Tocilizumab effect on rates of death, need for mechanical ventilation, and clinical improvement depending on combinations of possible outcomes predictors.

Outcomes	Tocilizumab	No Tocilizumab	p	OR (95%CI)
Baseline IL6 > 100 pg/mL and requiring normal or high-flow oxygen supplementation (5 or 6 scores in ordinal scale)				
n	53	34		
Death, n (%)	8 (15.1)	13 (38.2)	0.02	0.18 (0.06–0.52)
Mechanical ventilation, n (%)	8 (15.1)	7 (20.6)	0.57	0.68 (0.22–2.10)
Clinical improvement after 14 days, n (%)	20 (37.7)	10 (29.4)	0.49	1.45 (0.58–3.66)
Clinical improvement after 21 days, n (%)	33 (62.3)	13 (38.2)	0.047	2.66 (1.10–6.47)
Clinical improvement after 28 days, n (%)	38 (71.7)	16 (47.1)	0.02	2.85 (1.16–7.01)
Baseline IL6 > 100 pg/mL and SpO2 < 90%				
n	37	24		
Death, n (%)	4 (10.8)	12 (50.0)	<0.001	0.07 (0.02–0.27)
Mechanical ventilation, n (%)	2 (5.4)	7 (29.2)	0.02	0.14 (0.03–0.74)
Clinical improvement after 14 days, n (%)	12 (32.4)	3 (12.5)	0.12	3.36 (0.83–13.52)
Clinical improvement after 21 days, n (%)	24 (64.9)	6 (25.0)	0.004	5.53 (1.76–17.40)
Clinical improvement after 28 days, n (%)	28 (75.7)	9 (37.5)	0.004	5.18 (1.70–17.84)
Baseline IL6 > 100 pg/mL and CRP > 200 mg/L				
n	32	26		
Death, n (%)	5 (15.6)	7 (26.9)	0.34	0.50 (0.14–1.82)
Mechanical ventilation, n (%)	1 (3.1)	4 (15.4)	0.16	0.18 (0.02–1.70)
Clinical improvement after 14 days, n (%)	11 (34.4)	8 (30.8)	1.00	1.18 (0.39–3.57)
Clinical improvement after 21 days, n (%)	18 (56.3)	15 (57.7)	1.00	0.94 (0.33–2.68)
Clinical improvement after 28 days, n (%)	24 (75.0)	18 (69.2)	0.77	1.33 (0.42–4.23)
Baseline IL6 > 100 pg/mL and CRP > 200 mg/L and SpO2 < 90%				
n	21	13		
Death, n (%)	4 (19.0)	5 (38.5)	0.26	0.37 (0.08–1.80)
Mechanical ventilation, n (%)	1 (4.8)	3 (23.1)	0.27	0.17 (0.01–1.81)
Clinical improvement after 14 days, n (%)	6 (28.6)	3 (23.1)	1.00	1.33 (0.27–6.61)
Clinical improvement after 21 days, n (%)	11 (52.4)	5 (38.5)	0.49	1.76 (0.43–7.19)
Clinical improvement after 28 days, n (%)	15 (71.4)	8 (61.5)	0.71	1.56 (0.36–6.76)

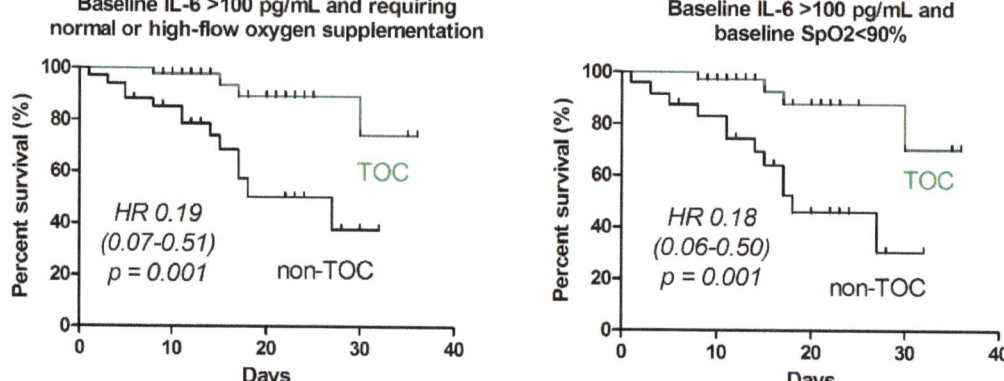

Figure 2. Kaplan–Meier graphs demonstrating the effect of tocilizumab versus no tocilizumab administration on patients' survival depending on baseline serum concentration of interleukin 6. The hazard ratios (HR) and their 95% confidence intervals are provided as well as the log-rank test p-values.

TOC

Adverse events related to therapy were infrequent and reported in 21.7% and 17.3% of patients in TOC and non-TOC arms, respectively. As shown in Table 5, the most frequent was an elevation of ALT activities, diarrhea, and prolonged QT interval. Prevalence of adverse events was similar in both arms (Table 5). No secondary infections were noticed in patients treated with TOC.

Table 5. Prevalence of adverse events.

Adverse Events	Tocilizumab	No Tocilizumab	p
n	170	655	
ALT elevation, n (%)	17 (10.0)	40 (6.1)	0.09
Diarrhea, n (%)	8 (4.7)	39 (5.9)	0.71
Prolonged QT interval, n (%)	3 (1.8)	11 (1.7)	1.00
Nausea, n (%)	2 (1.2)	12 (1.8)	0.75
Other, n (%)	7 (4.7)	11 (1.7)	0.07
All adverse events, n (%)	37 (21.7)	113 (17.3)	0.18

4. Discussion

Uncontrolled immune activation with high-level release of various pro-inflammatory cytokines is a hallmark of not only the lung damage but also multiorgan damage during later phases of COVID-19. It is usually termed as a "cytokine storm" and observed mainly during the second and third week of symptomatic disease in patients with severely impaired oxygen saturation [18]. Unsurprisingly, anti-cytokine agents including anti-IL-1R and anti-IL6R antagonists were among important candidates in the therapy of later stages of COVID-19. One of the rationales was a good suppressive effect of tocilizumab in cytokine release syndrome during CAR T-cells therapy [19]. Regardless of the pathophysiological link, various randomized and observational studies of TOC, while suggesting some benefit, did not bring clear evidence supporting its use in COVID-19. This may reflect the unique features of individual immune responses to pathogens, as well as the necessity of a complex and personalized approach in prescribing and timing immunomodulatory treatment.

Proposing clinical trial protocol taking such diversity into account proves to be challenging; thus, personalized medicine relies on observational research and real-life experiences.

Results of our real-world evidence study could not only potentially explain the lack of effect of TOC observed in other studies but also provide information on the optimal use of this agent. In our cohort, similar to the first two randomized controlled trials (RCT), TOC did not decrease overall mortality in hospitalized patients with COVID-19. In the first study by Stone JH et al. [14], 83% of 243 COVID-19 subjects requiring oxygen supplementation but not mechanical ventilation were randomized to TOC (8 mg/kg, single dose) or placebo. In this study, the hazard ratio (HR) for death was 0.83, which was not significant, with broad 95% confidence intervals (0.38 to 1.81, $p = 0.64$) suggesting heterogeneity of effect probably depending on other clinical variables not found in the publication. In another RCT by Hermine et al. [12] including 131 patients with COVID-19 pneumonia requiring oxygen supplementation but not mechanically ventilated, 64 were randomized to TOC (8 mg/kg, twice) or placebo. Likewise, the adjusted HR for 28-day mortality was 0.92 (90%CI 0.33–2.53). On the other hand, on day 14 in TOC-group, 12% fewer patients needed non-invasive or mechanical ventilation, or 12% less died (HR 0.58; 90%CI 0.33–1.00). Only the most recent and largest RCT by Salama et al. [13] showed a survival benefit in patients treated with TOC. In this study, 377 subjects with COVID-19 pneumonia, 64% requiring low-flow and 26% on non-invasive and high flow oxygen supplementation, were randomized to TOC (n = 259, 8 mg/kg, one or two doses) or placebo. By day 28, HR for mechanical ventilation or death was 0.56 (95%CI: 0.33–0.97, $p = 0.04$), while still the number of patients who died by that day of any reason was 10.4% in TOC group vs. 8.6% in the placebo group.

Summarizing all aforementioned randomized clinical trials despite a rather homogenous population included, which is patients with COVID-19 pneumonia mainly requiring oxygen supplementation but not ventilated, it was not possible to visualize the obvious survival benefit of TOC. Similarly in our study, the overall mortality was comparable between TOC and non-TOC patients (odds ratio, OR 1.05; 95%CI: 0.61–1.80). Furthermore, the group receiving TOC showed even lesser odds of clinical improvement after 14 and 21 days of therapy (OR 0.61 and 0.64, respectively), while it was comparable to the standard-of-care therapy at the end of observation, i.e., after 28 days (OR 0.87). On the other hand, only analyses in specific subgroups showed not only a survival benefit but also a more rapid clinical improvement in patients treated with TOC. It was quite striking that in previous studies, mortality HR had quite outsized confidence intervals, suggesting another factor playing the predictive role of TOC efficacy. Surprisingly enough, cited above RCT did not evaluate baseline IL-6 serum concentration even when TOC is aimed at blocking an IL-6 proinflammatory pathway. Indeed, we performed a detailed subgroup analysis aiming at the development of predictors of TOC response in COVID-19 subjects. Not unpredictably, the best response to TOC concerning decreasing 28-day mortality (OR = 0.27; 95%CI: 0.10–0.78, 11% vs. 31%, $p = 0.02$) was observed in subjects with baseline serum IL-6 > 100 pg/mL, while it was not observed in subject with baseline IL-6 50–100 pg/mL and below 50 pg/mL. Importantly, an IL-6 level of more than 100 pg/mL observed in approximately 18% of all studied patients possibly explain why the difference was not noted in overall studied groups in the aforementioned RCT but also in our study. This observation also underlines the pathogenetic complexity of cytokine imbalance during COVID-19. It is known that cytokine storm in COVID-19 consists of various, not necessarily overlapping, soluble immune mediators (SIMs) including IL-1β, IL-6, IL-8, and tumor necrosis factor-alpha (TNF-α) which could yield different predictive value [20]. Interestingly, Mathew et al. [21] in their elegant study had shown at least three different immunotypes of COVID-19, 1–3, depending on the cluster of differentiation of (CD)4+ cell, CD8+ cell, and B-cell, and plasmablasts activation/exhaustion, which was associated with different outcomes but also most likely with different levels of cytokines. Interestingly, despite baseline IL-6, the effect of TOC in our study did not depend on baseline CRP, D-dimer, or lymphocyte concentrations, which are also regarded as factors associated with prognosis [22].

Another important finding of our study was that the highest reduction in mortality, the need for mechanical ventilation, and best clinical improvement at day 28 in patients receiving TOC vs. standard-of-care (SOC) therapy was observed in patients with baseline IL-6 > 100 pg/mL and SpO2 < 90% (11 vs. 50%, 5 vs. 29%, and 75 vs. 37%, respectively), which was not the case in subjects with SpO2 ≥ 90%. This observation might further underline that in subjects with severe hypoxia, further deregulation between IL-6 levels and other cytokines is present and possibly IL-6 activation is deeper and not counterbalanced by regulatory mechanism, which could explain why the effect of TOC is more significant. In addition, in our study, correlation analyses showed the correlation pattern of IL-6 and some soluble immune mediators are different in patients with oxygen saturation lower and higher/equal to 90%.

The results of our study should be taken with some caution because of its retrospective real-world evidence design and because of the smaller number of participants in some subgroup analyses. Moreover, some patients in both arms received additional medication, which could affect the outcome of the disease. On the other hand, patients receiving TOC and non-TOC SOC therapies seem to be well balanced with regard to comorbidities and co-medications for COVID-19, and undoubtedly its advantage is the assessment of baseline serum IL-6 concentration. Indeed, while only one other single-center study showed a beneficial effect of TOC mainly in patients with higher IL-6 [23], our data in a real-world large dataset seems to guide the effective use of TOC in COVID-19. Safety profile of TOC in our study was good. Adverse events were infrequent and mild. However, risk of secondary infections should always be considered [24].

5. Conclusions

In conclusion, the possible benefit from the treatment of COVID-19 with tocilizumab can be achieved in selected subpopulations only. This regimen can reduce mortality and the need for mechanical ventilation in patients with a baseline concentration of interleukin 6 exceeding 100 pg/mL, particularly if they need oxygen supplementation due to oxygen saturation of ≤90%. Patients who worsened within the initial 7 days of hospitalization can also obtain some benefits from tocilizumab administration, but it should be clarified in further studies on a larger number of patients.

Author Contributions: R.F.—designed research, performed research, analyzed data, wrote majority of the article, performed the final submission. J.J. and J.P.—analyzed data, performed statistics, drawed figures, and wrote some parts of the article. D.Z.-M.—collected data, analyzed data, and wrote some parts of the article. M.R. (Magdalena Rogalska), T.Ł., A.B.-K., B.B., M.T.-Z., K.K., M.R. (Marta Rorat), P.L., D.K., J.K., P.P., A.P., I.M.-L., K.T., M.P., K.S.—collected data and analyzed data. All authors have read and agreed to the published version of the manuscript.

Funding: This research was funded by Medical Research Agency, grant number 2020/ABM/COVID19/PTEILCHZ and Polish Association of Epidemiologists and Infectiologists.

Institutional Review Board Statement: The study was conducted according to the guidelines of the Declaration of Helsinki, and approved by the Ethics Committee of Medical University of Białystok (29 October 2020, number APK.002.303.2020).

Informed Consent Statement: Informed consent was obtained from all subjects involved in the study.

Data Availability Statement: Data supporting reported results can be provided upon request from the corresponding author.

Conflicts of Interest: R.F. reports grants from Abbvie, Gilead, and Merck; personal fees from Gilead, Abbvie, Merck, and Roche; and non-financial support from Abbvie, Gilead, and Merck outside the submitted work. D.Z.M. and P.P. reports personal fees from Gilead and Abbvie, outside the submitted work. JJ reports personal fees from Gilead, Abbvie, Bausch Health, Merck, Promed, and Roche, and non-financial support from Abbvie, Gilead, and Merck outside the submitted work. K.S. reports personal fees from Gilead, Abbvie, and Merck, outside the submitted work. K.T. reports personal fees from Gilead, Abbvie, Merck, Promed, and Roche, and non-financial support from Abbvie, Gilead, and Merck outside the submitted work. J.K. reports personal fees from Gilead, Merck, ViiV, and Janssen outside the submitted work. IML reports personal fees from Gilead, Abbvie, and Pfizer. A.B.K., J.P., B.B., K.K., M.P., A.P., D.K., M.T.Z., C.I., MRog, and MRor declare no competing interests.

References

1. Mulangu, S.; Dodd, L.E.; Davey, R.T., Jr.; Mbaya, O.T.; Proschan, M.; Mukadi, D.; Manzo, M.L.; Nzolo, D.; Oloma, A.T.; Ibanda, A.; et al. A Randomized, Controlled Trial of Ebola Virus Disease Therapeutics. *N. Engl. J. Med.* **2019**, *381*, 2293–2303. [CrossRef]
2. Sheahan, T.P.; Sims, A.C.; Graham, R.L.; Menachery, V.D.; Gralinski, L.E.; Case, J.B.; Leist, S.R.; Krzysztof, P.; Feng, J.Y.; Trantcheva, I.; et al. Broad-spectrum antiviral GS-5734 inhibits both epidemic and zoonotic coronaviruses. *Sci. Transl. Med.* **2017**, *9*, eaal3653. [CrossRef]
3. Beigel, J.H.; Tomashek, K.M.; Dodd, L.E.; Mehta, A.K.; Zingman, B.S.; Kalil, A.C.; Hohmann, E.; Chu, H.Y.; Luetkemeyer, A.; Kline, S.; et al. Remdesivir for the Treatment of Covid-19—Preliminary Report. *N. Engl. J. Med.* **2020**, *383*, 1813–1826. [CrossRef]
4. Goldman, J.D.; Lye, D.C.; Hui, D.S.; Marks, K.M.; Bruno, R.; Montejano, R.; Spinner, C.D.; Galli, M.; Ahn, M.-Y.; Nahass, R.G.; et al. Remdesivir for 5 or 10 Days in Patients with Severe Covid-19. *N. Engl. J. Med.* **2020**, *83*, 1827–1837. [CrossRef]
5. Flisiak, R.; Zarębska-Michaluk, D.; Berkan-Kawińska, A.; Tudrujek-Zdunek, M.; Rogalska, M.; Piekarska, A.; Kozielewicz, D.; Kłos, K.; Rorat, M.; Bolewska, B.; et al. Remdesivir-based therapy improved recovery of patients with COVID-19 in the SARSTer multicentre, real-world study. *Pol. Arch. Intern. Med.* **2021**, *131*, 103–110.
6. Tang, N.; Bai, H.; Chen, X.; Gong, J.; Li, D.; Sun, Z. Anticoagulant treatment is associated with decreased mortality in severe coronavirus disease 2019 patients with coagulopathy. *J. Thromb. Haemost.* **2020**, *18*, 1094–1099. [CrossRef] [PubMed]
7. Horby, P.; Lim, W.S.; Emberson, J.R.; Mafham, M.; Bell, J.L.; Linsell, L.; Staplin, N.; Brightling, C.; Ustianowski, A.; Elmahi, E.; et al. Dexamethasone in hospitalized patients with Covid-19—preliminary report. *N. Engl. J. Med.* **2021**, *384*, 693–704. [PubMed]
8. Jose, R.J.; Manuel, A. COVID-19 cytokine storm: The interplay between inflammation and coagulation. *Lancet Respir. Med.* **2020**, *8*, e46–e47. [CrossRef]
9. Tomasiewicz, K.; Piekarska, A.; Stempkowska-Rejek, J.; Serafińska, S.; Gawkowska, A.; Parczewski, M.; Niścigorska-Olsen, J.; Łapiński, T.W.; Zarębska-Michaluk, D.; Kowalska, J.D.; et al. Tocilizumab for patients with severe COVID-19: A retrospective, multi-center study. *Expert Rev. AntiInfect. Ther.* **2021**, *19*, 93–100. [CrossRef] [PubMed]
10. Liu, B.; Li, M.; Zhou, Z.; Guan, X.; Xiang, Y. Can we use interleukin-6 (IL-6) blockade for coronavirus disease 2019 (COVID-19)-induced cytokine release syndrome (CRS)? *J. Autoimmun.* **2020**, *111*, 102452. [CrossRef]
11. Rosas, I.O.; Bräu, N.; Waters, M.; Go, R.C.; Hunter, B.D.; Bhagani, S.; Skiest, D.; Aziz, M.S.; Cooper, N.; Douglas, I.S.; et al. Tocilizumab in hospitalized patients with severe COVID-19 pneumonia. *N. Engl. J. Med.* **2021**. [CrossRef]
12. Hermine, O.; Mariette, X.; Tharaux, P.L.; Resche-Rigon, M.; Porcher, R.; Ravaud, P. Effect of Tocilizumab vs Usual Care in Adults Hospitalized With COVID-19 and Moderate or Severe Pneumonia: A Randomized Clinical Trial. *JAMA Intern. Med.* **2021**, *181*, 32–40. [CrossRef]
13. Salama, C.; Han, J.; Yau, L.; Reiss, W.G.; Kramer, B.; Neidhart, J.D.; Criner, G.J.; Kaplan-Lewis, E.; Baden, R.; Pandit, L.; et al. Tocilizumab in Patients Hospitalized with Covid-19 Pneumonia. *N. Engl. J. Med.* **2021**, *384*, 20–30. [CrossRef]
14. Stone, J.H.; Frigault, M.J.; Serling-Boyd, N.J.; Fernandes, A.D.; Harvey, L.; Foulkes, A.S.; Horick, N.K.; Healy, B.C.; Shah, R.; Bensaci, A.M.; et al. Efficacy of Tocilizumab in Patients Hospitalized with Covid-19. *N. Engl. J. Med.* **2020**, *383*, 2333–2344. [CrossRef]
15. Flisiak, R.; Horban, A.; Jaroszewicz, J.; Kozielewicz, D.; Pawłowska, M.; Parczewski, M.; Piekarska, A.; Simon, K.; Tomasiewicz, K.; Zarębska-Michaluk, D. Management of SARS-CoV-2 infection: Recommendations of the Polish Association of Epidemiologists and Infectiologists as of March 31, 2020. *Pol. Arch. Intern. Med.* **2020**, *130*, 352–357. [PubMed]
16. Flisiak, R.; Horban, A.; Jaroszewicz, J.; Kozielewicz, D.; Pawlowska, M.; Parczewski, M.; Piekarska, A.; Simon, K.; Tomasiewicz, K.; Zarebska-Michaluk, D. Management of SARS-CoV-2 infection: Recommendations of the Polish Association of Epidemiologists and Infectiologists. Annex no. 1 as of June 8, 2020. *Pol. Arch. Intern. Med.* **2020**, *130*, 557–558.
17. Flisiak, R.; Parczewski, M.; Horban, A.; Jaroszewicz, J.; Kozielewicz, D.; Pawłowska, M.; Piekarska, A.; Simon, K.; Tomasiewicz, K.; Zarębska-Michaluk, D. Management of SARS-CoV-2 infection: Recommendations of the Polish Association of Epidemiologists and Infectiologists. Annex no. 2 as of October 13, 2020. *Pol. Arch. Intern. Med.* **2020**, *130*, 915–918. [CrossRef] [PubMed]
18. Fajgenbaum, D.C.; June, C.H. Cytokine Storm. *N. Engl. J. Med.* **2020**, *383*, 2255–2273. [CrossRef] [PubMed]
19. Le, R.Q.; Li, L.; Yuan, W.; Shord, S.S.; Nie, L.; Habtemariam, B.A.; Przepiorka, D.; Farrell, A.T.; Pazdur, R. FDA Approval Summary: Tocilizumab for Treatment of Chimeric Antigen Receptor T Cell-Induced Severe or Life-Threatening Cytokine Release Syndrome. *Oncologist* **2018**, *23*, 943–947. [CrossRef]

20. Del Valle, D.M.; Kim-Schulze, S.; Huang, H.H.; Beckmann, N.D.; Nirenberg, S.; Wang, B.; Lavin, Y.; Swartz, T.H.; Madduri, D.; Stock, A.; et al. An inflammatory cytokine signature predicts COVID-19 severity and survival. *Nat. Med.* **2020**, *26*, 1636–1643. [CrossRef]
21. Mathew, D.; Giles, J.R.; Baxter, A.E.; Oldridge, D.A.; Greenplate, A.R.; Wu, J.E.; Alanio, C.; Kuri-Cervantes, L.; Pampena, M.B.; D'Andrea, K.; et al. Deep immune profiling of COVID-19 patients reveals distinct immunotypes with therapeutic implications. *Science* **2020**, *369*, eabc8511. [CrossRef]
22. Mueller, A.A.; Tamura, T.; Crowley, C.P.; DeGrado, J.R.; Haider, H.; Jezmir, J.L.; Keras, G.; Penn, E.H.; Massaro, A.F.; Kim, E.Y. Inflammatory biomarker trends predict respiratory decline in COVID-19 patients. *Cell Rep. Med.* **2020**, *1*, 100144. [CrossRef] [PubMed]
23. Galván-Román, J.M.; Rodríguez-García, S.C.; Roy-Vallejo, E.; Marcos-Jiménez, A.; Sánchez-Alonso, S.; Fernández-Díaz, C.; Alcaraz-Serna, A.; Mateu-Albero, T.; Rodríguez-Cortes, P.; Montes, N.; et al. IL-6 serum levels predict severity and response to tocilizumab in COVID-19: An observational study. *J. Allergy Clin. Immunol.* **2020**, *147*, 72–80. [CrossRef] [PubMed]
24. Deana, C.; Vetrugno, L.; Bassi, F.; De Monte, A. Tocilizumab administration in COVID-19 patients: Water on the fire or gasoline? *Med. Mycol. Case Rep.* **2021**, *31*, 32–34. [CrossRef] [PubMed]

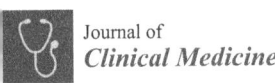

Journal of
Clinical Medicine

Review

The Use of Tocilizumab in Patients with COVID-19: A Systematic Review, Meta-Analysis and Trial Sequential Analysis of Randomized Controlled Studies

Alberto Enrico Maraolo [1], Anna Crispo [2,*], Michela Piezzo [3], Piergiacomo Di Gennaro [2], Maria Grazia Vitale [4], Domenico Mallardo [4], Luigi Ametrano [5], Egidio Celentano [2], Arturo Cuomo [6], Paolo A. Ascierto [4] and Marco Cascella [6]

1. First Division of Infectious Diseases, Cotugno Hospital, AORN dei Colli, 80131 Naples, Italy; albertomaraolo@mail.com
2. Epidemiology and Biostatistics Unit, Istituto Nazionale Tumori, IRCCS Fondazione G. Pascale, 80131 Naples, Italy; piergiacomo.digennaro@live.it (P.D.G.); e.celentano@istitutotumori.na.it (E.C.)
3. Department of Public Health and Infectious Diseases, Sapienza University of Rome, Viale del Policlinico 155, 00161 Rome, Italy; m.piezzo@breastunit.org
4. Department of Melanoma, Cancer Immunotherapy and Development Therapeutics, Istituto Nazionale Tumori, IRCCS Fondazione G. Pascale, 80131 Naples, Italy; dott.mariagrazia.vitale@gmail.com (M.G.V.); dome.mallardo@gmail.com (D.M.); paolo.ascierto@gmail.com (P.A.A.)
5. Department of Clinical Medicine and Surgery, Section of Infectious Diseases, University of Naples Federico II, 80131 Naples, Italy; luigi.ametrano@outlook.com
6. Division of Anesthesia and Pain Medicine, Istituto Nazionale Tumori, IRCCS Fondazione G. Pascale, 80131 Naples, Italy; a.cuomo@istitutotumori.na.it (A.C.); m.cascella@istitutotumori.na.it (M.C.)
* Correspondence: a.crispo@istitutotumori.na.it

Abstract: Background: Among the several therapeutic options assessed for the treatment of coronavirus disease 2019 (COVID-19), tocilizumab (TCZ), an antagonist of the interleukine-6 receptor, has emerged as a promising therapeutic choice, especially for the severe form of the disease. Proper synthesis of the available randomized clinical trials (RCTs) is needed to inform clinical practice. Methods: A systematic review with a meta-analysis of RCTs investigating the efficacy of TCZ in COVID-19 patients was conducted. PubMed, EMBASE, and the Cochrane COVID-19 Study Register were searched up until 30 April 2021. Results: The database search yielded 2885 records; 11 studies were considered eligible for full-text review, and nine met the inclusion criteria. Overall, 3358 patients composed the TCZ arm, and 3131 the comparator group. The main outcome was all-cause mortality at 28–30 days. Subgroup analyses according to trials' and patients' features were performed. A trial sequential analysis (TSA) was also carried out to minimize type I and type II errors. According to the fixed-effect model approach, TCZ was associated with a better survival odds ratio (OR) (0.84; 95% confidence interval (CI): 0.75–0.94; I^2: 24% (low heterogeneity)). The result was consistent in the subgroup of severe disease (OR: 0.83; 95% CI: 0.74–0.93; I^2: 53% (moderate heterogeneity)). However, the TSA illustrated that the required information size was not met unless the study that was the major source of heterogeneity was omitted. Conclusions: TCZ may represent an important weapon against severe COVID-19. Further studies are needed to consolidate this finding.

Keywords: COVID-19 pneumonia; tocilizumab; SARS-CoV-2; COVID-19; meta-analysis; trial sequential analysis

1. Introduction

Tocilizumab (TCZ) is a humanized monoclonal antibody that, via the binding to soluble and membrane interleukin (IL)-6 receptors, produces inhibition of the proinflammatory signals [1]. It is commonly used in several types of inflammatory arthritis, in Castleman's syndrome, and in cytokine release syndrome secondary to chimeric antigen receptor T cell therapies [2]. Given its ability to intercept proinflammatory cascades, TCZ is potentially useful in all clinical conditions produced by the dysregulation of inflammatory processes, especially when refractory to other approved treatments [3].

Although the precise pathogenesis of the coronavirus disease 2019 (COVID-19) pneumonia remains unsolved, evidence showed that within a complex cytokine storm scenario, SARS-CoV-2 provokes a dramatic increase in IL-6 levels [4]. Based on this evidence, it was suggested to use TCZ for improving the patients' outcomes in COVID-19 pneumonia [5]. Consequently, many clinical studies have been conducted to evaluate the efficacy of this treatment, and an increasing number of evidence-based medicine analyses can be found in the literature [6].

However, initial evidence syntheses failed to produce definitive results, especially owing to the conflicting findings emerging between observational studies and randomized clinical trials (RCTs) [7]. As matter of fact, in evaluating the effectiveness of drugs for the treatment of COVID-19, even in high-impact journals, the following methodological distortions were common among observational studies, particularly dealing with time-to-event analysis: immortal time bias, confounding bias, and competing risk bias [8].

Despite the rush for a game-changing treatment capable of significantly impacting the prognosis of COVID-19 patients, clinical practice must rely upon rock-solid evidence, and well-known RCTs are placed on the top of the hierarchy of evidence [9]. This is the rationale behind the choice to perform a systematic review and meta-analysis only focused on RCTs, involving the comparison of TCZ with placebo or standard of care (SoC), for the treatment of COVID-19.

2. Materials and Methods

This systematic review is PROSPERO registered (registration number: CRD42020226657) and complies with the Preferred Reporting Items for Systematic Reviews and Meta-Analyses (PRISMA) statement in its 2020 version (PRISMA Statement, Ottawa, ON, Canada) [10].

2.1. Search Strategy

PubMed, EMBASE, and the Cochrane COVID-19 Study Register were searched up until 30 April 2021 for RCTs to investigate the efficacy of TCZ in COVID-19 patients. The search was restricted to peer-reviewed articles. Neither geographical nor language restrictions were applied. The search strategies were designed by two researchers in the team (A.E.M., L.A.), using appropriate combinations of the following keywords through Boolean operators: "tocilizumab", "COVID-19", "SARS-CoV-2", "2019-nCoV", "novel coronavirus". Strategies for retrieving articles were adapted according to the databases' distinctive features. Specific details are provided in Supplementary Table S1. Manual checking of reference lists and citation tracking of included papers were undertaken in order to retrieve further articles.

2.2. Screening and Eligibility

Duplicate records were discarded by using the EndNote 20 reference managing software (Clarivate, Philadelphia, PA, USA) [11]. A two-step screening process for eligibility was carried out. First, two authors (M.D.G. and D.M.) excluded ineligible studies by screening titles and abstracts. Then, another couple of authors (A.C., M.P.) independently reviewed the full texts of potentially eligible studies for inclusion in the review. Disagreements were resolved through discussion and general consensus. Eligibility was assessed by resorting to the PICOS (population, intervention, comparators/controls, outcomes and study design) question format [11,12], as follows:

- Population: Patients affected by COVID-19.
- Intervention: Administration of tocilizumab, alone or in association with other drugs.
- Comparators/controls: SoC, placebo, or any kind of alternative interventions.
- Outcomes: The main outcome of interest was all-cause mortality reported using an intention-to-treat (not modified) method (28-/30-day mortality, in-hospital mortality,

overall survival according to the reported results). Secondary outcomes were represented by clinical success, time to recovery, rate of intensive care unit (ICU) admission, risk of mechanical ventilation requirement, duration of mechanical ventilation, length of stay (LOS), safety profile related to pharmacological intervention, toxicity, rate of secondary infection, and time to hospital discharge.
- Study design: Only RCTs were included.

Studies that did not fulfill the eligibility criteria were excluded. The minimum sample size required was at least 50 patients per arm.

2.3. Data Extraction

Two authors (A.C. and M.P.) independently abstracted data from each study and the data were subsequently double entered into a custom-made electronic database (an Excel spreadsheet) to eliminate data entry errors. Discrepancies were resolved by consensus, or with a third author (A.E.M.) if necessary. Data compilation used a standardized data extraction tool to report the following variables of interest: first author; country; sample size; main population features (e.g., age, gender, comorbidities); criteria of COVID-19 diagnosis; COVID-19 severity; setting (outpatient/in-patient, non-ICU/ICU); intervention characteristics (TCZ schedule, companion agent if present); comparator features; survival outcome measures such as number of deaths, odds ratios (ORs), and hazard ratios (HRs); and follow-up duration. Data regarding the main outcome were extracted for the whole study population and major subgroups of interest. When necessary, graphical data abstraction was conducted using open-source software. In addition, the full protocol of each study was consulted to verify the study objectives, population, and other relevant information regarding the study design and conduction.

2.4. Data Synthesis and Analysis

To obtain more appropriate estimates of the average treatment effect in the case of between-study heterogeneity, the pooled estimates of ORs with two-sided 95% CIs were computed for 28-day mortality. For this aim, a fixed-effect model according to the inverse-variance method [13], and the random-effect model of DerSimonian and Laird [14], were adopted. The assumption of homogeneity between studies was tested with Cochran's Q statistics, and the measure of the degree of inconsistency across studies was assessed with Higgins' I^2 index, quantifying heterogeneity as low, moderate, and high, with upper limits of 25, 50, and 75% for the I^2 values, respectively [15]. Predefined subgroups were analyzed to better understand if the treatment effect changed because of specific trial and patients characteristics. All results were displayed by specific forest plots. A p-value < 0.05 was considered statistically significant. Sensitivity analysis was carried out according to the leave-one-out cross validation method that calculates the pooled estimates omitting one study at a time, to capture some features of the included studies that are able to influence the pooled estimates. Funnel plots and regression tests, according to the method reported by Egger [16], were performed to assess the publication bias. Data analysis was performed using R 3.4.1 software packages (The R Foundation for Statistical Computing, Wien, Austria) [17,18]. The summary statistics to measure treatment effect were represented by the OR and presented along with appropriate 95% CI values.

Trial sequential analysis (TSA) was also performed for better interpreting the meta-analysis results, since it can minimize the risk of making a falsely positive/negative conclusion, thereby producing more conservative thresholds for statistical significance [19]. TSA combines conventional meta-analysis methodology with repeating significance testing methods applied to accumulating data in clinical trials. It calculates cumulative z-curves and uses the law of the iterated logarithm to penalize the Z value and to produce more conservative meta-analysis results [20]. TSA was performed using TSA software, version 0.9.5.10 Beta (Copenhagen trial unit, https://ctu.dk/tsa/, (accessed on 28 May 2021)).

2.5. Quality Appraisal

The Cochrane Collaboration tool for assessing risk of bias in RCTs was implemented to gauge the quality of the included studies [21]. The following items were evaluated: random sequence generation; allocation concealment; blinding of participants and personnel; blinding of outcome assessment; incomplete outcome data; selective reporting; and other potential sources of bias [21]. Risk of bias for each study was independently assessed by M.P. and P.D.G., and disagreements were discussed and resolved by consensus between both reviewers or by consultation with a third reviewer (A.C.).

3. Results

3.1. Study Selection and Characteristics

After de-duplication from an initial total of 2885 records, the titles and abstracts of 1589 studies were screened. Overall, 11 studies were considered eligible for full-text review, and nine met the inclusion criteria [22–30]. Figure 1 depicts the entire process of study identification, inclusion, and exclusion. Details of the included studies are available in Table 1. Overall, nine trials were included, enrolling 3358 patients in the TCZ group and 3131 subjects in the comparator group. Studies were conducted from March 2020 to early 2021 across several countries worldwide; all trials were multicenter. The enrolled patients suffered from moderate to critical disease, according to the definitions provided by the United States National Institutes of Health (NIH), as far as the clinical spectrum of SARS-CoV-2 infection is concerned [31]. Mortality was not always the primary endpoint but was assessed in all trials at 28 or 30 days except in one study, where researchers investigated in-hospital mortality [23]. Tocilizumab dosing was quite variable, ranging from 6 to 8 mg/kg, administered as a single dose or repeated short term.

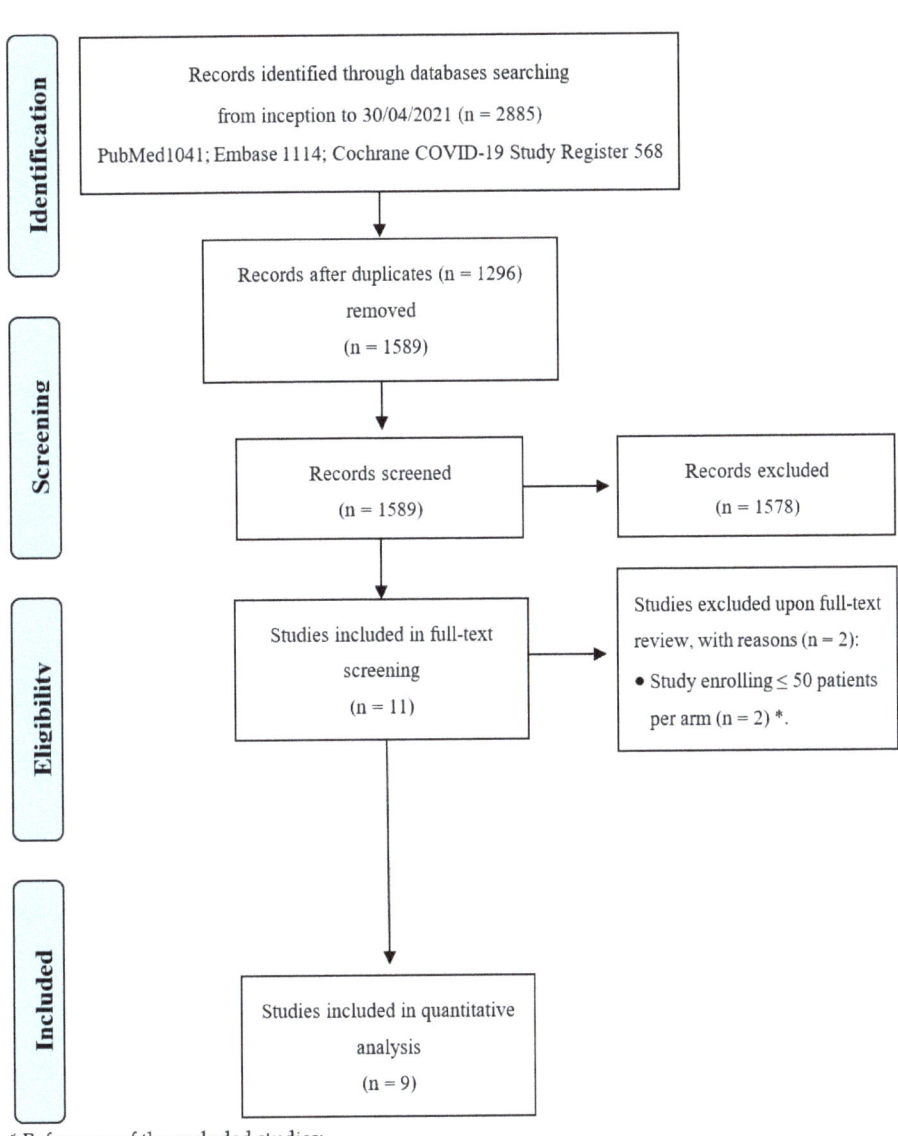

* References of the excluded studies:
1. Wang D, Fu B, Peng Z, et al. Tocilizumab in patients with moderate or severe COVID-19: a randomized, controlled, open-label, multicenter trial. Front Med 2021;15: 486-494.
2. Zhao H, Zhu Q, et al. Tocilizumab combined with favipiravir in the treatment of COVID-19: A multicenter trial in a small sample size. Biomed Pharmacother 2021;133: 110825.

Figure 1. PRISMA diagram: results of the literature search and flow diagram for the selection of eligible studies.

Table 1. Characteristics of included studies (only randomized controlled trials).

First Author/Study Name/Registration Number/Reference	Design and Country	Enrolment Dates	Recruitment Window	Inclusion Criteria	Mechanical Ventilation at Baseline (%)	Treatment Group versus Control Group (n)	Tocilizumab Dosing	Primary Outcome	Mortality
Hermine (CORIMUNO-TOCI 1) NCT04331808 [22]	Open label, multicenter (9 sites), France	31 March 2020 up to 18 April 2020	Within 72 h of SARS-CoV-2 diagnosis	Moderate, severe, or critical disease	0%	63 vs. 67	8 mg/Kg on day 1 (and 3 if necessary)	Scores > 5 on the WHO-CPS on day 4 and survival with no need of MV (including NIMV) at day 14	28 days
Gordon (REMAP-CAP) NCT02735707 [23]	Open label, multicenter (113 sites), international (6 countries)	19 April 2020 to 19 November 2020	Within 24 h of ICU admission	Critical disease	29.4%	353 vs. 402	8 mg/Kg (maximum 800 mg), repeated at 12–24 h if necessary	The number of respiratory and cardiovascular organ support-free days up to day 21	In-hospital
Rosas (COVACTA) NCT04320615 [24]	Double-blind, placebo-controlled, multicenter (62 sites), international (9 countries)	3 April 2020 up to 28 May 2020	Not specified	Severe or critical disease	37.5%	294 vs. 144	8 mg/Kg (maximum 800 mg), repeated at 8–24 h if necessary	Clinical status on a 7-category ordinal scale at day 28 (1, discharged/ready for discharge; 7, death)	28 days
Salama (EMPACTA) NCT04372186 [25]	Double-blind, placebo-controlled, multicenter (69 sites), international (6 countries)	14 May 2020 up to 18 August 2020	Within 48 h of hospital admission	Severe disease	0%	249 vs. 128	8 mg/Kg (maximum 800 mg), repeated at 8–24 h if necessary	Death or MV by day 28	28 days

Table 1. Cont.

First Author/Study Name/Registration Number/Reference	Design and Country	Enrolment Dates	Recruitment Window	Inclusion Criteria	Mechanical Ventilation at Baseline (%)	Treatment Group versus Control Group (n)	Tocilizumab Dosing	Primary Outcome	Mortality
Salvarani (RCT-TCZ-COVID-19) NCT04356355 [26]	Open label, multicenter (24 sites), Italy	31 March 2020 up to 11 June 2020	Not specified	Severe disease	0%	60 vs. 66	8 mg/Kg (maximum 800 mg), repeated at 12 h	Occurrence of the following events, whichever came first: • Admission to ICU with MV; • Death (any cause); • PaO_2/FiO_2 ratio less than 150 mmHg (confirmed within 4 h by a second examination)	30 days
Stone (BACC Bay) NCT04356937 [27]	Double-blind, placebo-controlled, multicenter (7 sites), United States	20 April 2020 up to 15 June 2020	Upon hospital admission	Severe disease	0%	161 vs. 81	8 mg/Kg as single dose	Intubation or death	28 days
Horby (RECOVERY) NCT04381936 [28]	Open label, multicenter (177 sites), United Kingdom	23 April 2020 up to 24 January 2021	Within 21 days of primary randomization	Severe and critical disease	14%	2022 vs. 2094	800 mg if weight > 90 kg; 600 mg if weight > 65 and ≤90 kg; 400 mg if weight > 40 and ≤65 kg; and 8 mg/kg if weight ≤ 40 kg; repeated at 12–24 h if necessary	All-cause mortality	28 days

Table 1. Cont.

First Author/Study Name/Registration Number/Reference	Design and Country	Enrolment Dates	Recruitment Window	Inclusion Criteria	Mechanical Ventilation at Baseline (%)	Treatment Group versus Control Group (n)	Tocilizumab Dosing	Primary Outcome	Mortality
Soin (COVINTOC) CTRI/2020/05/025369 [29]	Open label, multicenter (12 sites), India	30 May 2020 up to 21 August 2020	Upon hospital admission	Moderate and severe disease	5%	91 vs. 88	6 mg/Kg (maximum 480 mg), repeated within 12 h-7 days from the first dose	Proportion of patients with progression of COVID-19 from moderate to severe or from severe to death up to day 14	28 days
Veiga (TOCIBRAS) NCT04310228 [30]	Open label, multicenter (9 sites), Brazil	8 May 2020 up to 17 July 2020	Symptoms for more than 3 days	Severe and critical	16%	65 vs. 64	8 mg/Kg (maximum 800 mg) as single dose	Clinical status on a 7-category ordinal scale at day 15 (1, not admitted to hospital and with no limitation of activities; 7, death)	28 days

Legend: WHO-CPS, World Health Organization 10-point Clinical Progression Scale; MV, Mechanical ventilation; NIMV, non-invasive mechanical ventilation; ICU, intensive care unit; PaO_2/FiO_2 ratio, ratio of arterial oxygen partial pressure (PaO_2) to fractional inspired oxygen (FiO_2).

3.2. Risk of Bias

Since the majority of trials (6 out of 9) were open-label studies, performance bias and detection bias were classified as "high". The remaining components of risk, such as selection, attrition, and reporting bias, were classified as "low" for all trials included in this analysis. The risk-of-bias in each study is reported as Supplemental Figure S1.

3.3. Meta-Analysis of Main Outcome

All nine included RCTs concurred with the main analysis. The raw death rate was 24.8% in the TCZ group (835/3358) and 29.9% (935/3131) in the control group. According to the fixed-model approach, TCZ was associated with lower mortality in a statistically significant way (OR: 0.84; 95% CI: 0.75–0.94; I^2: 24% (low heterogeneity)). The results were consistent when implementing a random-effect model, although a widening of the CI was observed, including the vertical line (OR: 0.87; 95% CI: 0.71–1.07). All results related to the primary analysis are depicted in the forest plot presented in Figure 2.

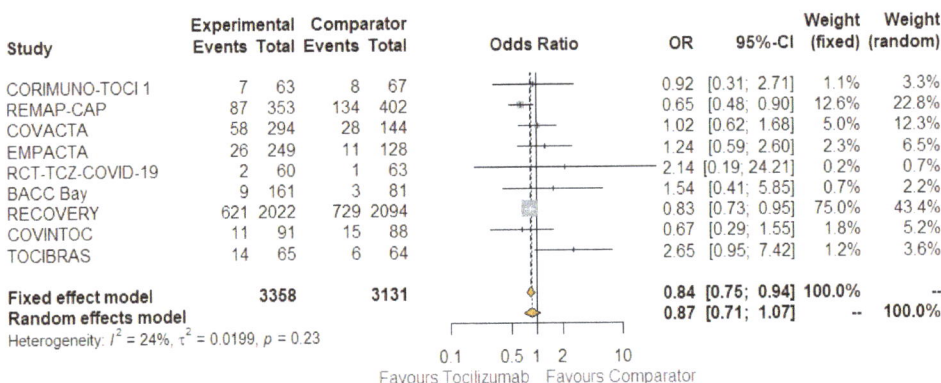

Figure 2. Overall meta-analysis of 28/30-day mortality. Abbreviations: OR, odds ratio; 95% CI, confidence intervals at 95%; Weight (fixed), weight of each study in a fixed-effect model; Weight (random), weight of each study in a random-effect model. Squares on the hazard ratio plot are proportional to the weight of each study; weighting is based on the inverse variance method.

3.4. Subgroup Analysis

Pre-planned key subgroup analyses were carried out to explore how the treatment effect varied across different subsets of studies or patients. When contrasting open label with placebo-controlled trials (Figure 3), the beneficial effect of TCZ on mortality was confirmed in the subgroup that included the first type of studies (OR: 0.82; 95% CI: 0.72–0.92; I^2: 36%; fixed-effect model), but the benefit disappeared in the other subgroup (OR: 1.12; 95% CI: 0.75–1.66; I^2: 0%; the results were the same according to fixed- and random-effect models), although not statistically significant. The results obtained when testing for subgroup difference were also not significant, so no interaction existed between the subtotal estimates for the subgroups.

Another subgroup analysis concerned the use of TCZ alone or with the SoC, in addition to the type of comparator: SoC with or without placebo (Figure 4). In the most numerous subgroup of TCZ versus SoC, even if including only three studies [22,25,27], the positive effect of TCZ on mortality was apparent (OR: 0.80; 95% CI: 0.71–0.91; I^2: 19%; with the fixed-effect model being the result of the overlapping of the random-effect model), in contrast to the other subgroups. The results obtained when testing for subgroup difference were not statistically significant.

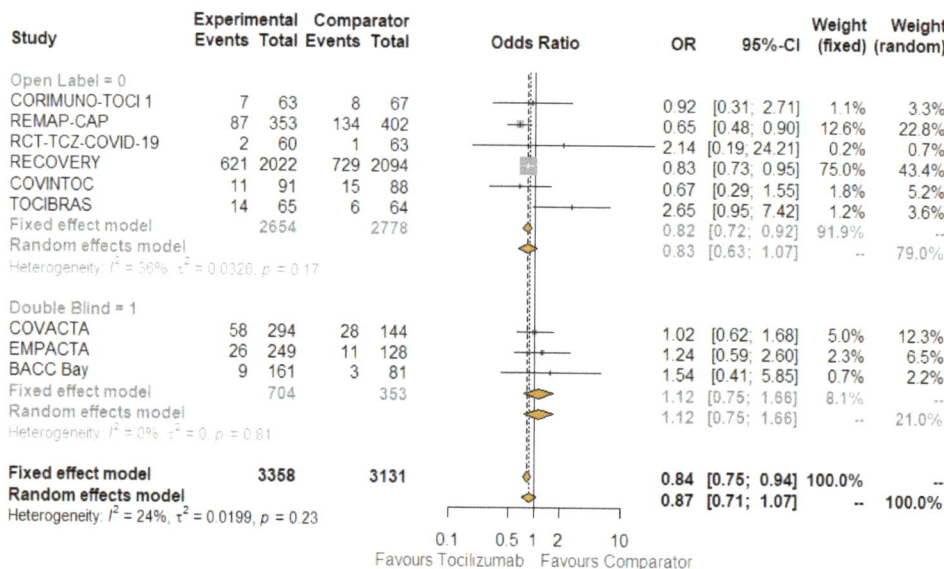

Figure 3. Meta-analysis of 28/30-day mortality in open-label vs. double blind studies. Abbreviations: OR: odds ratio; 95% CI, confidence intervals at 95%; Weight (fixed), weight of each study in a fixed-effect model; Weight (random), weight of each study in a random-effect model. Squares on the hazard ratio plot are proportional to the weight of each study; weighting is based on the inverse variance method.

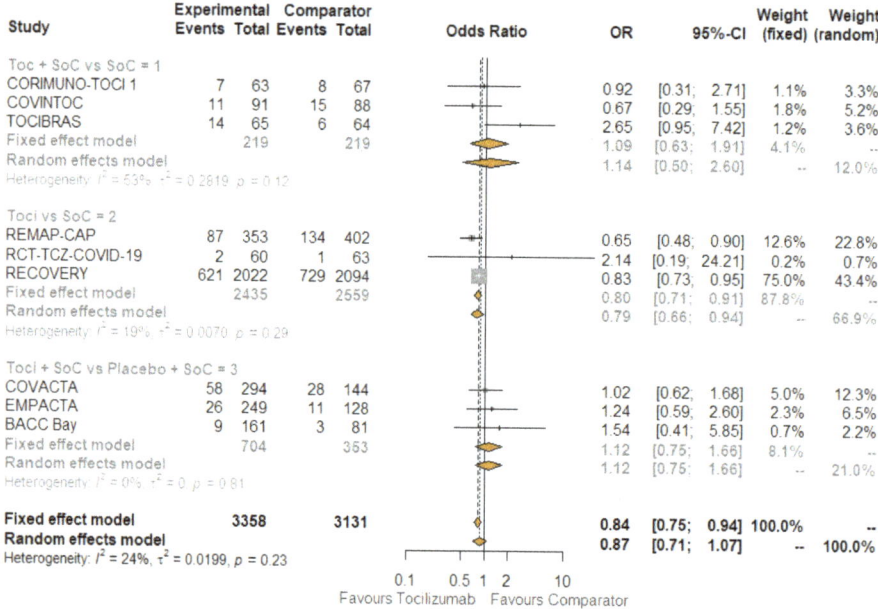

Figure 4. Pooled comparison of 28-day mortality according to treatment received. Abbreviations: Soc: standard of care; OR: odds ratio; 95% CI, confidence intervals at 95%; Weight (fixed), weight of each study in a fixed-effect model; Weight (random), weight of each study in a random-effect model. Squares on the hazard ratio plot are proportional to the weight of each study; weighting is based on the inverse variance method.

The last subgroup analysis involved the spectrum of disease severity, after extracting data on homogeneous categories of patients when data were available (Figure 5). The impact of TCZ in patients with moderate diseases seemed not to be clinically relevant (OR for mortality: 1.30; 95% CI: 0.64–2.64; I^2: 0%; these values were equal to the results of fixed-effect and random-effect analysis), whereas it appeared beneficial when considering severe/critical disease. Nevertheless, in this case, there was a discrepancy between the fixed-effect model (OR: 0.84; 95% CI: 0.75–0.94; I^2: 53%) and random-effect model (OR: 0.89; 95% CI: 0.71–1.18). No significant interaction existed between the subgroups when considering treatment effects.

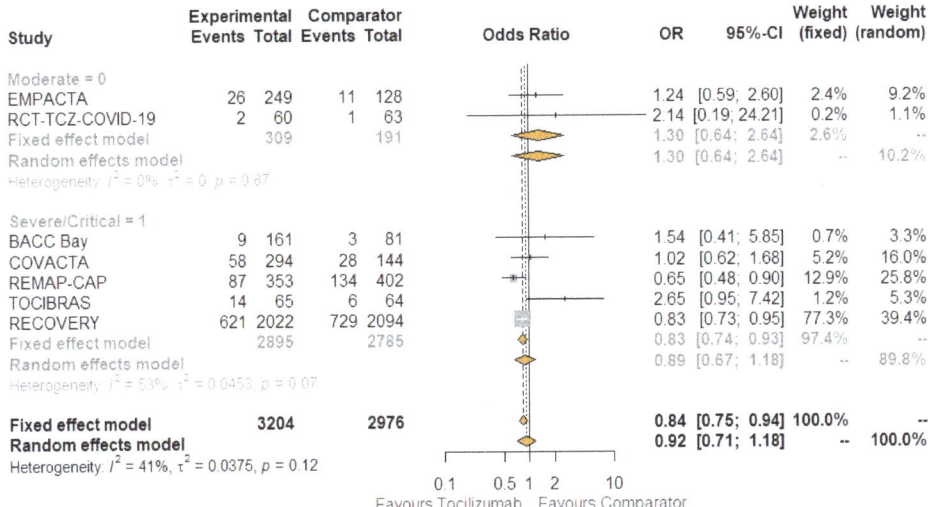

Figure 5. Pooled comparison of 28-day mortality according to disease status at baseline. Abbreviations: Soc: standard of care; OR: odds ratio; 95% CI, confidence intervals at 95%; Weight (fixed), weight of each study in a fixed-effect model; Weight (random), weight of each study in a random-effect model. Squares on the hazard ratio plot are proportional to the weight of each study; weighting is based on the inverse variance method.

3.5. Quality Appraisal and Publication Bias

The results of quality assessment are depicted in Figure S2: the major issues were related to open label studies [22,23,26,28–30] due to the lack of blinding. The results of stratifying studies according to this criterion (open label versus placebo-controlled) were already shown in Figure 3. The funnel plots of the primary outcomes of the studies are presented, along with the results of Egger's regression test ($p = 0.1441$), which suggest an absence of publication bias and small-study effects.

3.6. Sensitivity Analysis

In Table S2, the results of the sensitivity analysis are described. It was performed using the leave-one-out method and shows that the estimated pooled ORs, obtained excluding one study at time, are still consistent, even when omitting the study with the highest weight according to both the fixed-effect (75%) and random-effect 43.4%) models [28] (OR: 0.86; 95% CI: 0.68–1.07). This held true even when omitting the study that was apparently the major driver of heterogeneity, the TOCIBRAS study [30]: when it was excluded, the I^2 dropped to 0% and the OR for mortality associated with TCZ use was 0.82 (95% CI: 0.74–0.92).

3.7. Trial Sequential Analysis

In our trial sequential analysis, the type I error risk was set at α = 0.05 with a power of 0.80. In this condition, the required information size (RIS) for the meta-analyzed estimate was 7786, while our included number was 6489 subjects, even if the cumulative z-curve crossed above 1.96, which corresponded to the nominal threshold for statistical significance, demonstrating that the effect of tocilizumab seems to be more effective in reducing the 28/30-day mortality (Figure 6A). This conclusion was confirmed when omitting the TOCIBRAS trial, which was the major source of heterogeneity (Table S2), from TSA, since the cumulative z-curve also reached the RIS (Figure 6B).

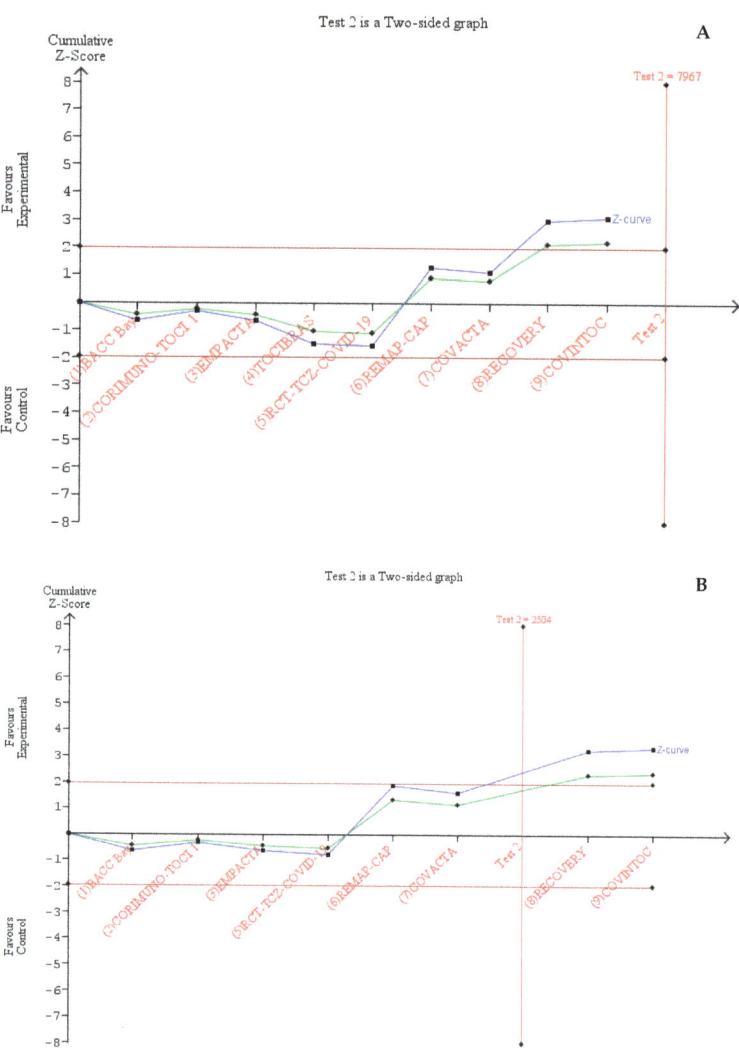

Figure 6. Trial Sequential analysis. (**A**) TSA of all trials included in meta-analysis. (**B**) TSA excluding the TOCIBRAS trial. The vertical red line represents the required information size to demonstrate or reject the hypothesis of a benefit from tocilizumab treatment, considering an alpha of 5% and a power of 80%. The blue line represents the cumulative z-curve, while the green line represents the cumulative z-curve (adjusted (penalized) according to law of the iterated logarithm).

4. Discussion

The results of our systematic review and meta-analyses are in line with the most recent development of the recommendations for COVID-19 treatment, which now include TCZ as an important option for patients with the severe or critical disease [32]. These data need to be put into context to understand how TCZ has become a potential life-saving agent in patients with SARS-CoV-2 infection.

Indeed, until mid-2021, the therapeutic armamentarium for patients with COVID-19 was quite bereft of effective weapons. Steroids, particularly dexamethasone, were the first class of drugs to show benefits in terms of the mortality of patients affected by severe SARS-CoV-2 infection [33]. Antiviral treatments failed to show any relevant impact on overall survival. This also applies to hydroxychloroquine/chloroquine [34], studies of which initially sparked much interest but, with the benefit of hindsight, appear to be biased by serious flaws inherent to the observational nature of these first studies [35], and more importantly to remdesivir, which has no or little effect on mortality [36] but might improve time to recovery and recovery rate [37]. As matter of fact, the window of opportunity for effective antiviral therapy is very narrow and it is open only in the early phase of the disease [38] when viral load peaks [39]. Afterward, the dysregulated hyperinflammatory response dominates in severe cases and is responsible for the most relevant manifestations [40]. Notably, although no single definition is widely accepted, the cytokine storm is an umbrella term encompassing many disorders whose shared hallmark is an immune dysregulation that potentially leads to multiorgan dysfunction [41]. The cytokine storm may be pathogen-induced, as seen in SARS-CoV-2 infection, iatrogenic, as observed in CAR (chimeric antigen receptor) T-cell therapy, or may ensue from autoimmune, neoplastic, or idiopathic causes [41].

Many factors contribute to the pathophysiology of the cytokine storm. Among the many stands is IL-6, whose circulating concentrations are known to be increased in many proinflammatory critical care syndromes, including COVID-19 [42]. It is a master cytokine, produced by—and acting on—immune and non-immune cells in multiple organ systems. IL-6 exerts pleiotropic effects, not only driving inflammation, fever, and carcinogenesis, but also regulating metabolism, bone turnover, and hematopoiesis, and thus, is fundamental for innate and adaptive immunity [42].

In light of its important physiological and anti-inflammatory functions, the blockade of IL-6 signaling might represent a double-edged sword but has turned out to be effective in some cytokine storm disorders, such as idiopathic multicentric Castleman's disease and CAR T-cell-induced cytokine release syndrome, through monoclonal antibodies that are directed at the IL-6 receptor (TCZ and sarilumab) or directly target IL-6 (siltuximab) [43].

Elevations in serum IL-6 levels in patients affected by severe COVID-19 have spurred a renewed interest in this cytokine as a therapeutic target in the broader context of the cytokine storm syndrome triggered by SARS-CoV-2 infection [5,44]. Despite the logistical difficulties, several studies have been conducted in a short time. Predictably, observational studies in particular suffered from relevant methodological limitations that threatened the validity of their conclusions [45]; moreover, they yielded inconsistent results when pooled with RCTs in evidence syntheses [46].

The need for high-quality data to inform clinical practice led to research efforts focusing only on RCTs. A Cochrane review published in March 2021 retrieved data up to the end of February [47], including eight RCTs investigating TCZ [22–29] and one RCT testing sarilumab [48], with pooling of the available information with respect to mortality. TCZ appeared to be effective in reducing 28-day mortality compared with SoC or placebo (relative risk: 0.89; 95% CI: 0.82 to 0.97; I^2: 0.0%), but the evidence was less certain when considering 60-day mortality, clinical improvement, and adverse events [47]. Remarkably, the largest trial, the RECOVERY study, was only in pre-print form at that time and its overall results were partially incomplete [28]. Several factors have been suggested to explain the differences in clinical outcomes highlighted by the Cochrane review. They include important differences in trial designs, the features of included patients, stages of disease, the use of co-interventions (e.g., the proportion of concomitant steroids), and the endpoint measurement scales [49].

The full publication of the RECOVERY trial [28] and the accumulation of further evidence regarding TCZ and other IL-6 blockers led to a prospective meta-analysis (on 27 RCTs) of utmost importance in June 2021. It showed that the use of IL-6 antagonists was associated with improved survival in COVID-19 patients, but the results were statistically significant only for TCZ (OR for mortality equal to 0.83; 95% CI: 0.74–0.92) [50]. Coherently with what was observed in the RECOVERY study, the subgroup of patients who received also corticosteroids appeared to benefit the most: the mortality risk was even lower (OR: 0.77; 95% CI: 0.68–0.87) [32]. On this basis, the World Health Organization (WHO) issued a strong recommendation on July 6 to use IL-6 blockers, specifically in patients with severe/critical disease [31]. This recommendation was maintained by the NIH guidelines with a specific indication in favor of TCZ plus steroids [51], confirming the setting of patients with severe COVID-19, and was in line with the recommendation of REMAP-CAP [23] in addition to RECOVERY [28], and was consistent with definitions of progressive disease and marked pro-inflammatory status based on concentrations of C-reactive protein (CRP) being higher than 75 mg/L, a threshold established in the RECOVERY study [28].

Our meta-analysis confirms the usefulness of TCZ in ameliorating the overall survival of COVID-19 patients, especially when burdened by severe (oxygen saturation < 90% on room air, respiratory rate > 30 breaths/min, signs of severe respiratory distress) or critical (acute respiratory distress syndrome, sepsis, septic shock, provision of life-sustaining therapies such as mechanical ventilation or vasopressor therapy) disease.

The strengths of our work are represented by protocol pre-registration, focusing on the most important and objective outcome (mortality), the inclusion of only RCTs published in full after peer-review and by the carrying out of TSA, a powerful tool for clinicians to assess the conclusiveness of meta-analyses that offers better control of type I (likelihood of overestimation) and type II (likelihood of underestimation) errors [52]. Taking into account only publications that appeared in peer-reviewed journals, we had the chance to compute analyses based on consolidated data, in contrast to the processes used in previous research syntheses that relied on preliminary results from pre-prints [7,53]. For instance, as to the primary outcome, early data related to the RECOVERY study described 596 events out of 2022 patients in the TCZ arm, and 694 deaths out of 2094 subjects in the comparator group [28]. The final results were 621/2022 and 729/2094, respectively [28]. Regarding TSA, the conventional meta-analysis demonstrated statistical significance since the z-curve exceeded the monitoring boundaries to reach the so-called 'area of benefit', although the TSA results demonstrated that the RIS value needed to detect or reject the anticipated effect with certainty (7967) was not reached. Interestingly, the only previous evidence regarding synthesis with the TSA of RCTs reached different conclusions, describing a cumulative z-curve not crossing the boundary of benefit but crossing the one for futility due to a RIS being estimated as equal to 5622 [53]. However, the TSA conducted by Snow and colleagues [53] was based on different raw numbers of events and participants; for instance, the preliminary results of RECOVERY [28], or the 90-day mortality results of for the REMAP-CAP trial [23], as well as those of other RCTs [26,27]. Nevertheless, in our study, a sensitivity analysis that excluded the TOCIBRAS trial [30], the paramount source of heterogeneity in the leave-one-out analysis (by omitting it, the I^2 dropped to 0%), showed that the boundary for futility was crossed. At any rate, definitive data from studies that are not still published, such as the REMDACTA trial that has enrolled patients affected by severe COVID-19 [54] and whose available results have been already included in the aforementioned prospective meta-analysis [50], are eagerly awaited since they may be conducive to a more informative TSA that can be used to establish whether additional studies are needed to confirm the usefulness of TCZ.

Of course, this study presents some limitations. In particular, owing to the publication of concurrent similar research syntheses [55,56], we did not explore secondary outcomes such as progression to mechanical ventilation, time to discharge, LOS, and safety profiles, which had already been addressed by previous works. Eventually, we did not perform meta-regression: in a preceding meta-analysis, there was no evidence of treatment effect modification by patient characteristics [57]. Nonetheless, conventional meta-analyses may be biased due to the ecological fallacy (also known as aggregation bias) since average patient characteristics are regressed against average trial outcomes; instead, individual patient characteristics should be regressed against the individual outcomes in the context of an individual patient data meta-analysis [58].

5. Conclusions

TCZ is one of the very few agents that has so far been found to favorably change the prognosis of patients with severe COVID-19 [59]. Nonetheless, additional RCTs are still needed to confirm this finding, upheld, beyond any reasonable doubt, by a strong biological rationale and by the data collected from completed RCTs, and to define the best schedule, in light of the different dosages administered across studies. Observational studies may have a complementary role, being instrumental in identifying adverse events and complications such as secondary bacterial infections that may develop after the usual follow-up of RCTs. Moreover, avenues for future research may be constituted by individual patient data meta-analyses and umbrella reviews. The former would allow the investigation of the effectiveness of treatment at the level of relevant patient subgroups. Granular data would permit a more precise understanding of the profile of the patients who would potentially benefit the most from the drug, besides the CRP threshold that is quite generic. The latter would allow the findings from multiple systematic reviews and meta-analyses about the review question to be compared and contrasted, and thus, would make it possible to present a wide picture of the available evidence, highlighting its consistency or potential discrepancies, in an attempt to explore and detail the underlying reasons for contradictory results.

Supplementary Materials: The following are available online at https://www.mdpi.com/article/10.3390/jcm10214935/s1, Figure S1: Risk of bias summary and risk of bias graph for selected studies: review authors' judgements about each risk of bias item for each included study, Figure S2: Begg's funnel plot and Egger's test for publication bias detection, Table S1: Full search strategy, Table S2: Sensitivity analysis, Table S3: PRISMA 2020 (Preferred Reporting Items for Systematic Review and Meta-Analysis) checklist.

Author Contributions: Conceptualization, A.E.M. and M.C.; methodology, A.E.M., A.C. (Anna Crispo), M.P. and M.C.; formal analysis, A.C. (Anna Crispo), M.P. and P.D.G.; data curation, A.C. (Anna Crispo), M.P., D.M., M.G.V. and L.A., writing—original draft preparation, A.E.M. and M.P.; writing—review and editing, A.E.M., A.C. (Anna Crispo), M.P., P.D.G., D.M., M.G.V., L.A., M.C., E.C., A.C. (Arturo Cuomo) and P.A.A.; supervision, A.C. (Arturo Cuomo) and P.A.A. All authors have read and agreed to the published version of the manuscript.

Funding: This research received no external funding.

Institutional Review Board Statement: No ethical approval was needed because data were retrieved and analyzed from previous published studies in which informed consent was obtained by primary investigators.

Informed Consent Statement: Not applicable.

Data Availability Statement: The datasets generated during the current meta-analysis are available from the corresponding author upon reasonable request. All data analyzed during this meta-analysis are included in the corresponding published articles, as reported in Table 1.

Acknowledgments: We sincerely thank Larry W. Tsay for sharing information regarding the clinical trial in which he was involved (the COVACTA study).

Conflicts of Interest: The authors declare no conflict of interest.

References

1. Sebba, A. Tocilizumab: The first interleukin-6-receptor inhibitor. *Am. J. Health Syst. Pharm.* **2008**, *65*, 1413–1418. [CrossRef] [PubMed]
2. Tanaka, T.; Narazaki, M.; Ogata, A.; Kishimoto, T. A New Era for the Treatment of Inflammatory Autoimmune Diseases by Interleukin-6 Blockade Strategy. *Semin. Immunol.* **2014**, *26*, 88–96. [CrossRef]
3. Rigal, J.; Pugnet, G.; Ciron, J.; Lépine, Z.; Biotti, D. Off-label use of tocilizumab in neuromyelitis optica spectrum disorders and MOG-antibody-associated diseases: A case-series. *Mult. Scler. Relat. Disord.* **2020**, *46*, 102483. [CrossRef]
4. Tang, Y.; Liu, J.; Zhang, D.; Xu, Z.; Ji, J.; Wen, C. Cytokine Storm in COVID-19: The Current Evidence and Treatment Strategies. *Front. Immunol.* **2020**, *11*, 1708. [CrossRef]
5. Buonaguro, F.M.; Puzanov, I.; Ascierto, P.A. Anti-IL6R role in treatment of COVID-19-related ARDS. *J. Transl. Med.* **2020**, *18*, 165. [CrossRef]
6. Alam, W.; Bizri, A.R. Efficacy of tocilizumab in COVID-19: A review of the current evidence. *Sci. Prog.* **2021**, *104*, 368504211030372. [CrossRef]
7. Tleyjeh, I.M.; Kashour, Z.; Damlaj, M.; Riaz, M.; Tlayjeh, H.; Altannir, M.; Altannir, Y.; Al-Tannir, M.; Tleyjeh, R.; Hassett, L.; et al. Efficacy and safety of tocilizumab in COVID-19 patients: A living systematic review and meta-analysis. *Clin. Microbiol. Infect.* **2021**, *27*, 215–227. [CrossRef] [PubMed]
8. Martinuka, O.; von Cube, M.; Wolkewitz, M. Methodological evaluation of bias in observational coronavirus disease 2019 studies on drug effectiveness. *Clin. Microbiol. Infect.* **2021**, *27*, 949–957. [CrossRef]
9. Deana, C. The COVID-19 pandemic: Is our medicine still evidence-based? *IR J. Med. Sci.* **2021**, *190*, 11–12. [CrossRef] [PubMed]
10. Page, M.J.; McKenzie, J.E.; Bossuyt, P.M.; Boutron, I.; Hoffmann, T.C.; Mulrow, C.; Shamseer, L.; Tetzlaff, J.M.; Akl, E.A.; Brennan, S.E.; et al. The PRISMA 2020 statement: An updated guideline for reporting systematic reviews. *BMJ* **2021**, *372*, n71. [CrossRef]
11. Bramer, W.M.; Milic, J.; Mast, F. Reviewing retrieved references for inclusion in systematic reviews using EndNote. *J. Med. Libr. Assoc.* **2017**, *105*, 84–87. [CrossRef] [PubMed]
12. Muka, T.; Glisic, M.; Milic, J.; Verhoog, S.; Bohlius, J.; Bramer, W.; Chowdhury, R.; Franco, O.H. A 24-step guide on how to design, conduct, and successfully publish a systematic review and meta-analysis in medical research. *Eur. J. Epidemiol.* **2020**, *35*, 49–60. [CrossRef]
13. Deeks, J.J.; Altman, D.G.; Bradburn, M.J. *Systematic Reviews in Health Care: Meta-Analysis in Context. Cap. 15*; John Wiley & Sons: Hoboken, NJ, USA, 2008.
14. Der Simonian, R.; Laird, N. Meta-analysis in clinical trials revisited. *Contemp. Clin. Trials* **2015**, *45*, 139–145. [CrossRef]
15. Higgins, J.P.; Thompson, S.G.; Deeks, J.J.; Altman, D.G. Measuring inconsistency in meta-analyses. *BMJ* **2003**, *327*, 557–560. [CrossRef] [PubMed]
16. Egger, M.; Davey Smith, G.; Schneider, M.; Minder, C. Bias in meta-analysis detected by a simple, graphical test. *BMJ* **1997**, *315*, 629–634. [CrossRef]
17. Shah, A.; Smith, A.F. Trial sequential analysis: Adding a new dimension to meta-analysis. *Anaesthesia* **2019**, *74*, 793–800. [CrossRef]
18. Schwarzer, G. General Package for Meta-Analysis. Available online: https://github.com/guido-s/meta (accessed on 1 June 2021).
19. Borm, G.F.; Donders, A.R. Updating meta-analyses leads to larger type I errors than publication bias. *J. Clin. Epidemiol.* **2009**, *62*, 825–830. [CrossRef]
20. Imberger, G.; Thorlund, K.; Gluud, C.; Wetterslev, J. False-positive findings in Cochrane meta-analyses with and without application of trial sequential analysis: An empirical review. *Br. Med. J. Open* **2016**, *6*, e011890. [CrossRef] [PubMed]
21. Higgins, J.P.; Altman, D.G.; Gøtzsche, P.C.; Jüni, P.; Moher, D.; Oxman, A.D.; Savovic, J.; Schulz, K.F.; Weeks, L.; Sterne, J.A.; et al. The Cochrane Collaboration's tool for assessing risk of bias in randomised trials. *BMJ* **2011**, *343*, d5928. [CrossRef]
22. Hermine, O.; Mariette, X.; Tharaux, P.L.; Resche-Rigon, M.; Porcher, R.; Ravaud, P.; CORIMUNO-19 Collaborative Group. Effect of tocilizumab vs. usual care in adults hospitalized with COVID-19 and moderate or severe pneumonia: A randomized clinical trial. *JAMA Intern. Med.* **2021**, *81*, 32–40. [CrossRef] [PubMed]
23. REMAP-CAP Investigators; Gordon, A.C.; Mouncey, P.R.; Al-Beidh, F.; Rowan, K.M.; Nichol, A.D.; Arabi, Y.M.; Annane, D.; Beane, A.; van Bentum-Puijk, W.; et al. Interleukin-6 Receptor Antagonists in Critically Ill Patients with Covid-19. *N. Engl. J. Med.* **2021**, *384*, 1491–1502. [CrossRef]
24. Rosas, I.O.; Bräu, N.; Waters, M.; Go, R.C.; Hunter, B.D.; Bhagani, S.; Skiest, D.; Aziz, M.S.; Cooper, N.; Douglas, I.S.; et al. Tocilizumab in Hospitalized Patients with Severe Covid-19 Pneumonia. *N. Engl. J. Med.* **2021**, *384*, 1503–1516. [CrossRef]
25. Salama, C.; Han, J.; Yau, L.; Reiss, W.G.; Kramer, B.; Neidhart, J.D.; Criner, G.J.; Kaplan-Lewis, E.; Baden, R.; Pandit, L.; et al. Tocilizumab in Patients Hospitalized with Covid-19 Pneumonia. *N. Engl. J. Med.* **2021**, *384*, 20–30. [CrossRef] [PubMed]
26. Salvarani, C.; Dolci, G.; Massari, M.; Merlo, D.F.; Cavuto, S.; Savoldi, L.; Bruzzi, P.; Boni, F.; Braglia, L.; Turrà, C.; et al. Effect of Tocilizumab vs Standard Care on Clinical Worsening in Patients Hospitalized With COVID-19 Pneumonia: A Randomized Clinical Trial. *JAMA Intern. Med.* **2021**, *181*, 24–31. [CrossRef]
27. Stone, J.H.; Frigault, M.J.; Serling-Boyd, N.J.; Fernandes, A.D.; Harvey, L.; Foulkes, A.S.; Horick, N.K.; Healy, B.C.; Shah, R.; Bensaci, A.M.; et al. Efficacy of Tocilizumab in Patients Hospitalized with Covid-19. *N. Engl. J. Med.* **2020**, *383*, 2333–2344. [CrossRef] [PubMed]
28. RECOVERY Collaborative Group. Tocilizumab in patients admitted to hospital with COVID-19 (RECOVERY): A randomised, controlled, open-label, platform trial. *Lancet* **2021**, *397*, 1637–1645. [CrossRef]

29. Soin, A.S.; Kumar, K.; Choudhary, N.S.; Sharma, P.; Mehta, Y.; Kataria, S.; Govil, D.; Deswal, V.; Chaudhry, D.; Singh, P.K.; et al. Tocilizumab plus standard care versus standard care in patients in India with moderate to severe COVID-19-associated cytokine release syndrome (COVINTOC): An open-label, multicentre, randomised, controlled, phase 3 trial. *Lancet Respir. Med.* **2021**, *9*, 511–521. [CrossRef]
30. Veiga, V.C.; Prats, J.A.G.G.; Farias, D.L.C.; Rosa, R.G.; Dourado, L.K.; Zampieri, F.G.; Machado, F.R.; Lopes, R.D.; Berwanger, O.; Azevedo, L.C.P.; et al. Effect of tocilizumab on clinical outcomes at 15 days in patients with severe or critical coronavirus disease 2019: Randomised controlled trial. *BMJ* **2021**, *20*, 372. [CrossRef]
31. NIH COVID-19 Treatment Guidelines. Clinical Spectrum of SARS-CoV-2 Infection. Available online: https://www.covid19treatmentguidelines.nih.gov/overview/clinical-spectrum/ (accessed on 10 August 2021).
32. WHO Therapeutics and COVID-19: Living Guidelines. 7.1 IL-6 Receptor Blockers. Available online: https://app.magicapp.org/#/guideline/nBkO1E/section/LrV7OL/ (accessed on 10 August 2021).
33. WHO Rapid Evidence Appraisal for COVID-19 Therapies (REACT) Working Group; Sterne, J.A.C.; Murthy, S.; Diaz, J.V.; Slutsky, A.S.; Villar, J.; Angus, D.C.; Annane, D.; Azevedo, L.C.P.; Berwanger, O.; et al. Association between Administration of Systemic Corticosteroids and Mortality Among Critically Ill Patients with COVID-19: A Meta-analysis. *JAMA* **2020**, *324*, 1330–1341. [CrossRef]
34. Maraolo, A.E.; Grossi, A. Safety of hydroxychloroquine for treatment or prevention of SARS-CoV-2 infection: A rapid systematic review and meta-analysis of randomized clinical trials. *Immun. Inflamm. Dis.* **2021**, *9*, 31–36. [CrossRef]
35. Renoux, C.; Azoulay, L.; Suissa, S. Biases in Evaluating the Safety and Effectiveness of Drugs for the Treatment of COVID-19: Designing Real-World Evidence Studies. *Am. J. Epidemiol.* **2021**, *190*, 1452–1456. [CrossRef]
36. Ansems, K.; Grundeis, F.; Dahms, K.; Mikolajewska, A.; Thieme, V.; Piechotta, V.; Metzendorf, M.-I.; Stegemann, M.; Benstoem, C.; Fichtner, F. Remdesivir for the treatment of COVID-19. *Cochrane Database Syst. Rev.* **2021**, *8*, CD014962. [CrossRef] [PubMed]
37. Kaka, A.S.; MacDonald, R.; Greer, N.; Vela, K.; Duan-Porter, W.; Obley, A.; Wilt, T.J. Major Update: Remdesivir for Adults with COVID-19: A Living Systematic Review and Meta-analysis for the American College of Physicians Practice Points. *Ann. Intern. Med.* **2021**, *174*, 663–672. [CrossRef] [PubMed]
38. Sundararaj Stanleyraj, J.; Sethuraman, N.; Gupta, R.; Thiruvoth, S.; Gupta, M.; Ryo, A. Treating COVID-19—Are we missing out the window of opportunity. *J. Antimicrob. Chemother.* **2020**, *76*, 283–285. [CrossRef]
39. Cevik, M.; Tate, M.; Lloyd, O.; Maraolo, A.E.; Schafers, J.; Ho, A. SARS-CoV-2, SARS-CoV, and MERS-CoV viral load dynamics, duration of viral shedding, and infectiousness: A systematic review and meta-analysis. *Lancet Microbe* **2021**, *2*, e13–e22. [CrossRef]
40. Gustine, J.N.; Jones, D. Immunopathology of Hyperinflammation in COVID-19. *Am. J. Pathol.* **2021**, *191*, 4–17. [CrossRef]
41. Fajgenbaum, D.C.; June, C.H. Cytokine Storm. *N. Engl. J. Med.* **2020**, *383*, 2255–2273. [CrossRef]
42. McElvaney, O.J.; Curley, G.F.; Rose-John, S.; McElvaney, N.G. Interleukin-6: Obstacles to targeting a complex cytokine in critical illness. *Lancet Respir. Med.* **2021**, *9*, 643–654. [CrossRef]
43. Kang, S.; Tanaka, T.; Narazaki, M.; Kishimoto, T. Targeting Interleukin-6 Signaling in Clinic. *Immunity* **2019**, *50*, 1007–1023. [CrossRef]
44. Montesarchio, V.; Parrela, R.; Iommelli, C.; Bianco, A.; Manzillo, E.; Fraġanza, F.; Palumbo, C.; Rea, G.; Murino, P.; De Rosa, R.; et al. Outcomes and biomarker analyses among patients with COVID-19 treated with interleukin 6 (IL-6) receptor antagonist sarilumab at a single institution in Italy. *J. Immunother. Cancer* **2020**, *8*, e001089. [CrossRef] [PubMed]
45. Tleyjeh, I.M.; Kashour, T.; Mandrekar, J.; Petitti, D.B. Overlooked Shortcomings of Observational Studies of Interventions in Coronavirus Disease 2019: An Illustrated Review for the Clinician. *Open Forum. Infect. Dis* **2021**, *8*, ofab317. [CrossRef]
46. Khan, F.A.; Stewart, I.; Fabbri, L.; Moss, S.; Robinson, K.; Smyth, A.R.; Jenkins, G. Systematic review and meta-analysis of anakinra, sarilumab, siltuximab and tocilizumab for COVID-19. *Thorax* **2021**, *76*, 907–919. [CrossRef] [PubMed]
47. Ghosn, L.; Chaimani, A.; Evrenoglou, T.; Davidson, M.; Graña, C.; Schmucker, C.; Bollig, C.; Henschke, N.; Sguassero, Y.; Nejstgaard, C.H.; et al. Interleukin-6 blocking agents for treating COVID-19: A living systematic review. *Cochrane Database Syst. Rev.* **2021**, *3*, CD013881. [CrossRef] [PubMed]
48. Lescure, F.X.; Honda, H.; Fowler, R.A.; Lazar, J.S.; Shi, G.; Wung, P.; Patel, N.; Hagino, O.; Sarilumab COVID-19 Global Study Group. Sarilumab in patients admitted to hospital with severe or critical COVID-19: A randomised, double-blind, placebo-controlled, phase 3 trial. *Lancet Respir. Med.* **2021**, *9*, 522–532. [CrossRef]
49. Angriman, F.; Ferreyro, B.L.; Burry, L.; Fan, E.; Ferguson, N.D.; Husain, S.; Keshavjee, S.H.; Lupia, E.; Munshi, L.; Renzi, S.; et al. Interleukin-6 receptor blockade in patients with COVID-19: Placing clinical trials intocontext. *Lancet Respir. Med.* **2021**, *9*, 655–664. [CrossRef]
50. WHO Rapid Evidence Appraisal for COVID-19 Therapies (REACT) Working Group; Shankar-Hari, M.; Vale, C.L.; Godolphin, P.J.; Fisher, D.; Higgins, J.P.T.; Spiga, F.; Savovic, J.; Tierney, J.; Baron, G.; et al. Association Between Administration of IL-6 Antagonists and Mortality Among Patients Hospitalized for COVID-19: A Meta-analysis. *JAMA* **2021**, *326*, 499–518. [CrossRef]
51. NIH COVID-19 Treatment Guidelines. Therapeutic Management of Hospitalized Adults with COVID-19. Available online: https://www.covid19treatmentguidelines.nih.gov/management/clinical-management/hospitalized-adults--therapeutic-management/ (accessed on 10 August 2021).
52. Kang, H. Trial sequential analysis: Novel approach for meta-analysis. *Anesth. Pain Med.* **2021**, *16*, 138–150. [CrossRef]

53. Snow, T.A.C.; Saleem, N.; Ambler, G.; Nastouli, E.; Singer, M.; Arulkumaran, N. Tocilizumab in COVID-19: A meta-analysis, trial sequential analysis, and meta-regression of randomized-controlled trials. *Intensive Care Med.* **2021**, *47*, 641–652. [CrossRef] [PubMed]
54. A Phase III, Randomized, Double-Blind, Multicenter Study to Evaluate the Efficacy and Safety of Remdesivir Plus Tocilizumab Compared with Remdesivir Plus Placebo in Hospitalized Patients with Severe COVID-19 Pneumonia. Available online: https://www.clinicaltrials.gov/ct2/show/NCT04409262 (accessed on 10 August 2021).
55. Klopfenstein, T.; Gendrin, V.; Gerazime, A.; Conrozier, T.; Balblanc, J.C.; Royer, P.Y.; Lohse, A.; Mezher, C.; Toko, L.; Guillochon, C.; et al. Systematic Review and Subgroup Meta-analysis of Randomized Trials to Determine Tocilizumab's Place in COVID-19 Pneumonia. *Infect. Dis. Ther.* **2021**, *10*, 1195–1213. [CrossRef]
56. Selvaraj, V.; Khan, M.S.; Bavishi, C.; Dapaah-Afriyie, K.; Finn, A.; Lal, A.; Mylonakis, E. Tocilizumab in Hospitalized Patients with COVID-19: A Meta Analysis of Randomized Controlled Trials. *Lung* **2021**, *199*, 239–248. [CrossRef]
57. Tharmarajah, E.; Buazon, A.; Patel, V.; Hannah, J.R.; Adas, M.; Allen, V.B.; Bechman, K.; Clarke, B.D.; Nagra, D.; Norton, S.; et al. IL-6 inhibition in the treatment of COVID-19: A meta-analysis and meta-regression. *J. Infect.* **2021**, *82*, 178–185. [CrossRef] [PubMed]
58. da Costa, B.R.; Sutton, A.J. A comparison of the statistical performance of different meta-analysis models for the synthesis of subgroup effects from randomized clinical trials. *BMC Med. Res. Methodol.* **2019**, *19*, 198. [CrossRef]
59. Ascierto, P.A.; Fu, B.; Wei, H. IL-6 modulation for COVID-19: The right patients at the right time? *J. Immunother. Cancer* **2021**, *9*, e002285. [CrossRef]

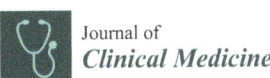

Systematic Review

Artificial Intelligence for COVID-19 Detection in Medical Imaging—Diagnostic Measures and Wasting—A Systematic Umbrella Review

Paweł Jemioło [1,*], Dawid Storman [2] and Patryk Orzechowski [1,3]

1. AGH University of Science and Technology, Faculty of Electrical Engineering, Automatics, Computer Science and Biomedical Engineering, al. A. Mickiewicza 30, 30-059 Krakow, Poland; patryk.orzechowski@gmail.com
2. Chair of Epidemiology and Preventive Medicine, Department of Hygiene and Dietetics, Jagiellonian University Medical College, ul. M. Kopernika 7, 31-034 Krakow, Poland; dawid.storman@doctoral.uj.edu.pl
3. Institute for Biomedical Informatics, University of Pennsylvania, 3700 Hamilton Walk, Philadelphia, PA 19104, USA
* Correspondence: pawljmlo@agh.edu.pl

Abstract: The COVID-19 pandemic has sparked a barrage of primary research and reviews. We investigated the publishing process, time and resource wasting, and assessed the methodological quality of the reviews on artificial intelligence techniques to diagnose COVID-19 in medical images. We searched nine databases from inception until 1 September 2020. Two independent reviewers did all steps of identification, extraction, and methodological credibility assessment of records. Out of 725 records, 22 reviews analysing 165 primary studies met the inclusion criteria. This review covers 174,277 participants in total, including 19,170 diagnosed with COVID-19. The methodological credibility of all eligible studies was rated as *critically low*: 95% of papers had significant flaws in reporting quality. On average, 7.24 (range: 0–45) new papers were included in each subsequent review, and 14% of studies did not include any new paper into consideration. Almost three-quarters of the studies included less than 10% of available studies. More than half of the reviews did not comment on the previously published reviews at all. Much wasting time and resources could be avoided if referring to previous reviews and following methodological guidelines. Such information chaos is alarming. It is high time to draw conclusions from what we experienced and prepare for future pandemics.

Keywords: COVID-19; diagnosis; artificial intelligence; medical imaging; systematic umbrella review; methodological credibility

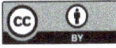

1. Introduction

In early December, 2019, a new coronavirus epidemic was identified in Wuhan [1]. Coronavirus disease 2019 (COVID-19) is a viral infection spread by direct contact with people experiencing the illness (from droplets generated by sneezing and coughing) or indirectly [2]. It is caused by Severe Acute Respiratory Syndrome Coronavirus 2 (SARS-CoV-2). As of 23 February 2022, over 420 million people have been diagnosed with COVID-19, with nearly 5.89 million associated deaths [3]. The consecutive waves of COVID-19 affected many societies, as well as scientific foundations and organisations [4–7]. On 30 January 2020, the World Health Organisation (WHO) issued a public health emergency of international concern (PHEIC) associated with COVID-19 and declared the state of a pandemic on 11 March 2020 [8].

Disease manifestation is variable, with some infected people remaining asymptomatic (even up to 57% [9]) and others suffering from mild (including fever, cough, and aches) to severe (involving lethargy with dyspnoea and increased respiratory rate) and critical manifestations (requiring mechanical ventilation). It may lead to serious neurological, musculoskeletal, or cerebrovascular disorders or may even progress to a life-threatening respiratory syndrome in some patients [10,11].

Moreover, in 80% of patients, COVID-19 may leave one or more long-lasting symptoms, with fatigue, headaches, attentional difficulties, anosmia, and memory loss manifesting the most frequently [12]. Wide-ranging longer-term morbidity has also been described in the absence of severe initial illnesses [13].

The essence of stopping the significant increase in morbidity is, in addition to treatment, quick diagnostics. The identification of those infected allows for better management of the pandemic (e.g., isolation, quarantine, hospital admission or admission to the intensive care unit) [14]. Understanding the accuracy of tests and diagnostic features seems essential to develop effective screening and management methods [15].

As the pandemic unfolded, many ways have been found to diagnose COVID-19. The primary method for diagnosing COVID-19 is Nucleic Acid Amplification Tests (NAATs). It utilises respiratory tract samples (mainly from the nasopharynx or oropharynx). However, some guidelines recommend nasal swabs [16], and some evidence suggests lower respiratory samples, such as sputum, may have higher sensitivity [17].

From the pandemic onset, chest radiography (X-ray) has been a helpful tool for COVID-19 diagnosis [18]. Nevertheless, even routine chest radiography does not confirm that the patient has COVID-19, especially early on [19], so diagnosing based on an X-ray is challenging. On the contrary, a computed tomography (CT) has been able to discover COVID-19 abnormalities with sensitivity exceeding 97% [20]. However, it was reported to have only 25% to 83% specificity for symptomatic patients [21]. Some evidence suggests it helps to detect COVID-19 earlier than manifested by the positive reverse transcription-polymerase chain reaction (RT-PCR) test [22,23]. Additionally, from the beginning of the pandemic, COVID-19 diagnosis based on ultrasound imaging proved to be of sensitivity and accuracy, which is similar to differentiating with CTs [24].

With the rising role of medical imaging as a diagnostic tool for COVID-19, a question arose if and to which extent automated tools could be included in clinical diagnosis. Up to this day, artificial intelligence (AI), or more specifically, deep learning (DL), have started to play an increasingly vital role in medicine [25]. AI can be employed in the first step of diagnosis, or the results it produces may be used to confirm hypotheses generated by clinicians. In some recent studies and clinical trials, AI has been demonstrated to match or even exceed the performance of expert radiologists, which could potentially offer expedited and less expensive diagnostics [26–31]. A study and meta-analysis by [32] with 31,587 identified and 82 included studies shows DL is even capable of slightly outperforming health care professionals in detecting diseases from medical images with a pooled sensitivity of 87% (vs. 86%) and a pooled specificity of 93% (vs. 91%), respectively.

Since the emergence of the COVID-19 pandemic, around 237,000 related papers (and growing) have been published [33,34]. The urgency of reporting novel findings and high pressure to publish COVID-19-related research quickly has been reported to lead to exceptions to high standards of quality [35,36], an increase in overlap [37], lowering methodological credibility of some of the articles [38], or even accepting papers with numerous analytical errors [39].

Almost two years after the pandemic onset, it is the right time to start drawing conclusions [40]. We should also pay attention to the mistakes we have committed and avoid them in the face of the upcoming threats. The current situation is an opportunity to learn lessons on dealing with crises.

This systematic umbrella review aims to screen reviews on AI techniques to diagnose COVID-19 in patients of any age and sex (both hospitalised and ambulatory) using medical images and assess their methodological quality. Additionally, our goal was to evaluate the research publishing process and the degree of overlap to assess the legitimacy of creating new works in the unfolding pandemic.

2. Materials and Methods

2.1. Data Sources and Searches

In order to determine whether there are any eligible papers, we conducted a pre-search in the middle of August 2020 via Google Scholar by browsing. Next, we searched seven article databases (MEDLINE, EMBASE, Web of Science, Scopus, dblp, Cochrane Library, IEEE Xplore) and two preprint databases (arXiv, OSF Preprints) from inception to 1 September 2020 using predefined search strategies. In developing the search strategy for MEDLINE, we combined the Medical Subject Headings (MeSH) and full-text words. In Text S1, we present the used strategies. No date or language restrictions were adopted. Additionally, we searched the references of included studies for eligible records.

2.2. Study Selection

We focused on any review (systematic or not) that includes primary studies utilising AI methods with medical imaging results to diagnose COVID-19. We were particularly interested in the performance of such classification systems, e.g., accuracy, sensitivity, specificity. Based on available guidelines [16], we excluded these primary studies that used reference standards other than assay types (NAATs, antigen tests, and antibody tests) from nasopharyngeal or oropharyngeal swab samples, nasal aspirate, nasal wash or saliva, sputum or tracheal aspirate, or bronchoalveolar lavage (BAL) [41].

Additionally, due to overlapping and double referencing of the post-conference articles (particular chapters), we excluded entire proceedings and post-conference books as they contain little information about the topics (presented in chapters) *per se*. However, we did not exclude reviews (chapters) as they were still present in our search.

The protocol of this review was published [42] and registered [43] on the OSF platform.

Using Endnote X8 (Clarivate Analytics ®) and Rayyan [44], we checked identified references for duplicates. P.J., D.S., and P.O. independently screened the remaining references using the latter application, and subsequently, independently assessed the full texts for meeting the inclusion criteria.

To improve the understanding of the criteria among the reviewers, we carried out pilot exercises before the screening of titles and abstracts and full texts assessment. We achieved consensus via discussion if any conflicts occurred.

2.3. Definitions

We defined the terms used in our eligibility criteria below. *Review* refers to a paper identified by authors as a review or a survey. *AI* refers to computer programs that can perform tasks as intelligent beings [45]. *COVID-19* refers to a disease caused by the SARS-CoV-2 virus [46]. *Imaging* refers to individuals' medical imaging results (e.g., CT scans, X-rays, ultrasound images) [47,48].

Diagnosis refers to the identification of an illness (here: COVID-19) [49]. *Performance metrics* refers to evaluating machine learning algorithms. These measures are utilised to juxtapose observed data (actual labels) with the predictions of the model [50].

2.4. Data Extraction and Quality Assessment

Before the extraction phase, we checked included preprints for peer-reviewed versions and included them, if available. We predefined an extraction form, and P.J. and D.S. collected all necessary data independently. We gathered information about authors, funding, population, models, outcomes—AI diagnostic metrics, and additional analyses.

We also extracted bibliometric data about publishing dates (availability), sending to the editors (first and last version), and acceptance in a journal or a conference of included reviews. Moreover, we checked the availability dates for primary studies.

To provide a common understanding of the criteria, we performed calibration exercises before data extraction and credibility assessment. When the conflict occurred, we discussed the final version.

P.J. and D.S. conducted quality evaluations independently. We assessed the methodological credibility using AMSTAR 2 [51] with critical items (2, 4, 7, 9, 11, 13, and 15), indicated as such by AMSTAR 2 authors, and not yet validated extended version of QASR [52].

The general quality across the study was evaluated as *critically low* when more than one item in a critical domain was considered a flaw [51].

In this paper, we concentrate only on the results of applying AMSTAR 2 (as it is suggested for evaluating systematic reviews [53]), while a full assessment of both instruments will be included in the next methodologically focused article.

Additionally, we assessed the quality of reporting in included studies using the Preferred Reporting Items for Systematic Reviews and Meta-analyses for Diagnostic Test Accuracy (PRISMA-DTA) checklist [54]. We rated each module on the 3-item scale: 0 (*no* with no compliance), 0.5 (*partial yes* with fragmentary compliance), 1 (*yes* with total compliance). Next, the results were summed, and the overall score was then assigned.

Based on the method of Li et al. [55] and taking into account two more items in the DTA extension [54] (comparing to the original instrument [56]), we differentiated the quality of reporting as follows:

- *Major flaws* when the final score was ≤ 17.0,
- *Minor flaws* when the final score was ≥ 17.5 and ≤ 23.0,
- *Minimal flaws* when the final score was ≥ 23.5.

In the case of reviews without meta-analysis, we lowered the cut-offs by 1 point following PRISMA-DTA [54].

2.5. Data Synthesis and Analysis

In this umbrella review, we focus on the descriptive summary of included papers regarding the quality and reporting on the most significant characteristics, such as population, models, interpretability, and outcomes.

We did not synthesise the results quantitatively because of the quality of included reviews, the agreement between them, and the percentage of non-reported data (data we intended to extract, e.g., accuracy of diagnostic methods or AI model type, see Section 3). Therefore, we do not present a subgroup analysis and investigation of heterogeneity, sensitivity, and publication bias analyses.

As for the in-depth characteristics, all the primary studies were divided into two groups: included in one review only and included in at least one review. The studies included in more than one review were analysed in 2 ways (A and B) considering *not reported* data. In analysis A, whenever *not reported* data from one review occurred together with a specific value from the other paper, we considered it *non-overlapping* and excluded it. In analysis B, we ignored *not reported* data and included the specific value. After the exclusion of non-overlapping data for continuous variables, we calculated the statistics, namely means with ranges.

For diagnostics metrics, we prepared the scatter plots. We considered data regardless of non-overlapping. Whenever disagreements between reviews occurred (in specific primary studies), we averaged the values. In case of lack of data (*not reported*), we provided two charts with modal imputation and without it.

From the above analyses, we excluded those primary studies, which included more than one DL model.

We analysed how extensive was the search performed by the authors of the reviews, i.e., percentage of the identified primary studies available up to the selected date. In the first case, we considered the reference date, by which we mean the day that the review was either received, accepted by the editors, or published. In the second analysis, we relaxed this condition to the date the last cited paper included in the review was available.

Investigating the citations between the reviews, we considered two different scenarios: citing only published reviews and citing both published and preprint versions.

We assessed inter-review agreement only if at least two different reviews included the same paper (and only one DL model). We determined the inter-review agreement as a percentage of overlapping values within all extracted data (text and non-text) and subgroups of characteristics (text and non-text) and outcomes. The text variables considered the dataset used, architecture, and post-processing. The inter-review agreement was assessed in 2 ways (analyses A and modified B—exclude a pair, instead of ignoring it).

All analyses were conducted using Python 3.7.10 (including libraries: Matplotlib 3.2.2, Seaborn 0.11.1, Pandas 1.1.5 and NumPy 1.19.5).

3. Results

3.1. Included Studies

After removing duplicates, we screened 725 studies, of which 33 were read in the form of full texts. In total, we included 22 reviews [57–78] for qualitative synthesis. We followed PRISMA guidelines [56]. The full study flow is presented in Figure 1.

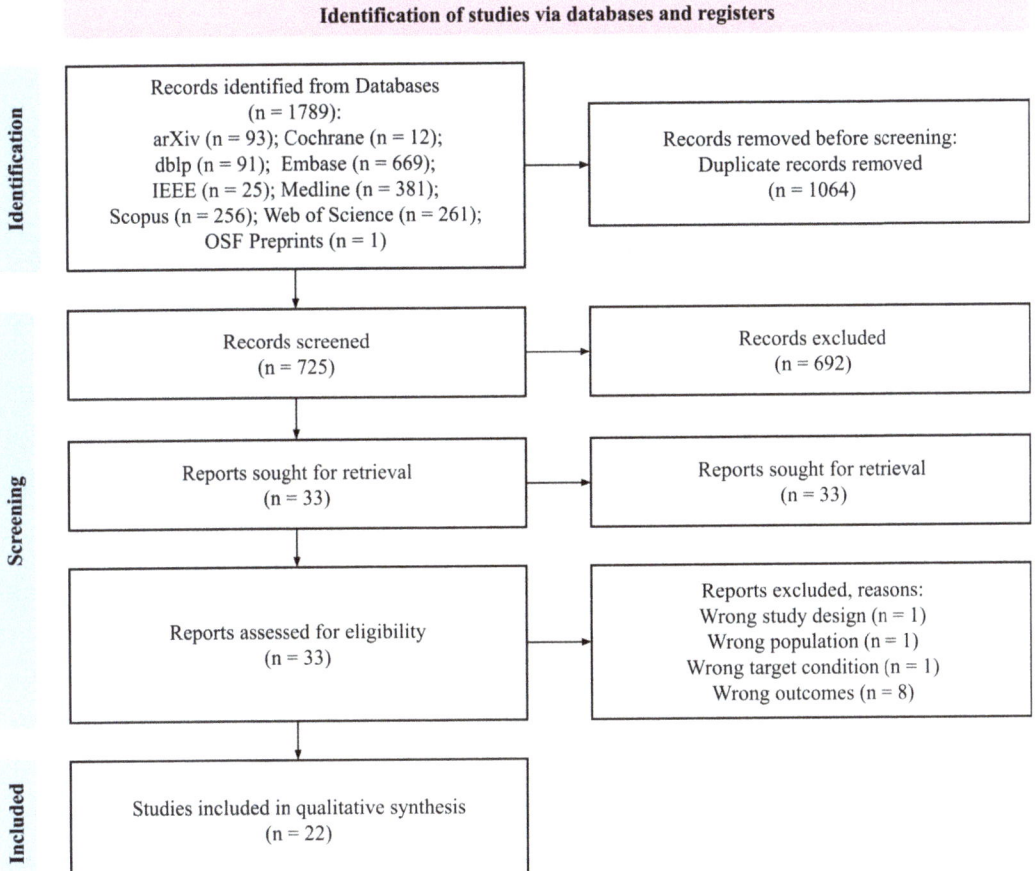

Figure 1. PRISMA flow chart.

The included and excluded studies (with reasons) are presented in Tables S1 and S2, respectively. The detailed characteristics of included reviews are shown in Table 1, while its extended version is ensured in Table S3.

We present the in-depth characteristics of primary studies in Table S4. Tables S5 and S6 focus on the non-overlapping between reviews and non-reporting in terms of specific extracted variables. Figures S1–S6 introduces visualised diagnostic metrics.

Table 1. Detailed characteristics of included reviews.

Variable	Number (Percentage)	Mean (Range) [2]
Number of reviews with the authors from a specific country		
United States of America	8 (18%)	NA
Australia	4 (9%)	NA
China	4 (9%)	NA
India	4 (9%)	NA
United Kingdom	3 (7%)	NA
Other	22 (49%)	NA
Total number of authors of the reviews	171	8 (1–43)
Type of publication		
Journal article (mean IF [1]: 4.14; range: 0–30.31)	13 (59%)	NA
IEEE Access	2 (9%)	NA
IEEE Reviews in Biomedical Engineering	2 (9%)	NA
Diagnostic and Interventional Imaging	2 (9%)	NA
Diabetes & Metabolic Syndrome: Clinical Research & Reviews	1 (5%)	NA
Applied Intelligence	1 (5%)	NA
British Medical Journal	1 (5%)	NA
Biosensors and Bioelectronics	1 (5%)	NA
Machine Vision and Applications	1 (5%)	NA
Current Problems in Diagnostic Radiology	1 (5%)	NA
Journal of the Indian Medical Association	1 (5%)	NA
Preprint article	8 (36%)	NA
Conference article	1 (5%)	NA
Was the review specified as systematic by the authors?		
No	20 (91%)	NA
Yes	2 (9%)	NA
Number of reviews that searched a given data source	50	5 (3–7)
arXiv	8 (36%)	NA
medRxiv	6 (27%)	NA
Pubmed/Medline	6 (27%)	NA
Google Scholar	6 (27%)	NA
bioRxiv	5 (23%)	NA
IEEE Xplore	3 (14%)	NA
Science Direct	3 (14%)	NA
ACM digital library	2 (9%)	NA
Springer	2 (9%)	NA
MICCAI conference	1 (5%)	NA
IPMI conference	1 (5%)	NA
Embase	1 (5%)	NA
Web of Science	1 (5%)	NA
Elsevier	1 (5%)	NA
Nature	1 (5%)	NA
Number of studies		
Reported by review authors as included	358	51 (20–107)
Applicable for this review question (total)	451	21 (1–106)
Applicable for this review question (unique only)	165	7.5 (0–11)

[1] Impact Factor; [2] Not Applicable.

None of the reviews provided information about ethnicity, smoking, and comorbidities. Only one review [68] reported on age and gender proportion as well as the study design of discussed primary papers. None of the studies conducted a meta-analysis, but one summarised the results with the use of averages [71].

The analysed reviews described 165 primary papers (on average: eight primary studies per review, range: 1–11). Of these, 138 of them were included in at least one review, of which 73 were included only in one. Only 27 of the primary studies considered more than one DL model for diagnosis.

3.2. Quality of Included Studies

The general quality of all included studies is *critically low* (see Figure 2). Six reviews [62–64,66,68,77] provided full information about sources of funding and conflict of interest. It was the most satisfied item. None of the studies provided a list of excluded papers, explanation of eligible study design, and sources of funding in included studies.

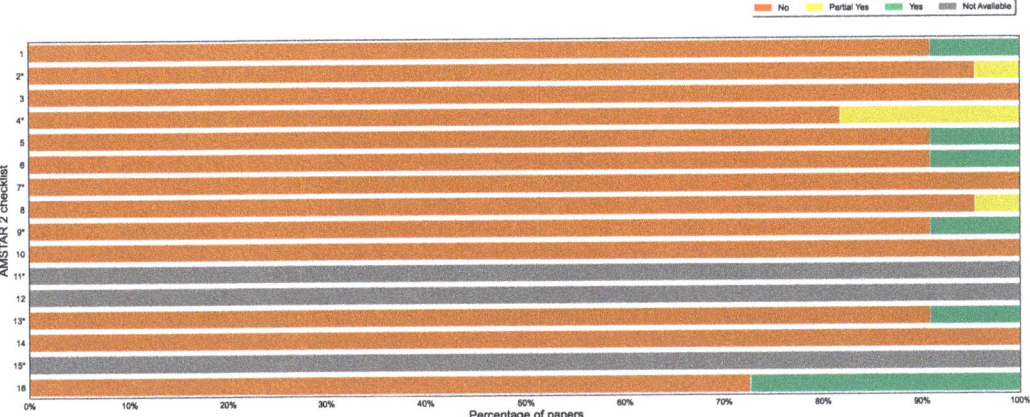

Figure 2. Quality graph: our judgements on each AMSTAR 2 item presented as the percentage of all the included studies; * denotes critical domains.

A heatmap with the authors' judgements regarding AMSTAR 2 items can be found in Figure S7. In Figure S8, we also included results per specific review.

In terms of reporting, *major flaws* are present among 21 of the included papers. Only one review [68] contains *minor flaws* (see Figures 3, S9 and S10). The most affected domains were those concerning additional analyses both in terms of methods and results (all reviews). Similarly, a summary of evidence was not reported in any review.

On the contrary, 12 of the included papers [57,59,62–64,66,68–71,77,78] reported fully on funding. Additionally, 11 reviews [57,58,60,65,66,69,70,72,73,76,77] and eight reviews [57,59,60,65–67,71,77] described the rationale and objectives in the introduction adequately. These were the most satisfied domains.

The mean overall score of reporting quality across the included reviews equals 6.23 (1.5–17.5). Across all items and studies, the most frequent score was 0 (*no*) with 67%; 19% of the time, we assessed the items as 0.5 (*partially yes*). A heatmap with all authors' judgements regarding PRISMA-DTA items can be found in Figure S9. In Figure S10, we also included summarised results per specific review.

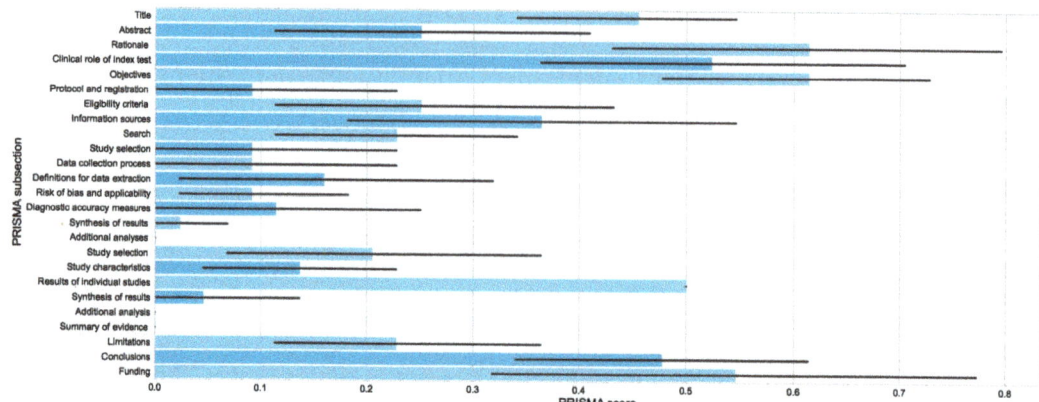

Figure 3. Quality of reporting graph: our judgements about each PRISMA-DTA item presented as averages (with 95% confidence intervals—black lines) across all included studies. Different shades of blue are used just to improve the chart's clarity.

3.3. Resources and Time Wasting Analyses

The included studies were published or available online without peer reviewing from 11 April 2020 to 12 October 2020 (see Figure S11). In Figure 4, we presented a cumulative chart of all 165 primary studies included in the discussed reviews.

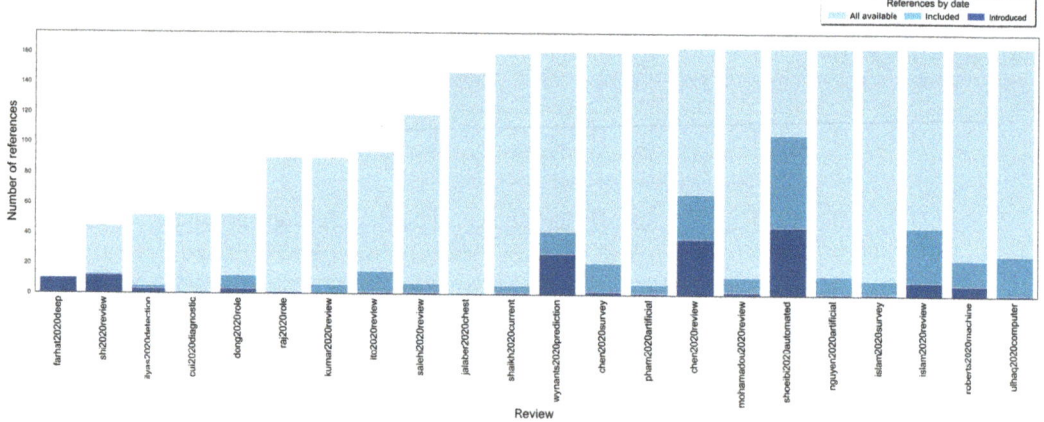

Figure 4. The cumulative chart of included, available (by the date), and introduced primary papers among discussed reviews.

The number of included interesting studies (related to our research question) in selected reviews ranged from 1 [62–64] to 106 [73]. Moreover, we present the percentage of articles introduced by (first appear in) a particular review. Figure S11 additionally depicts the appearance of included reviews and interesting primary studies over time.

Half (50%) of all (165) primary studies (the half-saturation constant) were included at least once before the end of July 2020. However, the same number of papers was available for inclusion three months earlier.

Next, we investigated the extent to which review authors performed the search. Regarding the reference date (see Figure S11), the mean percentage of the primary studies covered was 14% (1–64). When relaxed, the mean percentage of covered studies increased to 24% (1–65). More details about the search are presented in Table S7.

Out of all the studies, 14% did not include any new paper into consideration. The mean primary studies that were introduced by a particular review was 7.24 (0–45).

Analysing published versions of reviews only, the cross-citing equals 0.81 (0–4). Including also preprints, 1.1 (0–7) published papers or preprints were quoted by the authors of the subsequent reviews. Notably, 12 (55%) of reviews did not refer to any previously available ones at all.

Figures S12–S21 present results regarding the agreement between reviews (*pairs of reviews*) in the reporting of characteristics and outcomes.

4. Discussion

Generally, we report that the quality of the included reviews was *critically low*. Similar findings were found by Jung et al. [79], who observed lowered methodological credibility in 686 of 14,787 screened COVID-19 papers. Analyses of reviews on COVID-19 by Yu et al. [80] and Al-Ryalat et al. [81] also showed their unsatisfactory credibility. It adds on top of the generally low quality of reporting of DL performance from medical images, with a high risk of bias present in 58 out of 81 of the existing studies (72%) [82].

Poor quality is not related only to COVID-19 and AI. Still, it occurs in many fields such as bariatric surgery with up to 99% *critically low* articles [83], psychology with 95% of papers [84], or methodology where 53 out of 63 publications were of *critically low* quality [85].

What is more, we also noticed major flaws in reporting. Nagendran et al. [82] observed the same, but they used the original PRISMA instrument. In our research, three PRISMA-DTA domains were fully violated by all reviews. Although the authors focused on diagnostics, they poorly reported on accuracy measures and explicit description of the extraction process. None of the included studies performed a meta-analysis, similar to what Adadi et al. [86] found in their study.

The low credibility of evidence and flawed reporting (e.g., population characteristics) can be associated with a lack of knowledge of reporting standards and clinical practice or misunderstandings regarding AI methods and additional analyses.

We also observed multiple disagreements between the included reviews. However, excluding them from synthesis is associated with a vast information loss, e.g., the number of participants. Inconsistencies were also noticed in the reporting of DL architecture. For instance, the following names were used across multiple studies: *ResNet-18, ResNet18, resnet-18, 18-layer ResNet*. In some of the papers, the architecture was not reported at all. It made it challenging to group models into similar subsets. Some discrepancy was also observed in extracting the measurements of AI models performance, e.g., diagnostic effectiveness metrics. Such negligence may lead to further replicating the errors by subsequent studies and should be corrected before releasing the paper or soon after in an updated version or in an associated erratum.

Many of the reviews included in this paper did not strengthen the evidence on using AI in diagnosing COVID-19 from medical imaging. Those works have not identified and correctly cited pre-existing primary papers, which is deemed the essence of any research. Some of the potential explanations are that multiple similar studies might have been initiated around the same time, and prolonged review times impacted their content. Alternatively, the research objectives of some articles were broad enough to preclude a deeper analysis of the use of artificial intelligence in medical imaging.

Wasting may also (or in particular) be observed on the primary studies level. Failure to consider previous results may lead to publishing new papers describing models similar to those presented by other researchers. Shockingly, these newer DL architectures rely sometimes on fewer participants or COVID-19 cases, so they probably reflect reality less adequately. As researchers suggest, the amount of waste and poor biomedical research quality is staggering [35,87]. Papers that do not bring any additional evidence to the field can be considered redundant [88–91].

Proper reporting of deep learning performance from primary studies is challenging. Naudé [92] has pointed out some of the significant concerns regarding the adoption of AI in COVID-19 research, including data availability and its quality. Still, many studies do not ensure that the utilised code is open-source, which highly limits the reproducibility of their findings [93,94]. Therefore, we suggest sharing it so that you can react faster and more effectively from the perspective of the upcoming, similar breakdowns.

On average, when not considering credibility issues, the diagnostic metrics of described models exceed the human's ability to diagnose COVID-19 from medical imaging [32]. Sadly, no evidence of such an advantage could be transferred to any implications for practice because of not following reporting and quality instruments. It resembles a situation when a long jumper did not break the world record just because they stepped on the foul line.

4.1. Study Strengths and Limitations

Our umbrella review has the following strengths. First, the search strategy was comprehensive. It is based on adequate inclusion criteria related to the research question and spanned across a wide selection of existing data sources: papers and preprints. This selection was further expanded by searching the references of included papers to identify additional works. It is noteworthy that the searches were not limited in terms of format or language (we imposed no restrictions). The process of our review was rigorous as the study was preceded by the publication of protocol. We used the most up-to-date and applicable instruments to assess the credibility and quality of reporting—AMSTAR 2 and PRISMA with extension for DTA, respectively.

Nevertheless, these two have been designed for reviews in medicine and health sciences, where the formulation of the research question is structured, the methodology is validated, and the quantitative synthesis of results is popular.

It must be noted, though, that the vast majority of the included studies focused on a broader context than purely diagnosing COVID-19 from medical images.

In this study, we have also investigated wasting among the reviews. We based on the date of publishing of the last included primary study in a specific review. By doing so, we aimed at assessing the depth of the search performed by the authors. We assumed that if the authors included a given study, they should have had the required knowledge about all the papers available before it was released. This approach relaxes the strict requirement to include all the studies that appeared before the review was published and seems to measure the quality of the search more objectively.

The level of agreement between reviews differs remarkably depending on the extracted variable, so without comparing with the primary studies, we cannot be fully convinced of the data correctness reported in the reviews. In the assessment of the inter-review agreement, we considered only these reviews that included the same paper (and described one DL model).

5. Conclusions

The COVID-19 research is quickly moving forward. Each day hundreds of new papers are published [95–97]. As AI starts to play an increasingly important role in clinical practice [98,99], it is crucial to evaluate its performance correctly.

In this paper, we synthesised and assessed the quality of the 22 reviews that mention using AI on COVID-19 medical images. We reviewed them and critically assessed their reporting and credibility using well-established instruments such as PRISMA-DTA [54] and AMSTAR 2 [51].

We explored the beginning of the pandemic when much uncertainty and confusion existed in the world of science. It seems that the number of articles and the pace of their publishing during the future global outbreaks might be even faster. Thus, it is essential to draw the appropriate conclusions now and treat this *briefing* as an opportunity to optimise work and avoid wasting in publishing.

In order to accomplish this, we urge the authors of the reviews to use PRISMA [56] and AMSTAR 2 [51] and the authors of primary studies to follow appropriate tools [100,101].

It is high time to adopt best practices, improve the research quality, and apply higher scrutiny in filtering out non-constructive contributions.

Supplementary Materials: The following supporting information can be downloaded at: https://www.mdpi.com/article/10.3390/jcm11072054/s1, **Table S1**: Included studies with dates: first received, last received, accepted and published; **Table S2**: Exluded studies [102–112] with reasons; **Table S3**: Full characteristics of included reviews; **Table S4**: In-depth characteristics of primary studies; **Table S5**: Non-overlapping of in-depth characteristics variables; **Table S6**: Non-reporting of in-depth characteristics variables; **Figure S1**: CT-based COVID-19 diagnosis, without imputation; **Figure S2**: CT-based COVID-19 diagnosis, with modal imputation; **Figure S3**: X-Ray-based COVID-19 diagnosis, without imputation; **Figure S4**: X-Ray-based COVID-19 diagnosis, with modal imputation; **Figure S5**: COVID-19 diagnosis with full patients number data provided, without imputation; **Figure S6**: COVID-19 diagnosis with any patients number data provided, with modal imputation; **Figure S7**: Review authors' judgements about each AMSTAR 2 item across all included studies; * denotes critical items; **Figure S8**: AMSTAR 2 score in each included review; **Figure S9**: Review authors' judgements about each PRISMA-DTA item across all included studies; **Figure S10**: PRISMA-DTA score in each included review; **Figure S11**: Appearance of included reviews (vertical lines, reference date, see Table S1 and interesting primary studies (dots)); **Table S7**: Time and resource wasting statistics; **Figure S12**: Level of agreement based on overlapping in extracted data (characteristics only, without text data) between included reviews; analysis A; **Figure S13**: Level of agreement based on overlapping in extracted data (characteristics only) between included reviews; analysis A; **Figure S14**: Level of agreement based on overlapping in extracted data (outcomes only) between included reviews; analysis A; **Figure S15**: Level of agreement based on overlapping in extracted data (all variables, without text data) between included reviews; analysis A; **Figure S16**: Level of agreement based on overlapping in extracted data (all variables) between included reviews; analysis A; **Figure S17**: Level of agreement based on overlapping in extracted data (characteristics only, without text data) between included reviews; analysis B; **Figure S18**: Level of agreement based on overlapping in extracted data (characteristics only) between included reviews; analysis B; **Figure S19**: Level of agreement based on overlapping in extracted data (outcomes only) between included reviews; analysis B; **Figure S20**: Level of agreement based on overlapping in extracted data (all variables, without text data) between included reviews; analysis B; **Figure S21**: Level of agreement based on overlapping in extracted data (all variables) between included reviews; analysis B; **Text S1**: Search Strategies; PRISMA 2020 Checklist.

Author Contributions: Conceptualization, P.J., D.S., and P.O.; methodology, D.S. and P.J.; software, P.J. and P.O.; validation, P.J. and D.S.; formal analysis, P.J. and D.S.; investigation, P.J., D.S. and P.O.; resources, P.J.; data curation, P.J.; writing—original draft preparation, P.J., D.S. and P.O.; writing—review and editing, P.J., D.S. and P.O.; visualization, P.J. and P.O.; supervision, P.J.; project administration, P.J.; funding acquisition, P.J. All authors have read and agreed to the published version of the manuscript.

Funding: Research project supported by program *Excellence initiative— research university* for the University of Science and Technology. P.O. was supported by National Institutes of Health (grant number AI116794).

Institutional Review Board Statement: Not applicable.

Informed Consent Statement: Not applicable.

Data Availability Statement: Code used in this research is available on GitHub: https://github.com/pawljmlo/covid-ur-wasting (accessed on 25 March 2022). The data presented in this study are available on request from the corresponding author.

Conflicts of Interest: The authors declare no conflict of interest. The funders had no role in the design of the study; in the collection, analyses, or interpretation of data; in the writing of the manuscript, or in the decision to publish the results.

Abbreviations

The following abbreviations are used in this manuscript:

AI	artificial intelligence
BAL	bronchoalveolar lavage
COVID-19	Coronavirus disease 2019
CT	computed tomography
DL	deep learning
NAATs	Nucleic Acid Amplification Tests
PHEIC	public health emergency of international concern
X-ray	radiography
RT-PCR	reverse transcription-polymerase chain reaction
SARS-CoV-2	Severe Acute Respiratory Syndrome Coronavirus 2
WHO	World Health Organisation

References

1. Kahn, N. New virus Discovered by Chinese Scientists Investigating Pneumonia Outbreak 2020. Available online: https://www.wsj.com/articles/new-virus-discovered-by-chinese-scientists-investigating-pneumonia-outbreak-11578485668 (accessed on 23 February 2022).
2. World Health Organization. Report of the WHO-China Joint Mission on Coronavirus Disease 2019 (COVID-19). 2020. Available online: https://reliefweb.int/report/china/report-who-china-joint-mission-coronavirus-disease-2019-covid-19?gclid=EAIaIQobChMI2vX_nJro9gIVVj5gCh2LDQKuEAAYASAAEgLn9PD_BwE (accessed on 23 February 2022).
3. World Health Organization. WHO Coronavirus (COVID-19) Dashboard. 2020. Available online: https://covid19.who.int/ (accessed on 23 February 2022).
4. Simon, S.; Frank, B.J.; Aichmair, A.; Manolopoulos, P.P.; Dominkus, M.; Schernhammer, E.S.; Hofstaetter, J.G. Impact of the 1st and 2nd Wave of the COVID-19 Pandemic on Primary or Revision Total Hip and Knee Arthroplasty—A Cross-Sectional Single Center Study. *J. Clin. Med.* **2021**, *10*, 1260. [CrossRef] [PubMed]
5. Vahabi, N.; Salehi, M.; Duarte, J.D.; Mollalo, A.; Michailidis, G. County-level longitudinal clustering of COVID-19 mortality to incidence ratio in the United States. *Sci. Rep.* **2021**, *11*, 1–22. [CrossRef] [PubMed]
6. Saito, S.; Asai, Y.; Matsunaga, N.; Hayakawa, K.; Terada, M.; Ohtsu, H.; Tsuzuki, S.; Ohmagari, N. First and second COVID-19 waves in Japan: A comparison of disease severity and characteristics: Comparison of the two COVID-19 waves in Japan. *J. Infect. Dis.* **2020**, *82*, 84–123.
7. Coccia, M. The Effects of the First and Second Wave of COVID-19 Pandemic on Public Health. 2020. Available online: https://www.researchsquare.com/article/rs-110013/latest.pdf (accessed on 23 February 2022).
8. World Health Organization. World Health Organization coronavirus disease 2019 (COVID-19) Situation Report. 2020. Available online: https://apps.who.int/iris/handle/10665/331686 (accessed on 23 February 2022).
9. Kimball, A.; Hatfield, K.M.; Arons, M.; James, A.; Taylor, J.; Spicer, K.; Bardossy, A.C.; Oakley, L.P.; Tanwar, S.; Chisty, Z.; et al. Asymptomatic and presymptomatic SARS-CoV-2 infections in residents of a long-term care skilled nursing facility—King County, Washington, March 2020. *MMWR* **2020**, *69*, 377. [CrossRef] [PubMed]
10. Guan, W.j.; Ni, Z.y.; Hu, Y.; Liang, W.h.; Ou, C.q.; He, J.x.; Liu, L.; Shan, H.; Lei, C.l.; Hui, D.S.; et al. Clinical characteristics of coronavirus disease 2019 in China. *N. Engl. J. Med.* **2020**, *382*, 1708–1720. [CrossRef] [PubMed]
11. Le, T.T.; Gutiérrez-Sacristán, A.; Son, J.; Hong, C.; South, A.M.; Beaulieu-Jones, B.K.; Loh, N.H.W.; Luo, Y.; Morris, M.; Ngiam, K.Y.; et al. Multinational Prevalence of Neurological Phenotypes in Patients Hospitalized with COVID-19. *medRxiv* **2021**. [CrossRef]
12. Lopez-Leon, S.; Wegman-Ostrosky, T.; Perelman, C.; Sepulveda, R.; Rebolledo, P.A.; Cuapio, A.; Villapol, S. More than 50 Long-term effects of COVID-19: Asystematic review and meta-analysis. *SSRN* **2021**, *11*, 3769978.
13. Greenhalgh, T.; Knight, M.; Buxton, M.; Husain, L. Management of post-acute covid-19 in primary care. *BMJ* **2020**, *370*, m3026. [CrossRef]
14. Sun, Q.; Qiu, H.; Huang, M.; Yang, Y. Lower mortality of COVID-19 by early recognition and intervention: Experience from Jiangsu Province. *Ann. Intensive Care* **2020**, *10*, 1–4. [CrossRef] [PubMed]
15. Islam, N.; Salameh, J.P.; Leeflang, M.M.; Hooft, L.; McGrath, T.A.; Pol, C.B.; Frank, R.A.; Kazi, S.; Prager, R.; Hare, S.S.; et al. Thoracic Imaging Tests for the Diagnosis of COVID-19. *Cochrane Database Syst. Rev.* **2021**, CD013639. [CrossRef]
16. Centers for Disease Control and Prevention. Interim Guidelines for Collecting and Handling of Clinical Specimens for COVID-19 Testing. 2020. Available online: https:/cdc.gov/coronavirus/2019-nCoV/lab/guidelines-clinical-specimens.html/ (accessed on 23 February 2022).
17. Wang, W.; Xu, Y.; Gao, R.; Lu, R.; Han, K.; Wu, G.; Tan, W. Detection of SARS-CoV-2 in different types of clinical specimens. *JAMA* **2020**, *323*, 1843–1844. [CrossRef] [PubMed]
18. Smith, D.L.; Grenier, J.P.; Batte, C.; Spieler, B. A Characteristic Chest Radiographic Pattern in the Setting of COVID-19 Pandemic. *J. Thorac Imaging* **2020**, *2*, e200280. [CrossRef] [PubMed]

19. Cleverley, J.; Piper, J.; Jones, M.M. The role of chest radiography in confirming covid-19 pneumonia. *BMJ* **2020**, *370*. [CrossRef] [PubMed]
20. Kovács, A.; Palásti, P.; Veréb, D.; Bozsik, B.; Palkó, A.; Kincses, Z.T. The sensitivity and specificity of chest CT in the diagnosis of COVID-19. *Eur. Radiol.* **2020**, *31*, 1–6. [CrossRef] [PubMed]
21. Park, J.Y.; Freer, R.; Stevens, R.; Neil, S.; Jones, N. The Accuracy of Chest CT in the Diagnosis of COVID-19: An Umbrella Review. 2021. Available online: https://www.cebm.net/covid-19/the-accuracy-of-chest-ct-in-the-diagnosis-of-covid-19-an-umbrella-review/ (accessed on 23 February 2022).
22. Chua, F.; Armstrong-James, D.; Desai, S.R.; Barnett, J.; Kouranos, V.; Kon, O.M.; José, R.; Vancheeswaran, R.; Loebinger, M.R.; Wong, J.; et al. The role of CT in case ascertainment and management of COVID-19 pneumonia in the UK: Insights from high-incidence regions. *Lancet Respir. Med.* **2020**, *8*, 438–440. [CrossRef]
23. Ai, T.; Yang, Z.; Hou, H.; Zhan, C.; Chen, C.; Lv, W.; Tao, Q.; Sun, Z.; Xia, L. Correlation of chest CT and RT-PCR testing for coronavirus disease 2019 (COVID-19) in China: A report of 1014 cases. *Radiology* **2020**, *296*, E32–E40. [CrossRef] [PubMed]
24. Sultan, L.R.; Sehgal, C.M. A review of early experience in lung ultrasound in the diagnosis and management of COVID-19. *Ultrasound Med. Biol.* **2020**, *46*, 2530–2545. [CrossRef]
25. Ching, T.; Himmelstein, D.S.; Beaulieu-Jones, B.K.; Kalinin, A.A.; Do, B.T.; Way, G.P.; Ferrero, E.; Agapow, P.M.; Zietz, M.; Hoffman, M.M.; et al. Opportunities and obstacles for deep learning in biology and medicine. *J. R. Soc. Interface* **2018**, *15*, 20170387. [CrossRef] [PubMed]
26. Hosny, A.; Parmar, C.; Quackenbush, J.; Schwartz, L.H.; Aerts, H.J. Artificial intelligence in radiology. *Nat. Rev. Cancer* **2018**, *18*, 500–510. [CrossRef] [PubMed]
27. McBee, M.P.; Awan, O.A.; Colucci, A.T.; Ghobadi, C.W.; Kadom, N.; Kansagra, A.P.; Tridandapani, S.; Auffermann, W.F. Deep Learning in Radiology. *Acad. Radiol.* **2018**, *25*, 1472–1480. [CrossRef] [PubMed]
28. Wang, P.; Berzin, T.M.; Brown, J.R.G.; Bharadwaj, S.; Becq, A.; Xiao, X.; Liu, P.; Li, L.; Song, Y.; Zhang, D.; et al. Real-time automatic detection system increases colonoscopic polyp and adenoma detection rates: A prospective randomised controlled study. *Gut* **2019**, *68*, 1813–1819. [CrossRef] [PubMed]
29. Liu, X.; Faes, L.; Kale, A.U.; Wagner, S.K.; Fu, D.J.; Bruynseels, A.; Mahendiran, T.; Moraes, G.; Shamdas, M.; Kern, C.; et al. A comparison of deep learning performance against health-care professionals in detecting diseases from medical imaging: A systematic review and meta-analysis. *Lancet Digit. Health* **2019**, *1*, e271–e297. [CrossRef]
30. Loo, J.; Clemons, T.E.; Chew, E.Y.; Friedlander, M.; Jaffe, G.J.; Farsiu, S. Beyond performance metrics: Automatic deep learning retinal OCT analysis reproduces clinical trial outcome. *Ophthalmology* **2020**, *127*, 793–801. [CrossRef] [PubMed]
31. Bullock, J.; Luccioni, A.; Pham, K.H.; Lam, C.S.N.; Luengo-Oroz, M. Mapping the landscape of artificial intelligence applications against COVID-19. *J. Artif. Intell. Res.* **2020**, *69*, 807–845. [CrossRef]
32. Li, Y.; Cao, L.; Zhang, Z.; Hou, L.; Qin, Y.; Hui, X.; Li, J.; Zhao, H.; Cui, G.; Cui, X.; et al. Reporting and methodological quality of COVID-19 systematic reviews needs to be improved: An evidence mapping. *J. Clin. Epidemiol.* **2021**, *135*, 17–28. [CrossRef] [PubMed]
33. Chen, Q.; Allot, A.; Lu, Z. Keep up with the latest coronavirus research. *Nature* **2020**, *579*, 193. [CrossRef] [PubMed]
34. National Institutes of Health. COVID-19 Portfolio. 2020. Available online: https://icite.od.nih.gov/covid19/search/ (accessed on 23 February 2022).
35. Glasziou, P.P.; Sanders, S.; Hoffmann, T. Waste in COVID-19 Research. *BMJ* **2020**, *369*, m1847.
36. London, A.J.; Kimmelman, J. Against pandemic research exceptionalism. *Science* **2020**, *368*, 476–477. [CrossRef]
37. Quinn, T.J.; Burton, J.K.; Carter, B.; Cooper, N.; Dwan, K.; Field, R.; Freeman, S.C.; Geue, C.; Hsieh, P.H.; McGill, K.; et al. Following the science? Comparison of methodological and reporting quality of covid-19 and other research from the first wave of the pandemic. *BMC Med.* **2021**, *19*, 1–10. [CrossRef] [PubMed]
38. Mahase, E. Covid-19: 146 researchers raise concerns over chloroquine study that halted WHO trial. *BMJ* **2020**, *369*, 2197. [CrossRef] [PubMed]
39. Ioannidis, J.P. Coronavirus Disease 2019: The Harms of Exaggerated Information and Non-Evidence-Based Measures. *Eur. J. Clin. Invest.* **2020**, *50*, e13222. [CrossRef] [PubMed]
40. Osterholm, M.T. Preparing for the Next Pandemic. *N. Engl. J. Med.* **2005**, *352*, 1839–1842. [CrossRef] [PubMed]
41. The Coronaviridae Study Group of the International Committee on Taxonomy of Viruses. The species Severe acute respiratory syndrome-related coronavirus: Classifying 2019-nCoV and naming it SARS-CoV-2. *Nat. Microbiol.* **2020**, *5*, 536. [CrossRef] [PubMed]
42. Jemioło, P.; Storman, D.; Moore, J.H.; Orzechowski, P. Diagnosing COVID-19 from Medical Images with Artificial Intelligence—An Umbrella Survey. 2020. Available online: https://osf.io/kxrmh/ (accessed on 23 February 2022).
43. Jemioło, P.; Storman, D.; Moore, J.H.; Orzechowski, P. Diagnosing COVID-19 from Medical Images with Artificial Intelligence—An Umbrella Survey (Registration). 2020. Available online: https://osf.io/hkwfq/ (accessed on 23 February 2022).
44. Ouzzani, M.; Hammady, H.; Fedorowicz, Z.; Elmagarmid, A. Rayyan—A web and mobile app for systematic reviews. *Syst. Rev.* **2016**, *5*, 210. [CrossRef] [PubMed]
45. Copeland, B. Artificial Intelligence: Definition, Examples, and Applications. 2020. Available online: https://www.britannica.com/technology/artificial-intelligence (accessed on 23 February 2022).

46. Wang, L.; Wang, Y.; Ye, D.; Liu, Q. Review of the 2019 novel coronavirus (SARS-CoV-2) based on current evidence. *Int. J. Antimicrob. Agents* **2020**, *55*, 105948. [CrossRef] [PubMed]
47. Leondes, C.T. *Medical Imaging Systems Techniques and Applications: Computational Techniques*; CRC Press: Boca Raton, FL, USA, 1998; Volume 6.
48. Santosh, K.; Antani, S.; Guru, D.S.; Dey, N. *Medical Imaging: Artificial Intelligence, Image Recognition, and Machine Learning Techniques*; CRC Press: Boca Raton, FL, USA, 2019.
49. Cambridge Dictionary English Dictionary, Translations & Thesaurus. 2021. Available online: https://dictionary.cambridge.org/ (accessed on 23 February 2022).
50. Botchkarev, A. Performance Metrics (Error Measures) in Machine Learning Regression, Forecasting and Prognostics: Properties and Typology. *arXiv* **2018**, arXiv:1809.03006.
51. Shea, B.J.; Reeves, B.C.; Wells, G.; Thuku, M.; Hamel, C.; Moran, J.; Moher, D.; Tugwell, P.; Welch, V.; Kristjansson, E.; et al. AMSTAR 2: A critical appraisal tool for systematic reviews that include randomised or non-randomised studies of healthcare interventions, or both. *BMJ* **2017**, *358*, j4008. [CrossRef] [PubMed]
52. Jemioło, P.; Storman, D. Quality Assessment of Systematic Reviews (QASR). 2020. Available online: https://osf.io/dhtw3/ (accessed on 23 February 2022).
53. Lorenz, R.C.; Matthias, K.; Pieper, D.; Wegewitz, U.; Morche, J.; Nocon, M.; Rissling, O.; Schirm, J.; Jacobs, A. A psychometric study found AMSTAR 2 to be a valid and moderately reliable appraisal tool. *J. Clin. Epidemiol.* **2019**, *114*, 133–140. [CrossRef] [PubMed]
54. McInnes, M.D.; Moher, D.; Thombs, B.D.; McGrath, T.A.; Bossuyt, P.M.; Clifford, T.; Cohen, J.F.; Deeks, J.J.; Gatsonis, C.; Hooft, L.; et al. Preferred reporting items for a systematic review and meta-analysis of diagnostic test accuracy studies: The PRISMA-DTA statement. *JAMA* **2018**, *319*, 388–396. [CrossRef] [PubMed]
55. Li, J.l.; Ge, L.; Ma, J.c.; Zeng, Q.l.; Yao, L.; An, N.; Ding, J.x.; Gan, Y.h.; Tian, J.h. Quality of reporting of systematic reviews published in "evidence-based" Chinese journals. *Syst. Rev.* **2014**, *3*, 1–6. [CrossRef] [PubMed]
56. Page, M.J.; Moher, D.; Bossuyt, P.M.; Boutron, I.; Hoffmann, T.C.; Mulrow, C.D.; Shamseer, L.; Tetzlaff, J.M.; Akl, E.A.; Brennan, S.E.; et al. PRISMA 2020 explanation and elaboration: Updated guidance and exemplars for reporting systematic reviews. *BMJ* **2021**, *372*, n160. [CrossRef] [PubMed]
57. Shi, F.; Wang, J.; Shi, J.; Wu, Z.; Wang, Q.; Tang, Z.; He, K.; Shi, Y.; Shen, D. Review of artificial intelligence techniques in imaging data acquisition, segmentation and diagnosis for COVID-19. *IEEE Rev. Biomed. Eng.* **2020**, *14*. [CrossRef] [PubMed]
58. Ilyas, M.; Rehman, H.; Naït-Ali, A. Detection of covid-19 from chest X-ray images using artificial intelligence: An early review. *arXiv* **2020**, arXiv:2004.05436.
59. Dong, D.; Tang, Z.; Wang, S.; Hui, H.; Gong, L.; Lu, Y.; Xue, Z.; Liao, H.; Chen, F.; Yang, F.; et al. The role of imaging in the detection and management of COVID-19: A review. *IEEE Rev. Biomed. Eng.* **2020**, *14*. [CrossRef] [PubMed]
60. Ito, R.; Iwano, S.; Naganawa, S. A review on the use of artificial intelligence for medical imaging of the lungs of patients with coronavirus disease 2019. *Diagn. Interv. Radiol.* **2020**, *26*, 443. [CrossRef] [PubMed]
61. Kumar, A.; Gupta, P.K.; Srivastava, A. A review of modern technologies for tackling COVID-19 pandemic. *Diabetes Metab. Syndr.* **2020**, *14*, 569–573. [CrossRef]
62. Raj, V. Role of Chest Radiograph (CXR) in COVID-19 Diagnosis and Management. *J. Indian Med. Assoc.* **2020**, *118*, 14–19.
63. Cui, F.; Zhou, H.S. Diagnostic methods and potential portable biosensors for coronavirus disease 2019. *Biosens. Bioelectron.* **2020**, *165*, 112349. [CrossRef]
64. Jalaber, C.; Lapotre, T.; Morcet-Delattre, T.; Ribet, F.; Jouneau, S.; Lederlin, M. Chest CT in COVID-19 pneumonia: A review of current knowledge. *Diagn. Interv. Imaging* **2020**, *101*, 431–437. [CrossRef]
65. Salehi, A.W.; Baglat, P.; Gupta, G. Review on machine and deep learning models for the detection and prediction of Coronavirus. *Mater. Today Proc.* **2020**, *33*, 3896–3901. [CrossRef]
66. Farhat, H.; Sakr, G.E.; Kilany, R. Deep learning applications in pulmonary medical imaging: Recent updates and insights on COVID-19. *Mach. Vis. Appl.* **2020**, *31*, 1–42. [CrossRef] [PubMed]
67. Shaikh, F.; Anderson, M.; Sohail, M.R.; Mulero, F.; Awan, O.; Dupont-Roettger, D.; Kubassova, O.; Dehmeshki, J.; Bisdas, S. Current landscape of imaging and the potential role for artificial intelligence in the management of COVID-19. *Curr. Probl. Diagn. Radiol.* **2020**, *50*. [CrossRef] [PubMed]
68. Wynants, L.; Van Calster, B.; Collins, G.S.; Riley, R.D.; Heinze, G.; Schuit, E.; Bonten, M.M.; Dahly, D.L.; Damen, J.A.; Debray, T.P.; et al. Prediction models for diagnosis and prognosis of covid-19: Systematic review and critical appraisal. *BMJ* **2020**, *369*, 2204. [CrossRef] [PubMed]
69. Chen, J.; Li, K.; Zhang, Z.; Li, K.; Yu, P.S. A Survey on Applications of Artificial Intelligence in Fighting against COVID-19. *arXiv* **2020**, arXiv:2007.02202.
70. Pham, Q.V.; Nguyen, D.C.; Huynh-The, T.; Hwang, W.J.; Pathirana, P.N. Artificial Intelligence (AI) and Big Data for Coronavirus (COVID-19) Pandemic: A Survey on the State-of-the-Arts. *IEEE Access* **2020**, *8*, 130820–130839. [CrossRef] [PubMed]
71. Chen, D.; Ji, S.; Liu, F.; Li, Z.; Zhou, X. A review of Automated Diagnosis of COVID-19 Based on Scanning Images. *arXiv* **2020**, arXiv:2006.05245.
72. Mohamadou, Y.; Halidou, A.; Kapen, P.T. A review of mathematical modeling, artificial intelligence and datasets used in the study, prediction and management of COVID-19. *Appl. Intell.* **2020**, *50*, 3913–3925. [CrossRef]

73. Shoeibi, A.; Khodatars, M.; Alizadehsani, R.; Ghassemi, N.; Jafari, M.; Moridian, P.; Khadem, A.; Sadeghi, D.; Hussain, S.; Zare, A.; et al. Automated Detection and Forecasting of COVID-19 Using Deep Learning Techniques: A Review. *arXiv* **2020**, arXiv:2007.10785.
74. Nguyen, T.T. Artificial Intelligence in the Battle Against Coronavirus (COVID-19): A Survey and Future Research Directions. *arXiv* **2020**, arXiv:2008.07343.
75. Islam, M.N.; Inan, T.T.; Rafi, S.; Akter, S.S.; Sarker, I.H.; Islam, A. A Survey on the Use of AI and ML for Fighting the COVID-19 Pandemic. *arXiv* **2020**, arXiv:2008.07449.
76. Islam, M.M.; Karray, F.; Alhajj, R.; Zeng, J. A Review on Deep Learning Techniques for the Diagnosis of Novel Coronavirus (COVID-19). *IEEE Access* **2021**, *9*, 30551–30572. [CrossRef] [PubMed]
77. Roberts, M.; Driggs, D.; Thorpe, M.; Gilbey, J.; Yeung, M.; Ursprung, S.; Aviles-Rivero, A.I.; Etmann, C.; McCague, C.; Beer, L.; et al. Machine Learning for COVID-19 Detection and Prognostication Using Chest Radiographs and CT Scans: A Systematic Methodological Review. 2020. Available online: https://www.researchgate.net/publication/343689629_Machine_learning_for_COVID-19_detection_and_prognostication_using_chest_radiographs_and_CT_scans_a_systematic_methodological_review (accessed on 23 February 2022).
78. Ulhaq, A.; Born, J.; Khan, A.; Gomes, D.P.S.; Chakraborty, S.; Paul, M. Covid-19 control by computer vision approaches: A survey. *IEEE Access* **2020**, *8*, 179437–179456. [CrossRef] [PubMed]
79. Jung, R.G.; Di Santo, P.; Clifford, C.; Prosperi-Porta, G.; Skanes, S.; Hung, A.; Parlow, S.; Visintini, S.; Ramirez, F.D.; Simard, T.; et al. Methodological quality of COVID-19 clinical research. *Nat. Commun.* **2021**, *12*, 1–10. [CrossRef] [PubMed]
80. Yu, Y.; Shi, Q.; Zheng, P.; Gao, L.; Li, H.; Tao, P.; Gu, B.; Wang, D.; Chen, H. Assessment of the quality of systematic reviews on COVID-19: A comparative study of previous coronavirus outbreaks. *J. Med. Virol.* **2020**, *92*, 883–890. [CrossRef]
81. Al-Ryalat, N.; Al-Rashdan, O.; Alaaraj, B.; Toubasi, A.A.; Alsghaireen, H.; Yaseen, A.; Mesmar, A.; AlRyalat, S.A. Assessment of COVID-19-Related Meta-Analysis Reporting Quality. *Ir. J. Med. Sci.* **2021**, 1–5. [CrossRef]
82. Nagendran, M.; Chen, Y.; Lovejoy, C.A.; Gordon, A.C.; Komorowski, M.; Harvey, H.; Topol, E.J.; Ioannidis, J.P.; Collins, G.S.; Maruthappu, M. Artificial intelligence versus clinicians: Systematic review of design, reporting standards, and claims of deep learning studies. *BMJ* **2020**, *368*, m689. [CrossRef]
83. Storman, M.; Storman, D.; Jasinska, K.W.; Swierz, M.J.; Bala, M.M. The quality of systematic reviews/meta-analyses published in the field of bariatrics: A cross-sectional systematic survey using AMSTAR 2 and ROBIS. *Obes. Rev.* **2020**, *21*, e12994. [CrossRef]
84. Leclercq, V.; Beaudart, C.; Tirelli, E.; Bruyère, O. Psychometric measurements of AMSTAR 2 in a sample of meta-analyses indexed in PsycINFO. *J. Clin. Epidemiol.* **2020**, *119*, 144–145. [CrossRef]
85. Pieper, D.; Lorenz, R.C.; Rombey, T.; Jacobs, A.; Rissling, O.; Freitag, S.; Matthias, K. Authors should clearly report how they derived the overall rating when applying AMSTAR 2—A cross-sectional study. *J. Clin. Epidemiol.* **2021**, *129*, 97–103. [CrossRef]
86. Adadi, A.; Lahmer, M.; Nasiri, S. Artificial Intelligence and COVID-19: A Systematic Umbrella Review and Roads Ahead. *J. King Saud Univ. Comput. Inf. Sci.* **2021**. [CrossRef]
87. ESHRE Capri Workshop Group. Protect us from poor-quality medical research. *Hum. Reprod.* **2018**, *33*, 770–776. [CrossRef] [PubMed]
88. International Committee of Medical Journal Editors. Uniform requirements for manuscripts submitted to biomedical journals: Writing and editing for biomedical publication. *Indian J. Pharmacol.* **2006**, *38*, 149.
89. Johnson, C. Repetitive, duplicate, and redundant publications: A review for authors and readers. *J. Manipulative Physiol. Ther.* **2006**, *29*, 505–509. [CrossRef] [PubMed]
90. Yank, V.; Barnes, D. Consensus and contention regarding redundant publications in clinical research: Cross-sectional survey of editors and authors. *J. Med. Ethics* **2003**, *29*, 109–114. [CrossRef] [PubMed]
91. Huth, E.J. Repetitive and divided publication. In *Ethical Issues in Biomedical Publication*; JHU Press: Baltimore, MD, USA, 2000.
92. Naudé, W. Artificial intelligence vs COVID-19: Limitations, constraints and pitfalls. *AI Soc.* **2020**, *35*, 761–765. [CrossRef] [PubMed]
93. Corrado, E.M. The Importance of Open Access, Open Source, and Open Standards for Libraries. 2005. Available online: https://library.educause.edu/resources/2005/1/the-importance-of-open-access-open-source-and-open-standards-for-libraries (accessed on 23 February 2022).
94. Beaulieu-Jones, B.K.; Greene, C.S. Reproducibility of computational workflows is automated using continuous analysis. *Nat. Biotechnol.* **2017**, *35*, 342–346. [CrossRef]
95. Born, J.; Beymer, D.; Rajan, D.; Coy, A.; Mukherjee, V.V.; Manica, M.; Prasanna, P.; Ballah, D.; Guindy, M.; Shaham, D.; et al. On the role of artificial intelligence in medical imaging of covid-19. *Patterns* **2021**, *2*, 100269. [CrossRef]
96. Chee, M.L.; Ong, M.E.H.; Siddiqui, F.J.; Zhang, Z.; Lim, S.L.; Ho, A.F.W.; Liu, N. Artificial Intelligence Applications for COVID-19 in Intensive Care and Emergency Settings: A Systematic Review. *Int. J. Environ. Res. Public Health* **2021**, *18*, 4749. [CrossRef]
97. Syeda, H.B.; Syed, M.; Sexton, K.W.; Syed, S.; Begum, S.; Syed, F.; Prior, F.; Yu, F., Jr. Role of machine learning techniques to tackle the COVID-19 crisis: Systematic review. *JMIR Med. Inform* **2021**, *9*, e23811. [CrossRef]
98. Soltan, A.A.; Kouchaki, S.; Zhu, T.; Kiyasseh, D.; Taylor, T.; Hussain, Z.B.; Peto, T.; Brent, A.J.; Eyre, D.W.; Clifton, D.A. Rapid triage for COVID-19 using routine clinical data for patients attending hospital: Development and prospective validation of an artificial intelligence screening test. *Lancet Digit Health* **2021**, *3*, e78–e87. [CrossRef]
99. The Lancet Digital Health. Artificial intelligence for COVID-19: Saviour or saboteur? *Lancet Digit Health* **2021**, *3*, e1. [CrossRef]

100. Mongan, J.; Moy, L.; Kahn, C.E. Checklist for Artificial Intelligence in Medical Imaging (CLAIM): A Guide for Authors and Reviewers. *Radiol. Artif. Intell.* **2020**, *2*, e200029. [CrossRef] [PubMed]
101. Balsiger, F.; Jungo, A.; Chen, J.; Ezhov, I.; Liu, S.; Ma, J.; Paetzold, J.C.; Sekuboyina, A.; Shit, S.; Suter, Y.; et al. MICCAI Hackathon on Reproducibility, Diversity, and Selection of Papers. In Proceedings of the MICCAI Conference, Strasbourg, France, 27 September–1 October 2021.
102. Gil, D.; Díaz-Chito, K.; Sánchez, C.; Hern00E1ndez-Sabat00E9; A Early screening of sars-cov-2 by intelligent analysis of X-ray images. *arXiv* **2020**, arXiv:2005.13928.
103. Albahri, A.S.; Hamid, R.A.; Alwan, J.K.; Al-Qays, Z.; Zaidan, A.A.; Zaidan, B.B.; AlAmoodi, A.H.; Khlaf, J.M.; Almahdi, E.M.; Thabet, E.; et al. Role of biological Data Mining and Machine Learning Techniques in Detecting and Diagnosing the Novel Coronavirus (COVID-19): A Systematic Review. *J. Med. Syst.* **2020**, *44*, 122. [CrossRef]
104. Bressem, K.K.; Adams, L.C.; Erxleben, C.; Hamm, B.; Niehues, S.M.; Vahldiek, J.L. Comparing different deep learning architectures for classification of chest radiographs. *Sci. Rep.* **2020**, *10*, 13590. [CrossRef]
105. Chamola, V.; Hassija, V.; Gupta, V.; Guizani, M. A Comprehensive Review of the COVID-19 Pandemic and the Role of IoT, Drones, AI, Blockchain, and 5G in Managing its Impact. *IEEE Access* **2020**, *8*, 90225–90265. [CrossRef]
106. Bragazzi, N.L.; Dai, H.; Damiani, G.; Behzadifar, M.; Martini, M.; Wu, J. How Big Data and Artificial Intelligence Can Help Better Manage the COVID-19 Pandemic. *Int. J. Environ. Res. Public Health* **2020**, *17*, 3176. [CrossRef]
107. Nagpal, P.; Narayanasamy, S.; Garg, C.; Vidholia, A.; Guo, J.; Shin, K.M.; Lee, C.H.; Hoffman, E.A. Imaging of COVID-19 pneumonia: Patterns, pathogenesis, and advances. *Br. J. Radiol.* **2020**, *93*, 20200538. [CrossRef]
108. Bansal, A.; Padappayil, R.P.; Garg, C.; Singal, A.; Gupta, M.; Klein, A. Utility of Artificial Intelligence Amidst the COVID 19 Pandemic: A Review. *J. Med. Syst.* **2020**, *44*, 156. [CrossRef]
109. Rezaei, M.; Shahidi, M. Zero-shot learning and its applications from autonomous vehicles to COVID-19 diagnosis: A review. *Intell. Med.* **2020**, *3*, 100005. [CrossRef]
110. Kharat, A.; Duddalwar, V.; Saoji, K.; Gaikwad, A.; Kulkarni, V.; Naik, G.; Lokwani, R.; Kasliwal, S.; Kondal, S.; Gupte, T.; et al. Role of edge device and cloud machine learning in point-of-care solutions using imaging diagnostics for popula-tion screening. *arXiv* **2020**, arXiv:2006.13808.
111. Albahri, O.S.; Zaidan, A.A.; Albahri, A.S.; Zaidan, B.B.; Abdulkareem, K.H.; Al-Qaysi, Z.T.; Alamoodi, A.H.; Aleesa, A.M.; Chyad, M.A.; Alesa, R.M.; et al. Systematic review of artificial intelligence techniques in the detection and classification of COVID-19 medical images in terms of evaluation and benchmarking: Taxonomy analysis, challenges, future solutions and methodological aspects. *J. Infect. Public Health* **2020**, *13*, 1381–1396.
112. Manigandan, S.; Wu, M.-T.; Ponnusamy, V.K.; Raghavendra, V.B.; Pugazhendhi, A.; Brindhadevi, K. A systematic review on recent trends in transmission, diagnosis, prevention and imaging features of COVID-19. *Process Biochem.* **2020**, *98*, 233–240. [CrossRef]

MDPI
St. Alban-Anlage 66
4052 Basel
Switzerland
Tel. +41 61 683 77 34
Fax +41 61 302 89 18
www.mdpi.com

Journal of Clinical Medicine Editorial Office
E-mail: jcm@mdpi.com
www.mdpi.com/journal/jcm

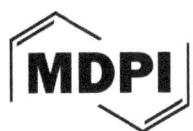